Women Medical Doctors in the
United States before the Civil War

Women Medical Doctors in the United States before the Civil War

A Biographical Dictionary

Edward C. Atwater

UNIVERSITY OF ROCHESTER PRESS

The University of Rochester Press gratefully acknowledges the Rare Books and Manuscripts Section of the Edward G. Miner Library, University of Rochester Medical Center, for its generous support of this publication.

First published 2016

University of Rochester Press
668 Mt. Hope Avenue, Rochester, NY 14620, USA
www.urpress.com
and Boydell & Brewer Limited
PO Box 9, Woodbridge, Suffolk IP12 3DF, UK
www.boydellandbrewer.com

ISBN-13: 978-1-58046-571-7

Library of Congress Cataloging-in-Publication Data

Names: Atwater, Edward C., author.
Title: Women medical doctors in the United States before the Civil War : a
    biographical dictionary / Edward C. Atwater.
Description: Rochester, NY : University of Rochester Press, 2016. | Includes
    bibliographical references and index.
Identifiers: LCCN 2016027494 | ISBN 9781580465717 (hardcover : alk. paper)
Subjects: | MESH: Physicians, Women | History, 19th Century | United States |
    Biography | Dictionary
Classification: LCC R692 | NLM WZ 150 | DDC 610.82—dc23 LC record
    available at https://lccn.loc.gov/2016027494

A catalogue record for this title is available from the British Library.

This publication is printed on acid-free paper.
Printed in the United States of America.

Contents

Photographs follow page 198.

Acknowledgments

This was an on and off project on which I worked over a period of more than forty years. The more recent availability online of the US decadal census records and the Internal Revenue rolls from the Civil War period, as well as other information now available on the Internet, made it possible to extend and expand the study, though it is still far from complete. Ideally, a personal visit to libraries and historical societies in each of the 170 or more communities served at one time or another by one of these doctors would be the way to go, but this method was not practical from a time or cost point of view.

I am greatly indebted to my friend and colleague Christopher Hoolihan, history of medicine librarian and archivist at the University of Rochester's Edward G. Miner Library, who thought the project worth doing, gave me continuing professional help, and repeatedly encouraged me to get to work when, as was frequently the case, I faltered. In addition to many suggestions, he undertook the monumental task of editing the bibliography and patiently dealt with many revisions of the manuscript. His colleague, Dennis Carr, interlibrary loan librarian, was able to find many obscure references I sought, as did his predecessor Sandra Charchalis. Nancy Bolger, professional editor and longtime friend, read every word and made many corrections that improved grammar and clarity of the text. Sonia Kane, Carrie Watterson, and Tracey Engel of the University of Rochester Press guided the book through the publication process.

I also visited and received help from staff members at the Rochester Public Library; the Boston Public Library; the New England Historic Genealogical Society Library; the New Hampshire State Library and the library of the New Hampshire Historical Society, both in Concord; the St. Albans (VT) Free Library; special collections at the Boston University Library, where records of the New England Female Medical College are housed; the Library Company of Philadelphia; the Pennsylvania Historical Society; the Grosvenor Collection at the Erie County Public Library; and the National Library of Medicine in Bethesda.

Elizabeth Carroll-Horrocks, head of special collections at the Massachusetts State Library, and her assistant, Silvia Meija, provided access to that library's extensive collection of Massachusetts city directories.

Matt Herbison, archivist, and Chrissie Landis, archives assistant, at Drexel University School of Medicine, where the records of the Woman's Medical College of Pennsylvania are now located, helped on several occasions, providing, among other things, Annie Stambach's married name (Galvin) and information about Margaret Phillips Richardson and Mary J. Scarlett-Dixon. Martha Gardner, assistant professor of history and social sciences at Massachusetts College of Pharmacy and Health Sciences University, was kind enough to lend me her notes made in preparation for writing her thesis on the graduates of New England Female Medical College, notes from which I learned especially about scholarship aid to students. She also directed me to Samuel Gregory's remarkable scrapbook that appears to include every Massachusetts newspaper clipping about the New England Female Medical College from 1847 to 1868. Devhra Bennett Jones, archivist at the Lloyd Library and Museum in Cincinnati, where the records of the Eclectic Medical Institute and the Eclectic College of Medicine are located, provided useful information, especially about Alice Stockham. Arlene Shaner, acting curator and reference librarian at the New York Academy of Medicine, made me copies of the *Biennial Catalogues* of the New York Hygeio-Therapeutic College. Clifford Hall, grandnephew of Susan Hall Barry and great-great-grandson of Eliza Hall McQuigg, made family materials available. Arthur Cleveland, great-grandson of Emeline Cleveland, gave me access to a collection of her papers.

The many librarians, archivists, curators, town historians, and genealogists who offered information about individual physicians I have tried to thank in each case. Their help was essential. The following is a list of many of these people: Patricia J. Albright, college archives librarian, Mt. Holyoke College, for information on Sophronia Fletcher and Mary Ann Brown Homer Arnold; Susan Bell, Putney Historical Society, Putney, Vermont, for information on Laura Marion Wheeler Fairchild Wheaton Plantz; the staffs of the Buswell Memorial Library, Wheaton College, Wheaton, Illinois, and the Cole Library, Cornell College, Mt. Vernon, Iowa, for information on Minerva Falley Hoes; Katharine M. Cartwright, Sharon, Massachusetts, for information on Susan Richards Capen; Joyce Carver, genealogist, Marshall, Michigan, for information on Salome Amy Slout Peterman; Freda Chabot, retired librarian, Fitchburg Public Library, for information on Sarah Cheny Reed Randall Brigham; Kathy Clair, director of the Reddick Public Library, Ottawa, Illinois, for information on Phebe Ann Shotwell; Mildred A. Coolidge, Hudson Historical Society, Hudson, Massachusetts, for information on Harriet S. Brigham; Patsy Copeland, Chief of Information Services, Tulane University Medical Center, for information on Elizabeth D. A. Magnus Cohen; Philip Crnkovich, Lancaster Public

Library, Lancaster, Pennsylvania, for information on H. W. Brinton Carter; Linda Crocker, chief genealogist, Seelye Genealogical Society, provided substantial information related to Finette Scott Seelye; Karen A. Culp, Tiffin-Seneca Public Library, Tiffin, Ohio, for information on Julia Rumsey; Jennifer Donaldson, archivist, Woodstock Historical Society, Woodstock, Vermont, for information on Marenda Briggs Randall; Tim Duerden, Delaware County (NY) Historical Society, for information on Olive Frisbie McCune; Edward Elsner, Oswego (NY) Public Library for information on S. G. F. Harrington; Edith Ford and Sandy Harmel, Cedar County Historical Society, Tipton, Iowa, for information on Lydia S. Campbell and for photographs of Savina Leah Fogle Williams' tombstone in the Clarence Cemetery; Joy Hennig, Local History Division, Worcester (MA) Public Library, for information on Betsey Russell Clark; Sharon Hess, Clinton Public Library, Clinton, Iowa, for information on Adeline Sadler Littlejohn; Jean C. Hillis, Persia, New York, town historian, for information on Laura A. Lord; Linda L. Homa, Union County Public Library, Lewisburg, Pennsylvania, for information on Sarah C. Kleckner Saltzgiver and on Mary Ellen Wolfe; JoAnne Jager, Lansing Public Library, Lansing, Michigan, for information on Augusta R. Montgomery Nelson; Virginia Johnson, Taunton (MA) Public Library, for information on Frances Sproat Cooke; Walter Kurth, Multnomah County Library, Portland, Oregon, for information on Augusta R. Montgomery Nelson; Helene J. Lindblad, Brimfield (MA) Public Library, for information on Mary Ann Brown Homer Arnold; Stephen Logsdon, archivist, Becker Library, Washington University School of Medicine, for checking the records of Washington University and the St. Louis Medical College regarding faculty appointments of Marion Augusta Fairchild; Daniel Lombardo, curator of Special Collections at Jones Library, Amherst, Massachusetts, for material on Ellen Herman Goodell Smith; the staff of Louisiana Division, New Orleans Public Library, for information about Elizabeth D. A. Magnus Cohen; Evelyn L. Lyman, director of the Swan Library, Albion, New York, for information on Elizabeth Josephine Vaile; Laurie L. McFadden, university archivist, Alfred University, Alfred, New York, for information on Susan Maxson Estee; Fauna Mihalko, Genealogy Department Madison-Jefferson Public Library, Madison, Indiana, for information on Elizabeth Jane Wiley Warren Corbett; Patty Mosher, archivist, Galesburg Public Library, Galesburg, Illinois, for information on Sarah Randall Humphrey; Elizabeth Murphy, research assistant, Tufts Library, Weymouth, Massachusetts, for information on Sarah Whitman Salisbury; Geraldine Noble, Warren County Historical Society, Lebanon, Ohio, for information on Rebecca L. Vancleve Anton; the staff of the Ohio Historical Center, Columbus, Ohio, for material on Laura Marion Wheeler Fairchild Wheaton Plantz; Marjory Allen Perez, Wayne County (NY) Historian, for information on DeLavenna Burroughs; Susan R. Perkins, Herkimer County (NY) Historical Society, for information on Olive Chesilla Arnold Wood; Ernest L. Plummer, president/archivist, Kennebec Historical Society, Augusta, Maine, and Kent London and Julie Lyon, Vassalborough (Maine) Historical Society, for information on Huldah Allen Page; the staff of the Quincy (IL) Public Library, for information on Marion Augusta Fairchild; Joyce Reynolds, Moores Memorial Library, Christiana, Pennsylvania, for information on Hannah Brinton Carter; Lisa Rixley, archivist, Dayton Metro Library, Dayton, Ohio, for information on Lovina Dolley Bacon Thomas; Delia A. Robinson, Town of Gaines (NY) historian, for information on Elizabeth Josephine Vaile; Diana P. Rofini, librarian, Chester County Historical Society, West Chester, Pennsylvania, for information on Sarah Ann Entrikin; Nancy McCraw Ross, Carnegie Librarian, Carnegie Center of the Brazos Valley, Bryan, Texas, for information on Mary T. Denton Butts; Victoria Schneiderman, head of reference, Medford Public Library, for searching local directories for Anna Sarah Angell Curtis; Sally Setzer, Lake City (Minnesota) Historical Society, for information on Catherine Josephine Underwood Jewell; Nancy Sherrill, Genealogy Library, Vigo County Public Library, Terre Haute, Indiana, for information on Angeline M. Lockwood Wilson Moore; Claudia Spencer, Atchison (KS) Public Library, for information on Olive Chesilla Arnold Wood; Mary Lou Sprague, Talcott Free Library, Rockton, Illinois, for information on Emily M. Smith Guthrie; Norman Thompson, Tri-State Corners Genealogical Society, Falls City Library and Arts Center, Falls City, Nebraska, for information on Olive A. Williams Maxson; Mary A. Throop, Geneva (NY) Public Library, for information on Mary Wright Pierson; Jeannette Voiland, Special Collections, Seattle Public Library, for information on Adaline Melinda Willis Weed; Irene Wainwright, Louisiana Division, New Orleans Public Library, for information on Frances Burritt; Doris W. Waters, Genealogy & Local History Division, Guernsey Memorial Library, Norwich, New York, for information on Elizabeth Taylor; Eleanora F. West, Fitchburg Historical Society, for information on Sarah Cheny Reed Randall Brigham; Robert Winder, Aurora (IL) Public Library, for information on Rhoda H. Hyde Williams Maxcy; Paul Woehrmann, Milwaukee Public Library, for information on Mary Ann Brown Homer Arnold; and Christopher Wood, Cleveland Public Library, who provided an obituary for Janet Baily Rabon.

My greatest thanks go to my wife, Ruth, who put up with my occasional periods of irascibility when things were not going well, but most of all with papers lying about, all over the house. She says I have a desk in every room. My son, Ned, refers to the main part of the operation in the cellar as "the Beast." Daughter Rebecca, once a professional editor, made suggestions about several parts of the manuscript over the years. All of my family, happily, will no longer be subjected to "progress" reports—glad that the project is finished, or as finished as I am able to make it.

I would be pleased to hear from any readers who can offer corrections or additional information or leads about any of these doctors. It is also my hope that some of these "lost women" will appeal to other writers as subjects worthy of more extensive research and fuller biographies.

Edward C. Atwater
Rochester, New York
October 2016

Introduction

Since the early 1970s, the number of women graduating from American medical schools has been about 40 percent of all graduates and more recently more than 50 percent of the total number, roughly in proportion to the number of applicants. The last all-male school (Dartmouth) and the last all-female school (Woman's Medical College of Pennsylvania) became coeducational in 1960 and 1970, respectively. This change from earlier times was seen in other professions as well, reflecting the evolution of society's view of a woman's place. Women have become more prominent in the ministry, the law, the business world, the sports world, even the military. Only the Roman Catholic priesthood remains unchanged. Women in medicine have come to parity with men not only in number but in stature as well.

During the century before 1970, the percentage of American medical students who were women remained relatively constant at a much lower level, about 4–5 percent and, as late as the 1970s, the position of women in the profession was quite different from what it is today. The woman doctor then was a second-class citizen, almost excluded from the more prestigious and lucrative crafts such as surgery and its subspecialties. Instead, pediatrics, obstetrics, gynecology, and psychiatry were thought to be fields in which a woman might appropriately work. Or she might seek employment in an institution such as a school or state hospital. Throughout this period, however, beginning in the middle 1870s, women doctors were increasingly offered medical society membership, though staff privileges for women at hospitals were uncommon until after the turn of the century.

It is a third, and still earlier, period that attracted my interest: from 1849, when the first doctor of medicine degree was conferred on a woman in the United States, until the beginning of the Civil War. During this thirteen-year span, more than 250 women received MD degrees from chartered medical schools in the United States. Several things distinguish the members of this cohort from those that followed. They were not primarily out to prove that women could "do it." They wanted especially to teach patients about their anatomy and physiology, about the "laws of life," about the prevention of sickness. In this they were missionaries and reformers, especially those from

Eclectic and hydropathic schools. As a group, they were older than were those who came after 1870, and many had considerable experience as teachers. Fifty percent of them were married before going to medical school. Some were widows with small children to support. In proportion to their numbers, Quakers were the predominant denomination, and several of them belonged to the liberal Longwood Progressive Friends Annual Meeting. Many were involved in the antislavery, woman's rights, and suffrage movements.

Some of these pioneer woman physicians are well known to us today and have been written about extensively—Elizabeth and Emily Blackwell, Emeline Horton Cleveland, Clemence Lozier, Ann Preston, Marie Zakrzewska, and others—primarily those who were part of the metropolitan medical professoriate—though even the accomplishments of these women have often been overshadowed by the reverence in which they are held as icons.

By contrast, those physicians who worked in the community, outside the hospital, were less apt to receive such recognition. There were exceptions to this, of course: Hannah Longshore in Philadelphia, Sarah Adamson Dolley in Rochester, and Mercy Bisbee-Jackson in Boston were prominent practitioners in their respective communities. A few, like Mary Edwards Walker, were sufficiently eccentric to attract attention to themselves. Still others, while not famous, are known to historians of medicine interested in the subject of female medical education. Most of these doctors, however, have passed into oblivion. Though almost all of them practiced medicine after graduating and became respected professionally in their communities, as a group they have not won the interest of historians.

There are several reasons for this neglect, one of the chief ones being the difficulty in tracking their later careers. Many of them practiced in small- or medium-sized towns where, in the course of successful professional careers, they became accepted as nothing out of the ordinary. They died, as did their male counterparts, with little notice attracted by their passing, except, perhaps, a brief death notice in the local newspaper. This notice was often not in the town in which they had practiced and were known, because they had moved to another location to live with children or a new husband. Many of them moved frequently, either within a community or from town to town.

In addition to this is the fact that medical school catalogs and census records of the period were rather imprecise in spelling names and recording middle initials. A surprising number of names of persons known to be living in the United States were not found in those census rolls. Also, there were no comprehensive national medical directories until the first edition of the Polk directory in 1886. (The Butler directories of 1874 and 1877 were less complete, gave little information but names, often only with initials, and listed names alphabetically by state without providing a comprehensive index.) By the time of the 1886 Polk directory, many of the pre–Civil War cohort had retired or died. An even more challenging problem was posed by the name changes that came with marriage. The practice then in vogue was for a woman to keep her maiden middle name rather than her maiden surname. This system further obscured a woman's identity and made it difficult to identify a woman once she married. Still another problem was that information about actual clinical practice was rarely found.

In spite of these impediments, it was possible to compile a roster of 280 women, each of whom received an MD degree from a chartered medical school in the United States between 1849 and 1861, inclusive. (Certain exceptions will be noted hereafter.) The reason for selecting 1861 as the end date, aside from the need to make some limit, and the fact that it was the start of a major social upheaval, was that the decade of the 1860s saw a sharp decline in the number of females matriculating at schools. The antimode was in 1863, when only fourteen women graduated. During the Civil War only New England Female Medical College, Penn Medical University (a now extinct Eclectic school in Philadelphia, not to be confused with the University of Pennsylvania), and the Female Medical College of Pennsylvania produced women doctors.

How was the roster constructed? The primary source used to identify these early woman doctors came from annual announcements and catalogs of medical schools. Because no complete set of these records exists at any institution, even the National Library of Medicine, it was necessary to piece the roster together with materials from several libraries. In cases where this source no longer exists or is incomplete (such as for Central Medical College in Rochester, Syracuse Medical College, Worcester Medical Institution, Penn Medical University in Philadelphia, New York Hygeio-Therapeutic College, Starling Medical College in Columbus, Ohio, and Graefenberg Medical Institute in Dadeville, Alabama), information was obtained from histories of those schools and from contemporary journals and newspapers. For Western Reserve University, Female Medical College of Pennsylvania, Eclectic Medical Institute, and Eclectic College of Medicine, both in Cincinnati, there are published general catalogs and histories. Frederick C. Waite's *History of the New England Female Medical College* has appendixes listing graduates of that school, as does Harold J. Abraham's *Extinct Medical Schools of Nineteenth-Century Philadelphia* for graduates of Penn Medical University. David H. Beckwith wrote a history of the Western Homoeopathic College, found in King's *History of Homoeopathy*.

Included on the roster are the names of graduates from any school with a charter from a state legislature giving it authority to award the degree doctor of medicine.[1] There were fourteen such schools that awarded medical degrees to women before 1862, six Regular (Geneva Medical Institution, Western Reserve, Female Medical College of Pennsylvania, New England Female Medical College, Starling Medical College, Graefenberg Medical Institution); six Eclectic (Central Medical College, Syracuse Medical College, Worcester Medical Institution, Penn Medical University, Eclectic Medical Institute, Eclectic College of Medicine); one homoeopathic (Western Homoeopathic College [with other names subsequently]); and one hydropathic or hygienic (New York Hygeio-Therapeutic College). In addition, graduates from these schools before they received their charters are also included. There were two such schools: New England Female Medical College and New York Hygeio-Therapeutic College. The New England school received its definitive charter on May 28, 1856, specifically authorizing it "to confer the usual degree of Doctor of Medicine." The original charter of that school (April 30, 1850) was less specific: the college was to provide "for the education of Midwives, Nurses, and Female Physicians, with all the powers and privileges, and subject to all the duties restrictions, and liabilities set forth . . . in the Revised Statutes" (Waite). There were eight graduates of this school before the 1856 charter. They are included here based on the fact that their curriculum was similar to that in later use, they were known throughout their careers as doctors of medicine, and newspaper accounts of the 1854 commencement said that graduates "received the degree Doctor of Medicine" from President Tyler, and, the following year, that the president "conferred the degree Doctor of Medicine" (Gregory scrapbook, 79, 89).

There were twenty-one graduates of the New York Hygeio-Therapeutic College between 1854 and February 7, 1857, when it received its charter from the state. They are included because their curriculum was similar to that which held later and because they, too, were recognized in their communities as doctors with professional training. Identifying graduates of this school with certainty was a problem. Only the 1853–54 and the 1860–61 catalogs list separately the names of those who actually graduated. The others record the names of all students in attendance. It was necessary to depend on reports of graduation in the *Water-Cure Journal*. Even here there were sometimes inconsistencies. Another hydropathic school, the American Hydropathic Institute, founded by Thomas Low Nichols and his wife Mary Gove Nichols, operated for two sessions in 1851 and 1852 in New York, was never chartered, and awarded diplomas to thirteen women and sixteen men. Except for three women who later received degrees from chartered schools (Esther C. Wileman, Harriet A. Judd [Sartain], and Harriet N. Austin), these graduates are not included here. For the record, a name list of graduates of the American Hydropathic Institute is provided in appendix B.

A word about these nineteenth-century "variant" medical systems, groups that members of the "Regular" profession viewed as sects and did their best to suppress. Each of these "alternative" groups viewed itself as bringing needed reform to medicine as practiced by the established system, protesting mainly against the aggressive therapeutic methods its practitioners were using. The secret of the reformers' success was that they usually did less harm to the patient than the Regulars were doing. The Eclectics, successors to the earlier botanic reformers, foreswore the use of mineral medicines—"mischievous" mercury, for example—and emphasized vegetable remedies. The homoeopathic system was based on the idea that "like cures like." Homoeopathic physicians used minute doses of a medication to treat a symptom in a sick patient that large doses would produce in a healthy person. Regardless of what else those minute doses may have done, they usually did less harm and let nature take its course. The hydropaths were believers in the efficacy of water, applied internally and externally. This therapy was to be accompanied by a hygienic daily regimen of exercise, a diet emphasizing vegetables, the avoidance of any excess, and abstinence from alcohol and tobacco. With the discovery of bacteria later in the century, the focus of medicine changed from symptomatic treatment to public health and prevention of disease, and therapeutic systems gradually faded from the scene.

In this study no distinction is made among graduates of the various medical denominations, because no clear distinction can be made regarding the quality of the curriculum or the educational experience each had. Anatomy, including dissection, and physiology were then the courses that might be considered "scientific." These courses were generally as rigorous at the "variant" as at the "regular" schools. Only certain aspects of therapeutics consistently deviated. Certainly no denominational discrimination can be justified on the record of subsequent performance. Based on recognition by both peers and by the public at large many of the graduates from the non-Regular schools more than matched their counterparts from the Regular schools. Some of the subsequently most notable physicians attended Eclectic schools. Of the thirty-eight women whose names are included in one or more of fourteen standard biographical reference books (see appendix C), twenty-three attended non-Regular medical schools.

Once the roster was established, the following information was sought: birth and death dates and locations; parents' names, backgrounds, and vocations; early education; name(s) of husband(s), date(s) of marriage(s), children; places and type of practice; religious denomination; nonmedical activities and contributions in the community. When sufficient data were available, a brief life narrative was constructed. Federal census records, now more conveniently digitized and available on the Internet, local directories, local histories, local historians, vital statistic records, genealogies, newspaper articles, and correspondence with descendants were some of the sources used. Disappointing was the almost complete lack of information about the nature of the doctors' clinical practices. In only a few cases was such information found. Medical society and medical school records (other than annual announcements and catalogs) were of little help. Few of these women were admitted to medical societies until the 1870s, and both medical society and medical school records before the end of the nineteenth century are notable for their sketchiness and carelessness, if they exist at all.

It has not been possible to trace all of the 280 graduates, and it is likely that some of them will remain forever lost. Of the 222 biographies presented here, many have substantial detail, while for a smaller group very little information was found. Fifty-eight are listed by name only. Errors will be found in the data. This assumption is based on the number of errors that were already discovered and corrected. When dealing with census data, one finds remarkable numbers of people with the same names. Census data are often careless about spelling of names, initials, and penmanship. They often label women, even those known to be practicing medicine, as "keeping house." Unless there was other confirmatory evidence that a woman practiced medicine, in a situation where a census listing was thought to be the person sought though she was denoted only as "keeping house," such data were not used.

There are several reasons for making the effort to find out what happened to these first woman doctors. One, of course, is simple curiosity. But, also, the answers to several questions were sought. What was the social and religious background of these earliest doctors? What motivated them to have careers in medicine? What did they do after receiving their degrees, both professionally and personally? Where did they do it? As a cohort, did they differ from those who succeeded them after 1870? What effect did their work have on the medical profession, the public, and on medical education in the years that came after? It was not possible to answer many of these questions with complete statistical analysis. There were sometimes sufficient data to provide reasonable impressions, at other times only the occasional testimonial.

Information on birthplace is available for 206 women. Not surprisingly, 85 percent were born in the Northeast (New England, New York, New Jersey, Pennsylvania, and Ohio). New York produced the largest number (49) but only two were born in New York City. Of the other 47, more than half (29) were born in Central or Western New York. There were 36 from Massachusetts, 31 from Pennsylvania, 13 each from Vermont and Ohio, 11 from New Hampshire, 9 from Maine, 6 each from Connecticut and New Jersey, 4 from Indiana, 3 from Rhode Island, and 1 from Illinois. Only 10 were born south of the Mason-Dixon Line: 4 in Maryland, 2 each in Virginia and Georgia, and 1 each from North Carolina and Alabama. Ten were born in England, 2 in Scotland, 2 in Prussia, and 1 each from Canada and Italy.

Denominationally, Quakers predominated, with other Protestants—Methodist, Baptist, and Congregational—also numerous. Based on the 182 women for whom data are available, the average age for the entire group at the time of graduation from medical school was 33.2 years (range 17–61). Thirty-five were in their forties and 8 were over fifty.

Of 209, 50 (24 percent) never married, 101 (49 percent) were married before going to medical school, 8 married while at school, usually to a classmate, and 50 (24 percent) married after becoming doctors. Twenty-four were widows, and at least one other anticipated widowhood when they matriculated. Still another had an invalid husband. A few became physicians in anticipation of divorce. Fifty-three of the 159 who married had a physician husband, exactly a third.

As a group these woman physicians were less prolific mothers than was common in their time: 183 women had at least 356 children (ascertainment surely not complete). Forty of those married had no children as far as could be determined, 59 had one or two children, 30 had three or four, 17 had five to seven children, and 7 had eight to twelve children. At least 40 of the women had one or more children under the age of eighteen when they went to medical school. At least 24 women had lost one or more children before seeking medical training.

One of the most frequent reasons for becoming a physician (although this statement is based on circumstantial evidence) was economic: recently a widow, with or without small children to support. Another common reason, judging from the circumstances surrounding matriculation, was the loss of one or more young children and, presumably, the hope of protecting the rest of the family—and the extension of this good motive to the rest of the community, the hope of offering better care than appeared otherwise to be available. For those who, for whatever reason, did not marry, a medical degree provided a livelihood. No doubt all of them were happy to prove that "women could do it," but that seems to have been a primary motivation for relatively few of them, though many were activists in their communities (and some on a wider stage). It was quite common for them to be involved in the abolition movement (especially Quakers), the temperance movement, the suffrage movement, the dress reform movement, and other woman's rights activities. Some, like the Blackwells and Dr. Zakrzewska, had the education of women as their goal. A larger group took to the public lecture circuit, teaching citizens, especially women, about the anatomy, physiology, and hygiene of their bodies. Some, like Drs. Lydia Folger Fowler, Susan Everett, and Anna Longshore-Potts, did this as a career, others more briefly, to establish their repute in a community (for example, Hannah Longshore). Most went out into small communities and took care of patients.

It seems both puzzling and remarkable that it was possible to document Civil War service for only 19 of the 222 women on whom some information was found. At least 3,000 women are known to have served as nurses to the Union armies. Why did not more of the woman doctors, deprived of commissions as officer doctors, serve as nurses?[2]

Opposition to the woman physician was strong at first, especially from male physicians. It is remarkable how quickly this attitude began to fade. Most woman doctors became accepted and respected in their communities, although sometimes they did not stay in the community of their first choice. In 1858, for example, the Philadelphia County Medical Society recommended that its members "withhold from the faculties and graduates of female medical colleges, all countenance and support, and that they cannot, consistently with sound medical ethics, consult or hold professional medical intercourse with their professors or alumni [*sic*]." The state society soon followed suit. It was but a little over a decade later (1871) that the state society rescinded its earlier proscription, though individual opposition, of course, continued. Probably the main reason for opposition was cultural: a woman's place was in the home. But another important factor was that woman doctors encroached on the midwifery business, which was then the constant, dependable source of physician income.

The ultimate professional success of women came partly from the fact that they took care of women and children primarily. Many women were more comfortable confiding in a woman physician, who they believed, probably correctly, better understood them. Also important was the fact that they were less aggressive therapeutically, depending heavily on simple remedies and emphasizing Nature over Art, thus doing less harm. Important, too, was that almost all the women doctors were interested in teaching their patients about their own anatomy and physiology and about hygiene. The male doctors seemed less concerned with this. Notable among the exceptions to this were the nineteenth-century popular medical authors, Frederick Hollick, MD, and Edward Bliss Foote, MD, whose books saw many editions.

Taken together, this pioneer group was rather remarkable, most of them small-town girls who had taught school and would continue to be teachers after becoming doctors. It was their interest in preventive medicine and their role as teachers about health matters that distinguished them most from their male colleagues. They wanted for themselves some wider educational experience and careers outside the home, whether demanded by economic necessity or by a desire to contribute to the community or both. They fought the prejudices of society and prevailed. The variety of their individual experiences may be of interest.

References: Medical Society of Pennsylvania, *A Brief History of Proceedings of the Medical Society of Pennsylvania, in the Years 1859, '60, '66, '67, '68, '70 and '71, to Procure the Recognition of Women Physicians by the Medical Profession of the State* (Philadelphia, 1888); New England Female Medical College, scrapbook of clippings from Massachusetts newspapers kept by Samuel Gregory, covering the period September 7, 1847–65, at the Francis A. Countway Library of Medicine, Harvard University; Frederick C. Waite, *History of the New England Female Medical College, 1848–1874* (Boston, 1950).

Notes

1. Exceptions to this are the two Eclectic schools in New York State (Rochester and Syracuse) whose authority rested on the General Incorporation Law of 1848. "Eclectic Medical colleges in our State have, up to this time, derived their authority to confer degrees from the provisions of a General Incorporation Law, which formed, we believe, a part of the new State Constitution adopted in 1848. This law in reality contemplated the incorporation of Benevolent, Religious and other similar societies; and hence its application to Medical Colleges was *constructive*, though not *forbidden*, and, according to good legal authorities, not really *constrained*" (*Union Journal of Medicine* editorial, January 1853). The stumbling block, of course, was opposition of the "regular" profession. The legislature finally passed a law in its 1852 winter session, broadening access to charters from the Board of Regents.

2. There were two exceptions to this restriction: Orie Moon, who had the rank of captain in the Confederate army and was said to be the only female officer in the South, and Mary Edwards Walker, who may or may not have had a commission in the Union army. When seeking a commission she was turned

down repeatedly, and she is not listed in the official *Roster of Regimental Surgeons and Assistant Surgeons during the War of the Rebellion* (Washington, 1883). However, Nixon D. Stewart, in his history of the Fifty-Second Ohio Volunteer Regiment, a unit to which Dr. Walker was at one time attached, states that she was a first lieutenant.

Excellent Miss Blackwell
(1821–1910)

In the middle of the nineteenth century, Western New York was a leading edge of American society. With the completion of the Erie Canal
in 1825, it became possible to travel from Buffalo on Lake Erie to New
York in relative comfort and to ship economically a ton of flour, milled
in Rochester from local wheat, to that city. The entire region prospered,
its population increased rapidly, and it acquired many of those things
that prosperity brings: fine houses, public buildings, educational institutions, industries, cultural activities, and social movements. Western New
York was where the action was. It is no coincidence that reformers, reviv-
als, and utopian experiments proliferated there.

It was on Wednesday, July 19, 1848, that one hundred women and
men gathered at the Wesleyan Chapel in the village of Seneca Falls to
formalize what was to become the women's rights movement. That day,
sixty-five women and thirty-two men signed the declaration. The previous fall, in the nearby village of Geneva, a young woman presented
herself for matriculation at the previously all-male Geneva Medical
Institution. No woman had ever been admitted to an American medical school. A little over a year later, having successfully completed two
lecture courses, participated in the dissection of a cadaver, and passed
examinations, Miss Elizabeth Blackwell was awarded the degree doctor
of medicine.

The Geneva school did not have another woman graduate until
after the Civil War and even refused admission to Emily Blackwell, Elizabeth's sister. The fact that the school had graduated the first woman
doctor was largely coincidence, as will be seen. However, the *idea* of
women becoming doctors was in the wind, and, during the two and
a half years after Miss Blackwell's achievement, four more women,
attending medical schools then in Rochester and Syracuse, became
doctors of medicine. In the next six months after that, women would
receive medical degrees from schools in Pennsylvania, Ohio, and Massachusetts, as well. Before 1862, in no more than a dozen years, at least
280 women had become doctors of medicine in the United States.

Born in England, daughter of a businessman and dissenter, Miss
Blackwell immigrated to the United States and had studied medicine

with several physicians and at Blockley Hospital in Philadelphia before coming to medical school in Geneva. Her motivation for a career in medicine seems to have had little or nothing to do with pioneering. Historian Elizabeth Thomson, in her biographical sketch of Elizabeth in *Notable American Women*, writes:

> The prospect of marriage . . . filled her with foreboding. From girl-hood she admitted she had been extremely susceptible to "the disturbing influence exercised by the other sex," but whenever she "became sufficiently intimate with any individual to be able to realize what a life association might mean," she "shrank from the prospect, disappointed or repelled." [She was once] strongly drawn to a well-educated suitor, but troubled by their lack of "close and ennobling companionship." When a woman friend urged her to study medicine, the idea was at first distasteful, for she "hated everything connected with the body" and from childhood had been "filled . . . with disgust" by "the physical structure of the body and its various ailments." [The quotations are from Blackwell's autobiography.]

After graduation, she had experience in the hospitals of London and Paris. She practiced medicine in New York City from 1851 to 1857, when she founded the New York Infirmary for Women and Children, and nine years later, a medical school for women in association with the infirmary, a school at which she was professor of hygiene, a position in which she remained only a year. In 1869, she returned to England, where she spent the rest of her life, and where she founded the National Health Society, and was professor of gynecology at New Hospital and London School of Medicine for Women for a year. Thereafter, she remained active in the field of hygienic reform.

The medical historian Regina Morantz, writing in the *Dictionary of American Medical Biography* nicely summarized her career and contributions: "First woman to graduate with a medical degree in the United States (1849). Indefatigable pioneer advocate of women's medical education. Founder of two exemplary and innovative institutions for the training of women in medicine. Outspoken proponent of social hygiene, sanitation, and preventive medicine. Opponent of vaccination, animal experimentation, and bacteriology. Important role model for generations of women physicians who followed her into the medical profession" (171–72).

Another major contribution that Blackwell made is, however, less often recognized. By her presence, she brought greater civility to the classroom than had previously existed. There exist firsthand (albeit retrospective) accounts of what life was like at both the Geneva Medical Institution and the adjacent smaller liberal arts college, then called

Geneva College and known today as Hobart College. Andrew D. White, a student at Geneva College and later the first president of Cornell University, recalled what it was like when he was a student in the 1840s. "There were," he wrote, "about forty students [at the arts college], the majority of them sons of wealthy churchmen, showing no inclination to work, and much tendency to dissipation." He said he never thereafter saw "so much carousing and wild dissipation as I then saw in this little church college of which the especial boast was that, owing to the small number of its students, it was able to exercise a direct Christian influence upon every young man committed to its care." White went on to describe "a professor, an excellent clergyman, buried under a heap of carpets, mattresses, counterpanes and blankets ... another clerical professor forced to retire through the panel of a door under a shower of lexicons, boots, and brushes ... the President himself, on one occasion, obliged to leave the lecture-room by a ladder from a window, and on another, kept at bay by a shower of beer bottles." Another pastime was rolling cannon balls down the dormitory corridors.

Another student of those days, William Combs, recalled the following prank: a number of students took a work horse and led it up into the belfry of the college building. "The horse went up easy enough, but he utterly refused to come down, and there he remained three or four days, the students caring for him, while an energetic search was being made for the stolen horse; finally he was found and it took six or eight men to get him from his new quarters." So much for the sons of churchmen.

At the medical school student behavior was not much different, and the enrollment was larger. Stephen Smith, a student at the school and later public health officer of New York City, described his class as numbering about 150 students, mostly young men from the neighboring towns, sons of farmers and tradesmen. "A more riotous and uncivil group of young men could not well be collected." On several occasions residents of the neighborhood had felt compelled to send written protests to the faculty, threatening to seek action to have the school closed if the disturbances did not cease. Smith related also that "during lectures it was often almost impossible to hear the professors owing to the confusion."

This was the setting into which Miss Blackwell brought herself. Smith was present the day of her arrival. One morning, he recalled:

> All unexpectedly, a lady entered the lecture-room with the professor; she was quite small of stature, plainly dressed, appeared diffident and retiring, but had a firm and determined expression of face. Her entrance into that Bedlam of confusion acted like magic upon every

student. Each hurriedly sought his seat, and the most absolute silence prevailed. For the first time a lecture was given without the slightest interruption, and every word could be heard as distinctly as it would if there had been but a single person in the room. The sudden transformation of this class from a band of lawless desperadoes to gentlemen, by the mere presence of a lady, proved to be permanent in its effects. A more orderly class of medical students was never seen than this, and it continued to be to the close of the term.

If Elizabeth Blackwell had accomplished nothing but this, it would have been a landmark in medical education.

Actually, it had been the faculty, not the students, who opposed the matriculation of a woman. Miss Blackwell's Philadelphia preceptor had written to twenty-nine schools seeking admission for his student and was refused by each one. The Geneva faculty, apparently not wanting to appear arbitrary, or perhaps hoping to incur student favor, submitted the proposal to the class with the single proviso that a favorable decision must be unanimous. Prior to the evening meeting at which the vote was to be taken and that every student attended, there were "uproarious demonstrations of favour." The assembled group drew up two resolutions approving the admission of Miss Blackwell. Following their presentation "the most extravagant speeches, which were enthusiastically cheered." The vote was 113 in favor, one opposed. This one nay brought "a general rush . . . for the corner of the room which emitted the voice, and the recalcitrant member was only too glad to acknowledge his error and record his vote in the affirmative."

Miss Blackwell (listed as Blackwill in the 1847–48 *Register of Geneva College*) received forthwith a letter from the dean, enclosing the resolutions (which Elizabeth later had copied on parchment and esteemed "one of my most valued possessions"). In her autobiography, Miss Blackwell describes her great relief and gratitude to providence at finally being accepted at a medical school. On November 4, she set out by rail from Philadelphia to Geneva, via New York City, arriving at her destination at 11 p.m. on Saturday, November 6. After interviews with the dean and other faculty members next day she was enrolled as student #130. She proceeded, forthwith, to find a room at a boarding house but three minutes' walk down the street from the school. Perhaps a bit lonesome and homesick, she later recalled that she "hung my room with dear mementoes of absent friends, and soon with hope and zeal and thankful feelings of rest I settled down to study."

School, of course, was already in session, the lectures having started almost a month earlier. The curriculum consisted of daily lectures in five subjects and a laboratory course in which the students, under the direction of a demonstrator, dissected a cadaver. This course in practical anatomy was the biggest stumbling block to having a woman in medical school. It involved dissection, in mixed company, of a naked body, including the genital organs. It was common, in spite of public statements to the contrary, for there to be, at least on occasion, a certain amount of levity in the dissecting room and, in fact, the professor himself was known as a bit of a jokester.

On the day of Miss Blackwell's arrival, the professor of anatomy, Dr. Webster, was away and the demonstrator was not sure whether he should allow Miss Blackwell to dissect. On top of this, she had no books and knew not where to get any. On the second morning, Dr. Webster appeared, "a fat little fairy . . . blunt in manner and very voluble." There followed a conversation among Dr. Webster, Dr. Lee, the dean, and Miss Blackwell as to whether she should include anatomical dissection in her course of study. Dr. Lee asked her whether she planned to practice surgery, to which Dr. Webster replied, "Why, of course she does. Think of the cases of femoral hernia; only think what a well-educated woman would do in a city like New York. Why, my dear sir, she'd have her hands full in no time; her success would be immense. Yes, yes, you'll go through the course, and get your diploma with great éclat, too. We'll give you the opportunities. You'll make a stir, I can tell you." Dr. Webster proceeded into the lecture room, leaving Miss Blackwell outside, read a letter from Miss Blackwell's preceptor, and received a round of applause. Miss Blackwell entered. Miss Blackwell later recalled that her fellow students were always gracious and courteous to her.

Subsequent to the lecture, Miss Blackwell stayed to observe "one of the most delicate operations in surgery," that illustrated the subject of the lecture. The following Monday, to her dismay, she was not allowed to attend a second operation but, upon writing to the professor, thereafter was regularly present. Though never explicitly stated, it was, presumably, dissection or operations involving the genitalia of either sex that were problematic. "A trying day. . . . That dissection was just as much as I could bear. Some of the students blushed, some were hysterical. . . . My delicacy was certainly shocked. . . . I had to . . . call on Christ to help me from smiling, for that would have ruined everything." The problem was ultimately resolved by having Elizabeth dissect with four of the "steadier students" in a separate room.

The remainder of the course apparently passed without notable event. Miss Blackwell wrote, "The behaviour of the medical class during the two years that I was with them was admirable. It was that of true Christian gentlemen." Miss Blackwell led a lonely life as far as one can tell, friendly but formal with faculty and students, befriending only her landlady, Mrs. Waller. From little bits in her diary and letters, it seems clear that she had no social interest in men. Her classmates, she wrote, "might be women or mummies for ought I care." The jollity and kindness of Professor Webster led her to the conclusion that "certainly I shall love fat men more than lean ones henceforth." As school recessed for the summer, one student asked her for the "honour of an occasional correspondence," and another said he was glad he had decided to return for the next course because she would be there too. She rebuffed both of these overtures, calling them "too funny." Earlier, she had written in her journal, "I must work by myself all life long."

There are also firsthand descriptions of Elizabeth's graduation. A local Geneva resident, twenty-five-year-old Margaret DeLancey, daughter of the Episcopal bishop of Western New York who was living in Geneva at the time, wrote to her sister-in-law, telling of the event that took place in the Presbyterian Church: "About half-past ten or eleven the procession entered the building. The Lioness of the day, Miss Blackwell met them at the door and entered with the Medical Students—without hat or shawl. She wore a black silk dress—and cape—lace collar and cuffs and her reddishly inclined hair was very nicely braided. She sat in a front side pew with old Mrs. Waller [her landlady] until she received her diploma." Except for the students the audience was made up mostly of women: "The ladies—carried the day! There was scarcely a coat—excepting the Students'—visible! Nothing but a vast expanse of woman's [*sic*] bonnets and curious eyes." The candidates came to the stage, four at a time, to receive their degrees. "Last of all came 'Domina Blackwell'! She ascended the steps. The President touched his cap and rose. You might have heard a pin drop. He stood while he conferred the degree on her, handed her the diploma and bowed, evidently expecting that she would bow also and retreat. Not so, however! She seemed embarrassed and after an effort, said to the Dr.—'I thank you Sir. It shall be the effort of my life, by God's blessing, to shed honor on this Diploma'—then bowed, blushing scarlet, left the stage and took her seat in the front pew among the Graduates amid the Enthusiastic applause of all present." She left the church on the arm of her brother, Henry Blackwell, who had come up from New York, put on her bonnet and shawl, and with her classmates was "turned adrift on the streams of time."

Bibliography:

Blackwell, Elizabeth. *Address on the Medical Education of Women. Dec. 27th, 1855.* New York, 1856. 16 pp.

———. *Counsel to Parents on the Moral Education of Their Children*. London, 1878. 96pp. There were at least eight London editions by 1913. American editions in 1879, 1880, 1881, 1883. Italian edition, 1882.

———. *Pioneer Work in Opening the Medical Profession to Women*. London, 1895.

———. *Essays on Medical Sociology*. 2 vols. London, 1902.

References:

Combs, William. *Reminiscences*. From a clipping: *Geneva (NY) Courier*, March 1890. Geneva Historical Society, Geneva, New York.

DeLancey, Margaret Munro. "Dr. Elizabeth Blackwell's Graduation—an Eyewitness Account," edited by Wendell Tripp. In *New York History*, Cooperstown, NY, April 1962 (vol. 43, no. 2), 182–85.

Johnston, Malcolm Sanders. *Elizabeth Blackwell and Her Alma Mater*. Geneva, NY, 1947.

Morantz, Regina. "Elizabeth Blackwell." In *Dictionary of American Medical Biography*. 2 vols., edited by Martin Kaufman et al. Westport, CT/London, c. 1984.

Smith, Stephen. *Random Recollections of a Long Life: Remarks at a Dinner Given to Commemorate the Speaker's Eighty-Eighth Birthday, February 19, 1911*. New York, 1911.

Thomson, Elizabeth. "Elizabeth Blackwell." In *Notable American Women 1607–1950: A Biographical Dictionary*. 3 vols. Cambridge, MA, 1971.

White, Andrew D. *Autobiography of Andrew Dickson White*. New York, 1905.

Biographical Dictionary
of 222 Graduates

Note: The biographies, except that of Elizabeth Blackwell, are arranged alphabetically by surname at the time of graduation from medical school. In eleven instances where the doctor was better known by an earlier name (e.g., Bisbee, Lozier) or a later name (e.g., Dolley, Homet, Peterman, Piersol, Sartain, Wilder, Wiley, Wilhite, Winslow) the entry is cross-referenced under that name in the index of names. The surname at the time of graduation is in capital letters. The maiden surname, if known, is printed in italics.

A

Lucy W. ABELL (1808–93)

Lucy Abell was born in 1808, probably in Boston. Of her family background, parents' names, childhood and early education, nothing is known. Sometime in the early 1840s she married a man named Abell with whom she had two children: Charles R. (b. ca. 1844), a boot and shoe dealer who later became a lawyer, and Edith (b. ca. 1846), who became a music teacher.

In 1856, at the age of forty-eight, and probably after the death of her husband, Lucy began the study of medicine at the New England Female Medical College. She soon transferred to the Woman's Medical Academy in Boston, founded by William Symington Brown. Brown had been on the faculty of the New England Female Medical College but left, apparently because he was an Eclectic and the only non-Regular member of the staff. Lucy soon transferred again, this time to Penn Medical University in Philadelphia, an Eclectic institution and the alma mater of Professor Brown. She received her medical degree in April 1860 from that school.

She returned to Boston and established a medical practice as a homoeopathic physician, and she was said to be one of the earliest, perhaps the earliest, woman physician to practice homoeopathy in New England. The 1866 Boston directory and the 1874 and 1877 Butler medical directories locate her at 173 Charles Street.

In 1875, Dr. Abell went abroad for an extended period and, on her return in 1878, established herself in Washington, DC. While in the capital, she organized a Ladies' Physiological Society. After 1882 she returned to New England, settling in Brookline, a suburb of Boston. According to her obituary in the *New England Medical Gazette*, she "to a great extent gave up active professional work" at that time. However, she is listed in the 1890 and 1893 Polk medical directories as a practicing physician. The 1889 Boston directory also lists her as a physician practicing at 178 Washington Street.

Dr. Abell died in Needham, Massachusetts, on December 3, 1893, at the age of eighty-five, after a short illness. Her obituary notes that she was "long known and honored in Boston and elsewhere as one of the pioneers of homoeopathy, and of women in medicine."

References: *Boston Almanac*, 1861, 1864, 1867–69, 1874, 1875; *Boston Business and Copartnership Directory*, 1863–64; *Boston Directory*, 1866; Butler, 1874, 1877; *Massachusetts Register*, 1867, 1872; Polk, 1890, 1893; *New England Business Directory*, 1865, 1868, 1875, 1877; Obituary, *New England Medical Gazette*, 1894, 29:50; US census, 1870, 1880.

Charlotte G. ADAMS (b. ca. 1824–89)

Charlotte Adams (her maiden name is not known) was born about 1824 in Massachusetts. Nothing is known of her background, childhood, or early education. Sometime before 1843, she married John L. Adams, a physician. In 1850, the couple was living in South Scituate, Massachusetts.

The Adamses had three children: Viola L. (b. 1843), Edelbert P. (b. 1846), and Charles J. (b. 1855). Since the name of Dr. John Adams does not appear in the 1860 census enumeration, it is probable that he had died. In the meantime, Charlotte and the children had moved to Roxbury, a Boston suburb, and Charlotte attended New England Female Medical College in 1852, transferring to the Female Medical College of Pennsylvania the following season. She received an MD degree in 1853. The move to the Philadelphia school may have been due to the fact that the New England school was not yet chartered to award medical degrees. Presumably, the fact that she was a widow with three young children to support was her motivation for becoming a doctor.

Boston directories list her as a female physician in 1852. She is not listed in 1851 or 1853. In 1854, she is listed as a physician or female physician at 258 Tremont; in 1856 and 1857, as Mrs. Charlotte G. Adams, MD, at 291 Tremont; and in 1858, 1860, and 1863 she was in

Roxbury. In 1863–64 she was back in Boston at 5 Exeter Place. It is documented that she practiced medicine in Boston or Roxbury for at least a dozen years.

Careful search of Boston and Massachusetts directories from 1866–75 does not find her name. She is not listed as a physician in Massachusetts in the 1874 and 1877 Butler medical directories or in the Polk US national medical directory for 1886. Whether she practiced medicine after 1864 is not known, but since her youngest child was only nine years old in 1864, it seems hard to believe she did not. The only death date that has been found comes from the 1890 *Annual Announcement* of the Woman's Medical College of Pennsylvania. In it she is said to have died in March 1889, location not specified. Since she is still listed as Charlotte Adams, she had probably not remarried. Her whereabouts and activities between 1864 and 1889 are not known.

References: Boston city directories, 1852–75; Butler, 1874, 1877; *Massachusetts State Record and Year Book of General Information*, vol. 3 (1849), vol. 4 (1850); *Massachusetts State Record, New England Register, and Year Book of General Information*, vol. 5 (1851); *New England Business Directory*, 1856; Polk, 1886; US census, 1850, 1860; Woman's Medical College of Pennsylvania, *Annual Announcement*, Philadelphia, 1890.

Harriet *ADAMS* (1828–86)

Born in London, England, on August 28, 1828, Miss Adams came to the United States sometime before 1850. The census that year lists her as living in Palmyra, New York, in a home occupied by two sisters who worked as milliners and their respective eighteen-year-old daughters who were then in school. A prominent local citizen is said to have played an important financial role in Miss Adams's immigration and her subsequent medical education. This was Pliny Sexton (d. 1881), a Quaker, whose Palmyra home was part of the Underground Railroad, a house next to which Miss Adams would later live, and in whose cemetery plot she would be buried. (The only known documentation of Mr. Sexton's sponsorship, likely though it seems, is a 1963 statement to Palmyra town historian Robert Lowe by the attorney for Mr. Sexton's son, Pliny T. Sexton, that this was so.)

Miss Adams graduated from what was then called the Female Medical College of Pennsylvania in March 1859, returned home to Palmyra, and practiced medicine there until her death at fifty-seven in 1886. Her office hours, at least in later years, were daily from 2 to 5 p.m. For a while, she continued to live with the milliner sisters until sometime before 1875 when she bought the house at 36 Main Street (now 330 Main Street), just east of Pliny Sexton's home. The 1875 census lists two other persons living with her at this address: a sixteen-year-old male servant and a forty-year-old medical student, Lovina Snow. Snow and Adams are buried next to each other in the Pliny Sexton plot in Palmyra Cemetery. Sometime before her death Dr. Adams was thrown from her carriage and was, thereafter, an invalid. One obituary says she died of a brain tumor, raising the question of whether a subdural hematoma might have followed the carriage accident.

References: New York State census, 1865, 1875; Obituary, *Palmyra Courier*, April 1, 1886; Obituary, *Rochester Democrat*, March 30, 1886; US census, 1870; Advertisement, *Wayne County Journal*, April 1, 1880; *Gazetteer and Business Directory of Wayne County*, Syracuse, NY, 1867–68.

Sarah Read *ADAMSON* Dolley (1829–1909)

Sarah Dolley, born Sarah Read Adamson, in Schuylkill Meeting, Pennsylvania, on March 11, 1829, was the second daughter and third of five children of Charles Adamson, local farmer and storekeeper, and Sarah Mary Corson. The Corson family was rather medical: two of Sarah's uncles were physicians, as were six of her fifty first cousins, several of whom, like Sarah, started their medical studies under the tutelage of Uncle Hiram Corson (MD, University of Pennsylvania, 1829) and who, with the exception of Sarah, all went on to graduate from the University of Pennsylvania medical school. Sarah, however, after preparation at Friends School in Philadelphia, and with Uncle Hiram's tutelage, was denied entrance at all Philadelphia medical schools. She applied to Central Medical College, a recently organized Eclectic school in Rochester, New York, attended that institution, and received an MD degree on February 20, 1851. She and her classmate Rachel Brooks Gleason (q.v.) were the third and fourth women to receive medical degrees in the United States (after Elizabeth Blackwell [q.v.] and Lydia Folger Fowler [q.v.]).

After graduating, she applied to the board of the Philadelphia Hospital for "such a position in the Blockley Hospital as will afford me the opportunity of seeing its practice to such an extent and under such conditions as may comport with the proper regulations of the institution." The committee to which the request was referred reported favorably on May 25, 1851, saying (as described by Lawrence) that the chief resident physician was to "assign her to such position as will best enable her to obtain the knowledge she desires without detriment to the institution." John Croskey, writing a history of Blockley Hospital a quarter century later, reports this same event with slight differences in the quoted words. Dr. Adamson was the first woman on the professional staff of that famous hospital.

On returning to Rochester, Dr. Adamson married one of her medical school professors, Lester C. Dolley, MD, described some years later by another woman physician, Marion Craig Potter, as "a very scholarly and cultured gentleman." Lester had been courting Sarah at least from the time of her graduation. Among the letters in the Sarah Dolley papers is one from Sarah's parents, Charles and Mary Adamson, in response to an earlier letter from Lester regarding his proposal to marry Sarah. Carefully worded, it does not mention that Sarah would be marrying "out of meeting" but rather expresses the belief that "parental care ought not to extend so far as to prevent the union of those sincerely attached to each other, unless it is known that there is well grounded reason for objection. . . . We have a great confidence in dear Sarah's prudence and ability to discern and discriminate between sincere and affected merrit [*sic*]." They express the hope that the couple will eventually move to Philadelphia.

Lester and Sarah were married the following year. After returning from their wedding trip to New York City, Sarah wrote her brother, "We had a fine time in New York, visited Greenwood cemtary [*sic*], the Hospitals on Blackwell's Island, called on Miss Blackwell, etc., etc." She and Lester had two children, one of whom, Charles Sumner Dolley, lived to adulthood and became a marine biologist. A grandson died during the First World War. A granddaughter, Charlotte, married the son of sculptor Augustus St. Gaudens.

Dr. Dolley practiced medicine in Rochester for the next fifty-seven years, first with her husband and, after his death from spinal fever in 1872, by herself, emphasizing the care of women and children. She went to Europe twice for postgraduate training in Paris and Vienna, and in 1873–74 served as professor of obstetrics at Woman's Medical College of Pennsylvania. She apparently did not enjoy her teaching experience but undertook it in order to substitute for her sick friend Emeline Horton Cleveland (q.v.), and to be with her son in Philadelphia as he prepared for college. In 1886, under her leadership, the women doctors of Rochester (by then twelve in number), disbarred from hospital practice, opened the Provident Dispensary on Front Street and organized their own professional group, the Practitioner's Society. This group was later renamed the Blackwell Society, which later evolved into the New York State Woman's Medical Society.

Dr. Dolley was not only a medical leader, recognized as such by her male colleagues; she showed leadership in many other community activities. Raised a Quaker, she was expelled for marrying out of meeting and became a Congregationalist, and later a Presbyterian.

Sarah died at eighty on December 27, 1909, and is buried in Mt. Hope Cemetery.

In 1942, toward the end of her own life, Dr. Marion Craig Potter, protégée of Dr. Dolley and herself professionally prominent, recalled the Drs. Dolley. Both Lester and Sarah "were prominent physicians in the city, keenly interested in church and civic matters." Potter remarked about Sarah that, "for a quiet little Quaker woman, she knew all the Aldermen and the City Fathers, and met them all with the arts of a politician. She brought about the appointment of a woman on the Staff of Rochester City [now General] Hospital" as well as membership in the County Medical Society, a woman in attendance at the Monroe County Insane Asylum (forerunner of Rochester State Hospital), "and through her influence the law was passed that every institution for women in New York State should have a woman physician on the staff."

> She was a friend of Clara Barton and secretary of the Rochester Chapter of the American Red Cross which was one of the early chapters. . . . She was secretary for years of a social group, known as The Ignorance Club. . . . She travelled in Europe with Frances Willard and when she and her friend Susan B. Anthony met they relapsed into their Quaker 'Thee and Thou.' . . . She had a merrie little chuckle when she surmounted a difficult problem. She was a great leader and as a pioneer physician blazed a trail worthy for all women to follow. She left a lasting influence for good.

Bibliography: *Closing Lecture to the Class of 1873–4, Delivered at the Woman's Medical College of Pennsylvania, March 5, 1874* (Philadelphia, 1874); *An Address at the Second Annual Meeting of the Women's Medical Society of New York State, Held in Rochester, N.Y., March 11, 1908* (Rochester, 1908); Manuscript journal, 1860, Edward G. Miner Library, Rochester, NY.

References: Hiram Corson, *A History of the Descendants of Benjamin Corson, Son of Cornelius Corssen of Staten Island, New York* (Philadelphia, 1896), 84–85; *Notable American Women*, 1:497–99; Ellen S. More, *Restoring the Balance* (Cambridge, MA: Harvard University Press, 1999); Jane Marsh Parker, *Rochester, a Story Historical* (Rochester, NY, 1884), 265; Marion Craig Potter, response to a toast by Dr. Marion Craig Potter, January 24, 1942, typescript in the archives of the Edward G. Miner Library, Rochester, NY; John W. Croskey, *History of Blockley* (Philadelphia: F. A. Davis, 1929); Charles Lawrence, *History of the Philadelphia Almshouses and Hospitals* (Philadelphia: Author, 1905); Charles and Mary Corson, ALS to Lester Dolley, July 8, 1851, correspondence of Sarah Dolley, Edward G. Miner Library, Rochester, NY; S. Dolley, letter to her brother, July 6, 1852, correspondence of Sarah Dolley.

Sarah E. ALLEN (b. ca. 1832)

Sarah Allen (maiden name not known) was born in Ohio about 1832. According to the 1850 census she was then living in Maquon, Knox County, Illinois, was eighteen years old, and had married a twenty-seven-year-old Ohio-born physician named Milville (or Melville) Allen within the year. Two different dates for the wedding are recorded: January 3 and February 8, 1850.

During the decade that followed, the newlyweds moved to Peoria, Illinois. Sarah had a daughter, Emma (b. 1851), and, later in the 1850s, attended Western Homoeopathic College in Cleveland, graduating in 1858 with an MD degree. (One source says it was a degree in obstetrics.) Melville had apparently done well financially: the 1860 census listed him as owning $32,000 in real estate (he had property worth only $250 in 1850). This was certainly not acquired through small-town medical practice. The family had domestic help, which may have provided care for the young daughter while Sarah was at medical school. In the 1860 census, both Sarah and her husband are listed as "physicians."

Whether Sarah ever practiced medicine is not known. By the time of the 1870 census the family had moved to Chicago, where it appears they were living in a hotel or boarding house with five other families. Neither Sarah nor Melville is listed as a physician; they are now both "at home." So, presumably, they were not practicing medicine.

No entry for them is found in the 1880 census, and the 1890 census records were destroyed in a fire. In 1900, Sarah and Melville, now sixty-seven and seventy-six, respectively, are living in Clearwater Harbor, Florida. Ten years later, they are still there; daughter Emma, then forty-five, has returned home, and thirty-nine-year-old James Davidson is living with them. It seems unlikely that Sarah practiced medicine or midwifery, and if she did, but briefly. No death date for her has been found.

References: US census, 1850, 1860, 1870, 1880, 1900, 1910.

Rachel Humphrey *ALLYN* (1810–1903)

Rachel Allyn was born April 25, 1810, in Charleston, a village in Vermont's Northeast Kingdom settled by her father, Abner Allyn. Abner and his wife, Anna Melvin, had eight children. Rachel was the third of the six who survived to adulthood and the third child born in Charleston.

Years later, in 1870, when all of her siblings were dead except her eldest brother, Alpha, Rachel recounted some of the family history.

She told the story of Alpha being lost in the woods on a cold and rainy November night when he was sixteen (and she eight), the frantic and ultimately successful search for him by neighbors from several surrounding communities, and the lifetime limitations he incurred as a result.

As a young woman Rachel became a teacher and was among the first group of young ladies to obtain the certificates of proficiency required under a new Vermont law. Later, she became a nurse and is listed as such in the 1855 Lowell, Massachusetts, directory. She attended New England Female Medical College in Boston but, with six other classmates, transferred to Worcester Medical College, either because the Boston school did not yet have a charter authorizing it to grant doctoral degrees or because the Worcester school was coed. In 1857, now forty-seven years old, she received an MD degree.

Rachel moved to Lowell, Massachusetts, with its large population of young women working in the cotton mills, where she practiced successfully for twenty-six years before retiring, at seventy-three, to her native community of East Charleston, Vermont. She is listed as a physician in various Lowell directories between 1864 and 1883, the *New England Business Directory* and the *Massachusetts Register* from 1864–65 through 1883. She died on July 11, 1903, at the age of ninety-three. According to her death certificate, the cause of death was carcinoma of the scalp.

References: Rachel H. Allyn, "An Incident in the Early History of the Town," *Vermont Historical Magazine*, 1877, 132–36; *International Genealogical Index*; Lowell directory, 1864–66, 1868, 1870, 1872, 1880, 1883; *Massachusetts Register*, 1867, 1872, 1878; *New England Business Directory*, 1860, 1865, 1875.

Anna N. *Smith* ANDERSON (b. ca. 1809)

Anna N. Smith was born in Massachusetts about 1809 and, in 1837, moved from Connecticut to Bristol, Pennsylvania, a village in Bucks County on the Delaware River northeast of Philadelphia, to take charge of the female department of the recently opened Bristol Public School (December 15, 1837). The school building had cost $6,000 and was the first public school in the area. Male students were supervised by James Anderson, whom Anna soon married. The couple had four children: Lukens (b. 1839), Alice Ann (b. 1841), Edward (b. 1843), and Henry (b. 1845).

In the early 1850s, then in her midforties and her children aged eight through fourteen, Anna matriculated at the Female Medical College of Pennsylvania and, in March 1853, received an MD degree. She practiced thereafter in Bristol where, according to Doron Green in his *History of Bristol Borough*, she "was successful in the treatment of her cases" (187–88). In none of the census reports (1860, 1870, 1880) is her occupation mentioned.

The family seems to have moved around a bit, probably because of James's work as a schoolmaster. The 1850 census places the Andersons in Middletown, Bucks County, where James is listed as a "college principal." The 1860 census finds the family in Moreland, Montgomery County, where James is a "teacher" and his son, Lukens, then twenty-one, a "druggist." In the 1870 census they are in Salem, a village in southern New Jersey, where James is a schoolteacher. By 1880, Anna and James, then seventy-two and seventy-three, respectively, were living in Rahway, New Jersey with their youngest son, Henry, and his three-year-old daughter, Anna. The child's mother had probably died. Whether Anna practiced medicine after she left Bristol is not known. Her date of death is also unknown.

References: J. M. Battle, *History of Bucks County, Pennsylvania* (Spartanburg, SC, 1985); Doron Green, *A History of Bristol Borough in the County of Bucks, State of Pennsylvania* (Camden, NJ, 1911); US census, 1850, 1860, 1870, 1880.

Anna Sarah *ANGELL* Curtis (b. 1825)

Nothing is known of Anna Sarah's parents, background, childhood, or early education. When she graduated with an MD degree from New England Female Medical College in 1858 she was a resident of Providence, Rhode Island. She had no scholarship support while at medical school. She had made contributions to the school, $20 in 1850, five years before matriculating, and again in 1855, the year she started school.

The *Progressive Annuals* for 1862, 1863, and 1864 list an Anna S. Curtis as a practicing physician in Medford, Massachusetts. No other Anna S. has been identified among woman physicians of the time, so it seems likely—but not proven—that Anna Angell married George Curtis, a shipbuilder. Since it nowhere specifies that Anna Curtis has an MD degree, we cannot be certain that Anna the physician is Anna the MD. Assuming they are the same, George was the son of a prominent Medford shipbuilder who lived with the young couple. According to the 1860 census, the three are living in the same household. George and Anna had no children.

The Medford city directories for 1868, 1870, 1876, 1880, and 1887 list no Anna Curtis (or Angell) and no George Curtis, which suggests that the Curtises moved away sometime between 1860 and 1868. It is not known where they went. Nor is it known that Anna Sarah ever practiced medicine. No record was found that she paid the physician tax during the Civil War.

The 1870, 1880, and 1900 census reports list an Anna S. A. Curtis as a resident of Bridgewater, New Jersey, a farming community about thirty miles west of Manhattan. In 1870, she is listed as a farmer, born in Rhode Island, with $8,000 in real estate and $2,000 in personal property. The only other household resident is a fifteen-year-old farm hand. The 1880 census report a similar situation. Anna, now a widow, is listed as "housekeeping," and the farmhand is now a "farmer." The 1900 census finds Anna living alone on the farm, which she owns free and clear. Was this Dr. Anna Sarah? Nowhere is it mentioned that she was a physician, though that does not rule out the possibility that she was. The name is correct, she was born in Rhode Island, and her age is reasonably close (ages are seldom accurate in census data). But why did she move to New Jersey? Though a widow in 1880, had she been divorced before that date? What ultimately happened to Anna Sarah Angell remains unclear.

References: *Medford Directory*, 1868, 1870, 1876, 1880, 1887; *Progressive Annual*, 1862, 1863, 1864; US census, 1860, 1870, 1880, 1900.

Rebecca L. *Vancleave* ANTON (1827–92)

Rebecca Anton was the first woman doctor in Warren County, Ohio. She practiced medicine in Lebanon, with her doctor husband, for thirty-three years. Lebanon, the county seat, a village of a few thousand, is about halfway between Dayton and Cincinnati. Born on January 6, 1827, she married Scottish-born James Anton, April 12, 1852. He received an MD degree from Eclectic Medical Institute in Cincinnati the following year. Rebecca graduated from the Eclectic College of Medicine (Cincinnati) in 1859. The couple moved to Lebanon and established their practices forthwith.

Some years later, in 1877, Rebecca received a second MD degree, this one from the Eclectic Medical College of the City of New York. Whether this was simply a refresher course or whether it had something to do with her daughter's rheumatoid arthritis is not known. Rebecca died in Lebanon, November 2, 1892. James died Lebanon, October 28, 1897, at seventy, having practiced medicine in Lebanon for over three decades. The couple had two children: F. Gaul (b. 1856), who sold insurance and, later in Chicago, real estate. Nellie (b. 1860) lived in Lebanon and died February 6, 1919.

References: Funeral notice of Mrs. Dr. R. V. Anton (printed card); *Beers' History of Warren County, Ohio* (Chicago, 1972), 307; US census, 1860, 1870, 1880, 1900, 1910; Obituary for James Anton, *Western Star* (Lebanon, OH), November 4, 1897.

Hannah Angeline *Batchelor* ARNOLD (1821–97)

Hannah was born October 29, 1821, in Upton, Massachusetts, and spent most of her life in nearby Wrentham (Norfolk Co.). Her parents were Otis Batchelor and Susana Buck, both natives of Upton. She was the youngest of at least seven children. Hannah probably moved to Wrentham after marrying carpenter James M. N. Arnold on August 30, 1840. The Arnolds had three children. The eldest, a boy, died in infancy. The second, Henrietta Lucy, born May 7, 1844, died at seven months. The last child, Sarah Amelia, born October 17, 1847, lived to adulthood and, for a while at least, taught school.

More than a decade after the birth of her last child, Hannah attended the New England Female Medical College in Boston, where she had a Massachusetts state scholarship for 1857–58 and 1859–61. In 1861, she received a medical degree. Thereafter, she probably practiced in Wrentham. In each US census—1850, 1860, and 1870—the family is found in Wrentham, though in none of those years is Hannah listed as a physician. Nor is she listed in Polk medical directories for 1886, 1890, or 1893. However, both the *Massachusetts Register* in 1867 (but not in 1872), and the *New England Business Directory* for 1868 (but not in 1875), list her as a practicing physician. She was still denoted a physician in the Massachusetts Vital Records at the time of her death. So, it appears that Dr. Arnold practiced medicine for several years after her graduation and possibly for as long as thirty-six years (1861–97) in Wrentham, or, more specifically, its suburb Sheldonville. She died November 13, 1897, of heart disease.

References: *International Genealogical Index; Massachusetts Register,* 1867, 1872; Massachusetts Vital Records, Wrentham, MA, 1897; *New England Business Directory,* 1865, 1868, 1875; US census, 1850, 1860, 1870.

Harriet Newell *AUSTIN* (1825–90)

Harriet Austin was born August 31, 1825, in Killingly, Windham County, Connecticut, the daughter of Joseph Austin and his wife Abigail Woodward. The family moved to the village of Moravia in central New York State when she was young. Her formal education was at local schools. She attended and on December 6, 1851, received a diploma after a three-month course at the American Hydropathic Institute, an unchartered school in Manhattan established by Mary Gove Nichols and her husband Thomas Low Nichols. There, she was one of nine women in a class of twenty. She and two of her classmates, Harriet A. Judd and Esther C. Wileman, later received MD degrees from other schools. Austin received an honorary medical degree from the New York Hygeio-Therapeutic College in 1859.

Austin started practice in Owasco, New York, a village about ten miles north of Moravia but was soon persuaded by James Caleb Jackson, one of the principals at the nearby Glen Haven Water-Cure to join that group. Orsemus and Rachel Gleason, who had been providing the patient care at Glen Haven, had recently left to establish themselves in Elmira. Jackson, who had been business manager, needed help, especially in providing care to women patients. This Austin did. During the next five or six years she grew in professional stature, wrote prolifically for the *Water-Cure Journal,* and edited a house organ called the *Letter Box.*

In 1858, Austin and Jackson joined F. Wilson Hurd to establish a new water-cure at Dansville, New York—Our Home on the Hillside—which was to become one of the most famous and long-surviving institutions of its kind. (It evolved into a sanitorium after the Civil War when hydropathy lost its popularity and continued operation until the Great Depression.) In a description of the move from Glen Haven to Dansville, Austin gives an idea of the daily regimen.

> I am in a transition state—passing from Glen Haven to *our new home* and tarrying on the way, as Jews tarried in their passage from Egypt to the *land of promise.* . . . I am staying with fifteen of our patients at a hotel in the pretty little village of Homer. . . . We are learning to be very comfortable, and very much at home. . . . I am cook, going into the kitchen daily and helping to get *up our* meals. We make excellent bread by stirring Graham flour into warm water until the batter is as thick as it can well be stirred, and then dropping on to baking tins in the form of common sized biscuits, and baking thirty to forty minutes in a hot oven. Also, by making a very stiff batter of Indian meal and boiling hot water, and spreading it on tins in cakes half to three quarters of an inch thick, and baking in a hot oven. We have very good pies, both of apple and pumpkin, the crust being made of Graham flour mixed with cream. We have nice baked potatoes and baked apples, we have tomatoes, berries, peaches, squashes, turnips, corn, and beans, all without any salt or vinegar, or pepper or butter. So you can see persons can *fare sumptuously* in a hotel, without eating the flesh of dead animals, or drinking tea or coffee.

Breakfast was at 8:30 a.m. and dinner at 3 p.m. After dinner they sang, read Scriptures, and "acknowledged that it is God who preserves our lives from destruction and saves our souls from death." Clearly, diet, religion, and presumably exercise were the regimen. The diet was as much what one avoided as what one ate.

At Our Home on the Hill, Austin was one-third owner along with Hurd and Giles Jackson, James Caleb's eldest son, and after Giles' premature death from tuberculosis in 1864, one-half owner. In 1868, she became senior partner in the operation. James Jackson, though clearly the dominant figure, was never an owner. At Our Home Austin cared for men as well as for women, edited the house organ, the *Laws of Life*, and wrote her classic on "How to Take Baths" (1861). In addition to her role as physician, Austin was a significant figure in the effort to reform women's clothing. She favored what she called the American costume—pants and long topcoat. She wrote several pamphlets on the subject: *The American Costume for Women*, *The American Costume; or, Woman's Right to Good Health*, and *Health Dress*. "Our issue," she wrote, "is with the mode in which *all* women dress . . . and we assert that their dress is at variance with the nature of their physical constitution, and so forbids a true physical development; that it is a positive and powerfully exciting cause of disease, that it is a main cause of the feebleness of women and girls."

In 1882, the main building of Our Home burned to the ground. James Caleb and Harriet retired from the enterprise and moved to North Adams, Massachusetts. Harriet died there April 27, 1891, at the age of sixty. After the death of her parents, Harriet had been adopted by James Jackson, who already had two sons. According to Albert Leffingwell, a nephew of James Jackson and, after 1882, a partner in what was then renamed the Sanitorium, the adoption really established a ménage à trois among Harriet, James, and his wife Lucretia. He claimed that Harriet was "the (unrecognized) second wife to J. C. J. . . . for nearly forty years." He also wrote that she was "in her old age robbed and died of grief" (Leffingwell Papers). Harriet Austin is buried in the Jackson plot at Greenmount Cemetery, North Dansville, next to James Caleb Jackson.

Bibliography: "Woman's Present and Future," *Water-Cure Journal*, September 1853, 57; *The American Costume for Women* (Dansville, NY: F. Wilson Hurd & Co., 1859); *The American Costume; or, Women's Right to Good Health* (Dansville, NY: F. Wilson Hurd & Co., 1861); *Health Dress* (Dansville, NY: Sanitarium Publishing Co., 1886); *How to Take Baths* (Dansville, NY: F. Wilson Hurd & Co., 1861); ed., *The Laws of Life* (Dansville,

1858–93); ed., *The Letter Box* (Glen Haven, NY, 1856–57); Twelve letters published in the *Water-Cure Journal,* December 1857–November 1858).

References: A. O. Bunnell, *History of Dansville, 1789–1902,* excerpted by Martha Treichler, s.v., "Dr. Harriet Newell Austin," *Find a Grave,* http://www.findagrave.com/cgi-bin/fg.cgi?page=gr&GRid= 87375989 (accessed May 19, 2016); Greenmount Cemetery, N. Dansville, NY; Biographical entry in *An Annotated Catalog of the Edward C. Atwater Collection of American Popular Medicine* (Rochester, NY: University of Rochester Press, 2001), 1:54–55; Papers of Albert J. Leffingwell, Edward G. Miner Library, Rochester, NY.

Minerva Jane *AVERELL* (1825–54)

Minerva Jane Averell was born April 2, 1825, the third of eight children of Canfield Averell and Lydia Jewett Stowell of Madrid, St. Lawrence County, New York. Both parents were pioneers of the area. Mrs. Averell had come to the area in 1814 by horseback from Plattsburg, where, at the time, her brother was running a hotel. She moved to Madrid after her marriage. By the 1850s, when Minerva went to medical school, an older sister and younger brother had already died (at twenty-three and eleven years of age).

Minerva Jane did well at Syracuse (New York, Eclectic) Medical School, one of two women graduating on February 16, 1854, and was second valedictorian of her class. In her valedictory address (printed in its entirety in *Syracuse Medical and Surgical Journal,* 1854) she gave justification for women entering the medical profession: "The physician is daily called upon to give instruction to his patients about the laws of health. It is one of woman's particular missions on earth, to teach—to instruct."

Upon graduation, it was announced in the journal that Dr. Averell would teach a "course of lectures to the ladies" during the spring term about to start on March 6, 1854. Unfortunately, her health failed, and she was "prostrated by that active scourge of our Northern Counties" (presumably tuberculosis). It is recorded in the family Bible that "for years she had experienced the premonitory symptoms of the disease. . . . On the 10th of June last, she was brought home from Dr. Halsted's Water Cure Establishment in Northampton, Mass. apparently in a dying state, after which she rapidly declined." She died about August 1, 1854, at home in Madrid, having never been able to practice medicine. Originally a Congregationalist, Averell's relationship with that denomination had lapsed. Her funeral was held at the Universalist Church. She was a member of the Knights of Jericho, a society that promoted total abstinence.

References: Averell family Bible; St. Lawrence County Historical Association, personal communication from John A. Baule, historian; *Syracuse Medical & Surgical Journal*, 1854.

B

Mary Malin *Evans* BAILY (1810–65)

Mary Evans, born 1810 to a prominent Paoli, Pennsylvania, family, was the eldest of three children. Her paternal grandfather, Joshua Evans, had bought five hundred acres from William Penn in 1719, where in 1761 he built an inn around which the village of Paoli formed, a community that later achieved prominence as the western terminus of main line commuter trains. Her father, Joshua Evans Jr., hotelkeeper and farmer, was a member of the Pennsylvania legislature and later, from 1829 to 1833, served in the US House of Representatives. Her mother's sister, Aunt Sally, was for many years postmistress of Paoli. Her brother, unmarried, succeeded his father as hotelkeeper and farmer and was also a partner in the Columbia Manufacturing Company. Her mother, Lydia, died when Mary was eight. There is little information about Mary's early life and education. (This sketch is based almost entirely on letters in the Evans family papers.)

On May 14, 1839, then twenty-nine, Mary and John Parker Baily were married. Baily, a local man, and third of twelve siblings, was already well acquainted with the Evans family and had often sought help from his future congressman father-in-law. In 1833, John offered thanks, again, for the favor "you did for me at a time when I felt deserted and alone in the world." On another occasion he asked for a reference when seeking a job in the War Department and still later, in 1836, when applying for a commission as captain. In February 1842, now married three years, he started reading law with a firm in Pittsburgh, having been turned down by the Cincinnati firm he preferred. In a letter to Aunt Sally, February 28, 1844, Mary wrote, "We talked some about going to housekeeping, but that has blown over—we can live much pleasanter and cheaper by Boarding." In 1844, Baily was admitted to the bar.

Two years later (1846) things were not going well. Mary wrote her brother in confidence, "Mr. Baily is dissatisfied with me, that I have a portion of my furniture at Paoli . . . ," and so on. By June 1850, she wrote brother John several letters about getting back her "fortune" of $3,000 from Mr. Baily. This was money she had inherited from her father, who had died in 1846. Mary wanted to invest it in railroad stock and have the income go to "our common fund." The Bailys lived together until August 12, 1851.

On August 24, 1851, at age forty-one, Mary matriculated at the Troy Female Seminary, Troy, New York, later better known as Emma Willard after its founder and longtime principal. Mary was a "student," not a "pupil," and therefore not "under rules." She was not a graduate. The following year she entered Eclectic Medical Institute in Cincinnati. To her brother, she reported finding a boarding house for five dollars a week, including fuel (bituminous coal) and light, but was less happy about the cistern water supply: "[I] hope it will not be my unfortunate condition to have no other but this solution of mud, alias, River water to drink" (November 21, 1852). Her roommate, introduced by Professor Buchanan, was Julia Rumsey (q.v.) from Avoca, New York. The professor was "a kind of father all around." With Julia, she attended the Unitarian Church regularly. She wrote home that she would take the dissection course. Three months later (February 1853) she was about to start her second course, though it was a month sooner than she wanted to, and asked her brother for another draft of $100 or $120—"the latter sum is all my income until October."

In February 1853, Mary wrote, "I am making respectable progress under instruction from the different 'Chairs' and each claim[s] the same attention—but Anatomy and Physiology are the two subjects which I expect to make most available in my plans, if I assume to have any in regard to the future. I cannot graduate under three Courses of Lectures—which will bring me to this time next year—I hope my health will bear me on without faltering, but this is a sorry climate." A week or so later she was planning a trip to St. Louis: "The recreation may perhaps benefit me—renew me for the succeeding duty that awaits, for I know increased application rather than less will be incumbent on those who wish to possess a Certificate of Examination."

In August, she wrote to her brother, John, "I am going to the Clinical Institute—at stated times during the week—and come home and read. When meal hours arrive we form a pleasant table circle—formed of three teachers, 2 female medical students—and two old bachelors— one a printer, a smatterer in Divinity, and Hypochondriac; the other, a plain businessman—a master painter, which is good business in Cincinnati." She went on to say, "I feel as tho' I am gradually being drawn into the Medical Profession—perhaps it may subside—I do not know—but if I do locate myself to practice medicine it will be in the city of Troy." And a month later she wrote, "I have no fixed plans for the future beyond that of making use of my mind . . . also laying some claims to usefulness. . . . [I] continue to feel that the Troy Female Seminary will be the finale of my career."

Sometime before June 1853, John Baily and Mary were divorced. "I feel glad . . . that I am out of my bondage, although I believe some unions are genial, free and happy, and I congratulate such—my experiment has been sufficient." A few months later, writing to Aunt Sally in regard to a relative's newborn daughter: "I have ceased to regret that I have never held a noble boy of my own in my embracing arms—but I have not ceased to remember how religiously I aspired to that ideal joy." She expressed thanks that "the enlightened laws of my native state [gave] me an avenue of relief, by giving a wife the control of her own property" (October 9, 1853).

Mary did not like Cincinnati. In July 1853 she wrote, "I would not make Cincinnati my residence if a bounty were dependent on it—it is seated in what was a whole range of frog ponds—with a chain of hills shutting it in." In March 1854, she received an MD degree from Eclectic Medical Institute and returned to Troy, hoping to be offered a professorship of anatomy and physiology by the Willards. She was not. At least one reason was that the position was not full time and she would have been required to fulfill additional teaching duties. This she was unwilling to do.

During the year and a half she remained at Troy, she applied for a position as resident physician at a women's hospital in New York City, but the post went to a male doctor. She wrote to her brother, sounding him out on the possibility of her coming to live with him and of succeeding Aunt Sally as Paoli postmistress, a suggestion he deftly deflected. In 1856, she did return to Paoli, and, a couple of years later, she attended the Female Medical College of Pennsylvania, where she received a second doctor of medicine degree in 1859. She went back to Troy for a couple of years. On April 10, 1861, she wrote her brother that she was living beyond her means and wanted to return home. In 1864, fifty-four years old, she wrote, "I am not well, sick in body and mind and long for rest . . . I could almost say eternal rest." She died the following year. It does not appear that she ever practiced medicine.

References: Evans Family Papers 1709–1928, Library of Virginia, Richmond, VA, miscellaneous reels #4173, 4174, 4175, 4183.

Clemence Sophia *Harned* Lozier BAKER (1813–88)

Clemence Harned Baker founded the first medical school in New York State exclusively for women, the New York Medical College and Hospital for Women. She was born December 11, 1813, in Plainfield, New Jersey, the thirteenth and youngest child of David Harned, a Methodist, and Hannah Walker, a Quaker. Her formal education at Plainfield Academy ended when she was sixteen and married Abraham Witton

Lozier, a New York carpenter and builder. Of their children, only the youngest survived to adulthood, Abraham Witton Lozier Jr., and he became a physician. Abraham Sr. sickened and died in 1837, when Clemence was twenty-four. For several years before she was widowed, Clemence had run a school for sixty girls in her home. The curriculum included anatomy, physiology and hygiene—quite unusual for the day. She also held meetings there for the "promotion of holiness." During the 1840s she was an active member of the New York Female Moral Reform Society, a group whose goal was to prevent prostitution.

Encouraged by an older brother who was a physician, Clemence began reading medical books. She married John Baker and moved to Albany, but the marriage did not work out. Perhaps for this reason she moved to Webster, a village in Western New York, near Rochester. Here, she lectured on physiology and hygiene at a local church and soon enrolled at Central Medical College, a recently organized Eclectic institution in Rochester. In March 1853, she graduated with highest honors from the school, which by then had moved to Syracuse. The new doctor set up practice in New York City. The following advertisement appeared in the January 1855 *Water-Cure Journal*: "Mrs. C. S. Baker, M.D. graduate, Lying-In Institute, 201 W. 36th St. She also consults with and visits patients at their residences."

According to a memorial written by her son, she soon had a large practice, and, by the mid-1860s, her income was approaching $25,000 a year. Emboldened by an 1860 article written by Elizabeth Cady Stanton, Clemence sought and, on April 27, 1861, was granted a divorce from her husband. Thereafter she called herself Clemence Lozier.

Her home lectures on anatomy and physiology, and the Medical Library Association she organized so her students could read books about their health, led her to the idea of establishing a medical school for women. With the help of Mrs. Stanton, she lobbied the New York State Legislature and, in spite of fierce opposition, received a charter for the New York Medical College and Hospital for Women on July 14, 1863. It was the first medical school in New York City that accepted women as students. Dr. Lozier was president and clinical professor of diseases of women and children. She also performed a substantial amount of surgery at the hospital. After a tour of the hospitals of Europe in 1867, she returned and reorganized her own school. Within twenty years there were more than two hundred graduates of the institution. In the late 1870s, the school and hospital, against the advice of Dr. Lozier, moved to new and more elegant quarters, which led to financial problems. Lozier, a major contributor to the organization, was forced to declare bankruptcy in 1878. She continued her medical practice thereafter.

Dr. Lozier was very active in the woman's suffrage movement, both locally and nationally, was a substantial supporter of Susan B. Anthony's weekly publication *Revolution* (1868–70), and worked for women's education, sanitary reform, international arbitration, and better treatment of Indians and of prisoners. Earlier, she had worked to abolish slavery. Clemence Lozier died of heart disease at seventy-four on April 26, 1888, and is buried in Brooklyn's Greenwood Cemetery. Forty-eight graduates of the school, six of them her relatives, attended her funeral.

Bibliography: C. S. Lozier, *Child-Birth Made Easy* (New York, 1870); *Care of Children* (New York, 1871); C. S. Lozier, "The Care of Little Children," *Herald of Health,* January 1872, 18–22; C. S. Lozier, Madeleine Vinton Dahlgren, et al., *Arguments before the Committee on Privileges and Elections of the United States Senate, in Behalf of a Sixteenth Amendment to the Constitution of the United States, Prohibiting the Several States from Disenfranchising United States Citizens on Account of Sex,* January 11 and 12, 1878; *Spada barns behandling* (Stockholm, 1914).

References: Butler, 1874, 1877; *Notable American Women,* 440–42; William H. King, *History of Homoeopathy and Its Institutions in America* (New York, 1905), 3:125–36, 151–55; Abraham W. Lozier, *In Memoriam: Mrs. Clemence Sophia Lozier, MD* (New York, 1888); Polk, 1886; Obituary, *New York Times,* April 28, 1888.

Elizabeth Hannah *BATES* (b. ca. 1832–98)

An only child, Elizabeth Bates was born about 1832 in Charlemont, Franklin County, Massachusetts, to William Bates and Frances Lee Hanners. Her father was a physician. "Being somewhat delicate in health as a child, she was early inured to open air life, riding on horseback, or driving with her father on his professional rounds. Her lessons were often studied in the carriage as she accompanied him." Later, she attended Troy Female Seminary (Emma Willard) for two years, graduating in 1850. (The description of her childhood is found in the history of that school.) Returning home, she studied medicine with her father for two years and then matriculated at the Female Medical College of Pennsylvania. She was one of four graduates in the Class of 1854.

Dr. Bates started practice in Charlemont, "confining attention to diseases of women and children." In 1861, she moved to Owego, New York, where, for the next twenty-six years, she practiced medicine. At first, she was opposed by local physicians, but later she was admitted to the local medical society. An advertisement (one-third page) in an Owego directory reads:

Miss E. H. Bates, M.D. No. 11 Park St., Owego. Graduate of Woman's Medical College Philadelphia. Class 1854. Particular attention given to chronic diseases. Also, Diseases peculiar to women and children. Office hours, from 12 to 1 and 6 to 7 p.m. Also, Agent for Mutual Life Ins. Co., of New York. Assets, $40,000,000!

In 1887, she retired and settled in Portchester, New York, where she became involved in various community activities. Her special interest was the Congregational Church, to the building of whose present edifice she was a substantial contributor. According to her obituary, as a member of the Board of Health, "Dr. Bates was one of the most competent and thorough secretaries the Board ever had. She did more to have the orders of the Health Board obeyed and observed than any one that had ever served in the position."

Dr. Bates died at her home on April 5, 1898, of "hemorrhage, disease of the heart, peritonitis, etc.," having been unwell for some time. The funeral was held at her home the next day. An excerpt from the homily given by her pastor, the Rev. Mr. Hunt, who was apparently well acquainted with her, gives some interesting insights into her character. He mentions "her keen sense of justice and propriety. . . [her] high sense of moral and professional honor. . . . We may well preface our remarks with the reflection that Dr. Bates, like us all, had her personal peculiarities. Any one who had not learned the simple but often time difficult lesson of taking account of the personal equation in human character and experience with charity, and patience, and wisdom, and goodwill, was not prepared to deal with her, or justly to estimate her life." He continued, "Her opinions might differ from those of others . . . but she was not intolerant of a wise, conscientious, kind opponent. She was a friend 'to tie to' so long as she discerned in you the spirit of truth and good will. Human infirmities may have seemed to give the lie with this, but we cannot resist the conviction of her fairness and faithfulness of intention."

The Congregational Church, of which she had been a major financial supporter, giving land valued at $6,000 on which the present building sat, was surprised when her will was probated a month later. She left her entire estate ($135,000) to the University of Michigan for the purpose of establishing the Bates Professorship of the Diseases of Women and Children, provided that women were accepted as students in the school on the same basis as men. Though such a chair, by then, already existed, the university was happy to accept the bequest "for regular expenses of the department," an arrangement which, if it ignored donor intent, was, in the absence of any relatives to complain, apparently acceptable. (Dr. Bates's original intention of giving the money to

Harvard Medical School was probably aborted by Harvard's continued refusal to accept female matriculants.)

The bequest to the university "caused much wonderment here," reported the *Port Chester Journal.* The local citizenry could not understand why the cagy Dr. Bates had not even left outright to the church a $1,900 mortgage she held on it. Instead, she made the gift conditional: the church had to raise enough to pay off all other indebtedness in order to receive the gift. Dr. Bates is buried in Oneonta, New York.

References: Mrs. A. W. Fairbanks, ed., *Emma Willard and Her Pupils; or, Fifty Years of Troy Female Seminary 1822–1872* (New York: published by Mrs. Russell Sage, ca. 1898); Timothy R. B. Johnson, "Doctor Elizabeth Bates and Her Professorship of the Diseases of Women and Children at the University of Michigan" (Ann Arbor, ca. 1997); *New York Times*, May 4, 1898. p. 3, col. 2 [regarding legacy to the university]; *New York Times*, June 21, 1899, p. 6, col. 7; Obituary, *Portchester Journal*, April 14, 1898; *Portchester Journal*, May 12, 1898.

Elizabeth R. *Price* BAUGH (1825–89)

Elizabeth Price was born March 16, 1825, in Coventry, Pennsylvania, the second of six children (three girls, three boys) of William Price and his wife Lydia Urner, both Pennsylvania natives. Her father was a farmer and a member of the Pennsylvania state assembly during the years 1844 and 1845. The family was of German origin, the name Price being derived from Preisz. In June 1847, Elizabeth married Franklin Baugh (b. 1825), a Philadelphia attorney. They soon had four children: Aridne (b. March 4, 1848), Clementine (b. March 29, 1849), Horace L. (b. November 15, 1850), and Alice B. In 1850, the family was living at Spring Garden, Ward 1, Philadelphia.

In 1857, Elizabeth graduated from the Female Medical College of Pennsylvania with an MD degree. Her children all would have been under the age of ten at the time, so this feat was probably made possible with the help of a domestic. The 1850 census lists a fifteen-year-old Elizabeth Fry in the family. The 1870 census reports Elizabeth Baugh as a physician living in North Coventry, Chester County, Pennsylvania (PO Pottstown). All the children but Clementine were at home; Aridne, twenty-two, had no occupation; Horace, nineteen, was a carpenter; Alice, eighteen, was a schoolteacher. Franklin, not enumerated, was probably in Philadelphia. The 1880 census lists Elizabeth as a widow (Franklin died February 14, 1878, at the age of fifty-two). She is designated as "keeping house," not as a physician. Now, daughter Clementine is living with her. Whether Elizabeth practiced medicine for a short period or only when the occasion called for it is not clear. The Baugh genealogy says she was active in practice. Elizabeth died September 9, 1889.

References: US census, 1850, 1870, 1880; George F. P. Wanger, *A Genealogy of the Descendants of Rev. Jacob Price Evangelist—Pioneer* (Harrisburg, 1926).

Emily Norton *BELDEN* Taylor McCabe (1837–86)

Emily Belden was born in 1837 in Lenox, Massachusetts, the third daughter and third of six children (four females, two males) of Albert G. Belden, a farmer, and his wife, Olivia Norton. The three older girls were all baptized on December 11, 1839, at the Church on the Hill (Congregational), the oldest parish in Lenox. No information has been found about her childhood and schooling. In 1858, age twenty-one, she graduated from the New England Female Medical College in Boston with an MD degree. She must have attended three lecture courses because she had a Massachusetts scholarship for each year from 1855 to 1858.

The *Progressive Annuals* for 1862, 1863, and 1864 list her as a physician in Lenox. In 1864, she became resident physician and teacher of physiology at Mt. Holyoke Female Seminary, a post she held until 1868. During the 1864–65 school year she was also professor of obstetrics and diseases of women and children at her medical alma mater.

Unlike her predecessor at Holyoke, Sophronia Fletcher (q.v.), Dr. Belden was quite popular with the students. One of them, Isabella Collins Thomas (a woman from Fairport, New York, and recently married), wrote in a letter to her husband on September 27, 1864, "Visit to doctress Miss Belden; graduated from medical college in Boston five years ago; prescribed sarsaparilla, one teaspoon before each meal." Another student, Hettie M. Dodd, wrote in her diary on January 22, 1868, "Gertie feeling wretched. . . . Miss Belden ordered mustard powders." Hettie also wrote about physiology instruction: "Commenced review physiology. I don't believe I shall ever forget the bones or muscles. Miss Belden has drilled us so much on them." A few weeks later, on March 26, "Physiology is over with! Glory, Glory Hallelujah! I'm all through." (Hitchcock's *Physiology* was the textbook they used. Professor Hitchcock, president of nearby Amherst, served on the Board of Trustees at Holyoke until his death in 1864. As early as the 1840s he had given lectures, with a manikin, at Holyoke.)

In 1867, at the request of the seminary's trustees, Dr. Belden sent them some recommendations for changes at the seminary "for the promotion of the health of the family. . . . It is absolutely necessary that we have more vegetables and fruit; and a greater variety of food in general. That there should be some substitute for warm biscuit at breakfast. Occasionally we should have fresh fruit as second course for dinner in place of puddings. During the past term the flour, butter, molasses and cooking sugar has been very poor. It is necessary that more Graham flour and corn meal be provided and better tea for the sick department."

Following her resignation from the staff of Mt. Holyoke in 1868, Emily practiced medicine in the surrounding South Hadley area. She remained in touch with the college: "March 13th [1869] Miss Belden and Miss Stevens have been making us a visit which we have greatly enjoyed. They left this morning. We are thankful that Miss Belden's stay here has been so pleasant, as during her previous visit last summer in consequence of Miss Noble's severe illness, Miss Belden having consented to take the entire responsibility of her case, found the weeks she spent here full of care and anxiety while we learned anew to prize her efficient and invaluable aid in the sick room" (*Journal*, 40).

On May 11, 1869, in Lenox, she married Albert W. Taylor, a thirty-year-old dentist living and practicing in Minneapolis, where Emily moved forthwith. Back at Holyoke a friend wrote wistfully that she was now "too far away for our beloved physician to come to our aid in times of emergency as she has done during the two years since she resigned her position in the Seminary" (ibid., 53).

Sometime during the eighteen years between 1869 and 1887, Dr. Taylor died and Emily married John McCabe; he died in 1886. No evidence has documented that Emily practiced medicine after moving to Minneapolis. She is not listed in the 1874 or 1877 Butler medical directories or the 1886 Polk directory. However, the 1871 Minneapolis city directory lists her as Mrs. Dr. A. H. Taylor in the alphabetical section. This "beloved physician" died in 1886.

References: E. N. Belden, Undated letter [1867] to the Trustees of Mt. Holyoke Seminary, Williston Memorial Library, Mt. Holyoke College (South Hadley, MA); Hettie M. Dodd, typescript excerpts from the diary of Hettie M. Dodd, Mt. Holyoke, 1871, Williston Memorial Library; Excerpts from *Mt. Holyoke Journal Notebook* XI LD 7093.65.1869, Williston Memorial Library; Mt. Holyoke Female Seminary, *Twenty-Eighth Annual Catalogue, 1864–65* (Northampton, MA, 1865); Mt. Holyoke Female Seminary, *Twenty-Ninth Annual Catalogue*, 1865–66; *Progressive Annual*, 1862, 1863, 1864; Isabella Collins Thomas, letter from Mt. Holyoke to her husband, Walter, September 27, 1864, Williston Memorial Library; Mount Holyoke College, *General Catalogue of the Officers and Students . . . 1837–1911* (South Hadley, MA, 1911).

Julia Ann *Bridgeham* BEVERLY (b. ca. 1814–76)

Julia was born in Massachusetts about 1814, the daughter of Nathaniel Bridgeham and his wife Nancy. Nothing is known of her childhood and education. In 1833, or thereabouts, she married George Beverly, of Providence, Rhode Island. George was listed as being a painter in the 1850 census and as a sign painter in the 1860 census. The Beverlys had three sons, George, Frederic, and Albert.

In the early 1850s, when she was in her late thirties, and with two of her boys under twelve, Julia enrolled at the Female Medical College of Pennsylvania in Philadelphia. After three courses and a thesis entitled "A Disquisition on Iron," she graduated with an MD degree in March 1853 and returned to Providence, where she went into practice. That the Beverly family was intrigued by this event can be found in interfamily correspondence. "What do you think of Julia's becoming an M.D. She was so possessed to learn that George consented to let her. She thinks she shall have much practice in this city. I hope she may for it is very expensive qualifying herself for practice."

Though her name is not found in any of the medical directories of the period, she is listed as a practicing physician in the 1864 *Progressive Annual* and in the *New England Business Directory* for 1865 and 1875, in both of which she is denoted a homoeopath. Her name is also found on the 1862 IRS tax roll as having paid the ten-dollar fee as a physician. In her obituary she is noted as "MD."

Julia's name is not listed with the George Beverly family in the 1860 or 1870 census, and in the 1865 Rhode Island State census her name appears alone, suggesting that she and George had separated. (George, who may have remarried to a woman named Adelia [see 1870 census] died January 30, 1888.) Dr. Beverly died November 14, 1876, at the age of sixty-one. Her funeral took place at the New Jerusalem Church, Providence.

References: Obituary, *Evening Bulletin* (Providence), November 15, 1876; Obituary, *Providence Journal*, November 16, 1876; Rhode Island State census, 1855; Norma Adams Price, "The Family of Pardon Mawney Beverly of Providence, Rhode Island and Illinois" (Tempe, AZ, 1980); *New England Business Directory*, 1865, 1875; US census, 1850, 1860, 1870, 1880; US Internal Revenue Service tax roll, Providence, RI, 1862.

Hannah *BIRDSALL* Armstrong (ca. 1825–1909)

Hannah Birdsall was born about 1822 in Maryland, according to the 1880 census. Nothing has been found about her background, parents, childhood, or early education. She became the second wife of Dr. William Armstrong, a man eighteen years her senior. Whether they had children or he had children by his first wife, Anna, has not been determined. William Armstrong died November 3, 1887.

In the late 1850s, Hannah attended Penn Medical University and, in 1859, graduated with an MD degree. Little evidence has been found that she practiced medicine thereafter. Though she is listed in the *Progressive Annual* for 1864 as a practicing physician in Philadelphia, her name does not appear as a practicing physician in any of the medical directories or Philadelphia directories consulted, nor does her death notice denote her as MD. The 1880 census describes her occupation as "gentlewoman."

Philadelphia newspapers relate only that she was executrix of her husband's estate (*Philadelphia Inquirer*); he had died two years earlier. She sold a Pine Street property, probably her home, in 1903 (*Philadelphia Inquirer*). Hannah died August 20, 1909, at the age of eighty-four years. Her funeral was held at the M. E. Home, Belmont and Edgerley, and she was buried in Woodlands Cemetery.

References: Philadelphia city directories 1888, 1894; *Philadelphia Inquirer*, February 28, 1889 [executrix]; *Philadelphia Inquirer*, February 9, 1903 [property sale]; Obituary, *Philadelphia Inquirer*, August 23, 1909; *Progressive Annual*, 1864; US census, 1880.

Emily *BLACKWELL* (1826–1910)

Emily Blackwell was born October 8, 1826, in Bristol, England, the fourth daughter and sixth of nine surviving children of Samuel Blackwell and his wife, Hannah Lane. Samuel was a sugar refiner, dissenter, and reformer. When Emily was five the family moved from England to New Jersey, and thence to Cincinnati, where Samuel died in 1838 when Emily was twelve. Emily's sister Elizabeth, three and a half years her senior, would be the first woman to receive a medical degree in the United States.

Emily was a big girl, red haired, a good student, but very shy. She was fond of scientific subjects and decided on medicine as a career, a plan that Elizabeth encouraged, though warning her of the "social and professional antagonism" she would encounter. Emily taught school for a while—she did not enjoy it—to earn money for her medical education. Turned down by eleven medical schools to which she had applied for admission, she was admitted to and matriculated at Rush Medical College in Chicago but was not allowed to return for the second year, after the Illinois Medical Society censured the school for accepting a woman as student. Instead, she went to Western Reserve in Cleveland, where she graduated with honors in 1854. Off to Edinburgh for further training, she spent a year with Sir James Y. Simpson, from whom she learned a lot and through whom she gained access to clinics and hospitals in London, Paris, Berlin, and Dresden.

In 1856, after two years' experience in Europe, Emily returned to New York to join her sister, who had established a dispensary for women there. Elizabeth had also bought a house in which she rented out all the rooms as a source of income, making it necessary for her and Emily to sleep in the attic and cook and eat their meals in the cellar. With backing from Quaker friends, the dispensary soon became a hospital, chartered by the state as the New York Infirmary for Women and Children, an institution that offered both patient care and training opportunities for women physicians.

In 1858, Elizabeth went to Europe for a year, leaving Emily in charge. During the year, she and one of the trustees went to Albany, where they persuaded the legislature to provide $1,000 a year taxpayer support for the enterprise and with it, of course, gained official recognition. The infirmary grew steadily, moving twice to larger quarters (in 1860 and in 1874). In 1860, 130 patients were treated in hospital and 3,550 in the dispensary; by 1876, 7,549 were being treated.

The year before she moved permanently to England (1869), Elizabeth established a medical school in association with the hospital and dispensary, the Woman's Medical College of the New York Infirmary. With Elizabeth gone, Emily ran the two institutions for the next thirty years, as director of the hospital and professor of obstetrics and diseases of women and children, as well as dean of the medical school. A leader in innovation, the school required (as did others) a three-year graded course in 1876 and four years in 1893. The school year was extended to eight months in 1877. In 1866, medical social service was established—a "sanitary visitor" made the rounds of the tenement houses. A nurse training school, established in 1858, was periodically expanded and became increasingly demanding.

The Woman's Medical College graduated 364 physicians in its thirty-year existence. In her valedictory address to the school's thirty-first and final graduating class (1899), Dr. Blackwell reviewed the school's history and the progress in woman's medical education. The school at the infirmary, though totally destroyed by fire in 1897, had been completely rebuilt and its financial situation was the soundest it had ever been.

But the wave of the future was coeducation in Emily's view. (This had been true from the beginning, but all attempts to achieve it had been rebuffed.) Now, Johns Hopkins had opened (1893) as a fully coeducational institution, and Cornell was about to do the same in New York City. This is what the Blackwells had wanted from the beginning.

Thirty years earlier, there had been talk of such a plan. Cornell's president, Andrew D. White, two prominent New York physicians, Stephen Smith and Willard Parker, and Samuel Willits, president of the New York Infirmary Medical School, met at the Blackwell house—they all knew each other—to discuss such a plan, but the Cornell trustees decided they could not afford to start a medical school in New York. Now it was going to happen.

In 1898, Cornell University Medical College, located in New York, began accepting women, and Emily transferred her students to Cornell the following year. With the transfer of its students to Cornell, the infirmary school would adapt its new building to hospital use and would concentrate henceforth on graduate clinical education for women, something that was greatly needed but largely unavailable, since few women were offered staff positions at hospitals.

In 1882, Emily and her longtime friend Elizabeth Cushier, a gynecological surgeon at the hospital, started living together in what Elizabeth Thomson, writing in 1971, called a "close and devoted companionship." Regina Morantz-Sanchez, writing almost thirty years later, was able to call it a "Boston marriage." The couple lived together for eighteen years. Emily had an adopted daughter, Anna, as well. In summers, the family went to York Cliffs, Maine, where they had a summer home and where Emily would die with enterocolitis September 7, 1910, at the age of seventy-three. After a Unitarian service in Boston, her ashes were buried at Chilmark on Martha's Vineyard, where her daughter's family and other Blackwells had settled.

In the opinion of historian Frederick C. Waite, Emily was the physician, the clinician; her sister Elizabeth the reformer. This view was upheld by historian Elizabeth Thomson and others. Emily's practice was confined to the hospital and dispensary. She was described by students who knew her as of "commanding presence, noble face, and having a low, calm voice of uncanny quality." Wrote another student, "Although Dr. Emily Blackwell's contribution to the success of the New York Infirmary was not so spectacular as that of her older sister, she still brought to this young hospital and college an executive and medical ability that was unsurpassed by the best medical men of the day."

Bibliography: With Elizabeth Blackwell, "Medicine as a Profession for Women" (New York, 1860); *Address on the Medical Education of Women* (New York, 1864); *Women in the Regular Medical Profession: Report of the Association for the Advancement of Medical Education for women. . . .* (March 26, 1878, New York); *Address Delivered by Emily Blackwell at the Thirty-First Commencement of the Woman's Medical College of the New York Infirmary for Women and Children* (May 25, 1899).

References: *American National Biography*, 2:894–95; *Notable American Women*, 1:165–67.

Lucinda M. *Browne* BOWDITCH (1812–97)

Lucinda was born in Brentwood, Rockingham County, New Hampshire, December 17, 1812, the daughter of Josiah Brown (*sic*) and Anna Tuck. Nothing is known of her childhood or early education. About 1833, she married Joseph Bowditch and probably went at that time to live in Fairfax, a village of 2,111 inhabitants (1850) in Franklin County in northwestern Vermont. Though her residence in Fairfax is documented no earlier than the 1850 census, all her children were born in Vermont. The couple had four children: James S. (b. 1835), Anna (b. 1841), Josiah B. (b. 1843), and Roger W. (b. 1847). The family probably lived in Fairfax for at least forty years (1833–74). Joseph is listed as a justice in 1864. An 1857 plat map shows the house of J. Bowdish to be on Main Street at the western edge of the village next to the Congregational Church. Curiously, the family name was spelled Bowdish in all local directories of the period.

About 1860, when she was forty-eight years old and her youngest child thirteen, Lucinda went to Penn Medical University in Philadelphia and, in 1861, graduated with an MD degree. She returned to Fairfax and practiced medicine there. She is listed as a physician in *Walton's Vermont Register* from 1863 until 1874 and in the 1876 edition of the *Vermont Business Directory*. Her name appears on the 1865 IRS tax roll, probably as a physician, but this is not specified, nor is the amount of the tax she paid. Sometime between 1864 and 1870 husband Joseph died. His name does not appear in the 1870 census or those thereafter, and Lucinda is listed as a widow. In 1870, Lucinda owned $6,000 in real estate and had $1,300 in personal assets.

By 1880, Lucinda, Anna, and Roger had moved to Boston, where Lucinda is listed in the annual directory as a physician, living at 4 Myrtle Place, Roxbury. She lived at this address for the rest of her life and probably continued to practice medicine; her name is found in 1882, 1886, 1889, and 1895 Boston directories and in the 1886 and 1890 Polk medical directories, in each instance as a physician. The family name was spelled Bowditch after the move to Boston. Lucinda died at her home on May 4, 1897, at the age of eighty-four.

Note: Though Dr. Bowditch is listed as "Louisa M." in Abraham's enumeration of Penn Medical University graduates, no such person has been found. It has been presumed here that Lucinda and Louisa are the same person. Lucinda is denoted an Eclectic physician as early as 1864. Unless she received an MD degree in 1862 or 1863 (of which no record has been found) she must be Louisa. That the Bowdishes and the Bowditches are the same persons is clear since the names of children Anna and Roger appear in both listings.

References: Harold J. Abrahams, *Extinct Medical Schools of Nineteenth-Century Philadelphia* (Philadelphia, 1966); *Boston Almanac & Business Directory*, 1882, 1886, 1889, 1895; Bruce Weir, Internet posting on ancestry.com, "New England Bowditches," March 14, 2003, http:// boards.ancestry.com/surnames.bowditch/37.1/mb.ashx [birthplace, date, parents' names of Lucinda Bowditch] (accessed May 19, 2016); Polk, 1886, 1890; US census, 1850, 1860, 1870, 1880; US Internal Revenue Service tax roll for 1865; *Vermont Business Directory for 1876*; *Walton's Vermont Register & Farmer's Almanac*, 1863–74.

Mary Elizabeth *BREED* Welch (1830–82)

Mary Breed was born July 16, 1830, in Lynn, Massachusetts. Her father was a well-known lumber dealer in that town. As a young woman, Mary taught school in Lynn. In 1852, she graduated from Mt. Holyoke Seminary. Years later, a classmate remembered her as "a bright and beautiful woman, full of enthusiasm for her chosen profession" (obit.). That profession was medicine, and Mary went on to New England Female Medical College in Boston, where she was supported by a Massachusetts scholarship and from which institution she graduated in 1857 with an MD degree.

At medical school she wrote her thesis on the water-cure, an interest she continued by spending a year at Glen Haven Water-Cure in central New York State's Cortland County, where James Caleb Jackson and Harriet Austin (q.v.), who later established the famous water-cure Our Home on the Hill in Dansville, New York, and Silas and Rachel Brooks Gleason (q.v.), who operated a similar institution in Elmira, New York, had been before her. From there she went to the Hospital for Women in New York City, established by the Blackwell sisters (q.v.), where she worked for two years (1858–60). This was followed by a year (1861) at New England Hospital for Women and Children, recently established by Marie Zakrzewska (q.v.). Clearly, she was very well educated and trained for the profession.

Dr. Breed went to Fond du Lac, Wisconsin, to establish practice and stayed for two years. It is not known why she chose this location, but it apparently did not prove to her liking. She returned to Lynn in 1863. She, or Martha Flanders (q.v.), who came that same year, was the first woman doctor in that community but was soon followed by Esther Hill Hawks (q.v.). For the next nineteen years until her death she practiced medicine there with "particular attention paid to diseases of women" (1875 Lynn directory advertisement). She is also listed as a physician in 1868 and 1878–79 directories for nearby Salem, Massachusetts. She was a member of the New England Hospital Medical Society in Boston and was a corresponding member of the Gynecological Society of Boston.

In 1869, she married George O. Welch of Lynn, a Scottish-born taxidermist. They had no children. The Welches were reasonably well off. The 1870 census lists George as having $8,000 in real estate and $4,000 in personal property. Active in matters other than her profession, she was a supporter of the antislavery cause and belonged to the Lynn Suffrage Club. She was a reader not only of medicine, in which she kept current, but of literature as well. She belonged to the Chapin Club, the Saturday Reading Club, and the Lynn Woman's Club. She was a member of the Free Church at the Oxford Street Chapel and, later, of the Free Religious Association. At one time, Dr. Welch had large real estate holdings, but most were lost in a depression. Mary Breed Welch died silver haired but young, on June 21, 1882, of a stroke. She was fifty-one. In her obituary she was described as "very competent, eminently successful and popular . . . a loyal and devoted wife, an obliging neighbor, a sympathetic and generous friend."

References: *Essex County Directory*, 1866; *International Genealogical Index*; *Massachusetts Business Directory*, 1875; *New England Business Directory*, 1868, 1871; Obituary from an unidentified and undated newspaper, Lynn Historical Society, Lynn, MA; US census, 1870.

Harriet Sophia *BRIGHAM* (1823–1912)

When Harriet Sophia Brigham graduated from New England Female Medical College, she was a resident of Bolton, Massachusetts. The following biographical sketch is based on information about a Harriet Sophia Brigham, who was born in nearby Marlboro and who died in Hudson. These three Massachusetts communities are all within ten miles of one another. It seems almost certain that these two persons are one. However, there is nowhere mention that the person being here described was a physician or had gone to medical school. In census records she is always described as a teacher.

Harriet Brigham was born in Marlborough, Massachusetts, on September 14, 1823, the fourth of six children of Otis Brigham and his wife Lucy Stratton. Lucy died when the children were quite young, and they were each placed in various homes in the community. Harriet went to the home of the Rev. Mr. Alden in Marlborough. She attended the State Normal School in Framingham, became a teacher, and taught the rest of her professional life, successively in Marlborough and Sterling, Massachusetts; Auburn and Kansas City, Kansas; and later, for many years, at the State Reform Schools for boys in St. Louis, Missouri, and Pontiac, Illinois.

Assuming her to be "our" Harriet Brigham, she attended New England Female Medical College, where she had a scholarship from the Commonwealth, and received an MD degree in 1857 when she was thirty-four. No evidence has been found to suggest she practiced medicine. Possibly she taught anatomy and physiology, or, perhaps, she sought the relatively inexpensive "higher" education medical school then provided. In the late 1880s she gave up teaching and for nine years lived in the West and later in Florida. In 1896, then seventy-three, she moved back to Hudson and lived thereafter with her nephew, Walter R. Coolidge. She died in Hudson, August 16, 1912, at the age of eighty-eight. She never married.

References: Personal communication from Mildred A. Coolidge, Hudson Historical Society, Hudson, MA; Obituary, *Hudson News-Enterprise*, August 23, 1912; US census, 1850, 1880, 1900, 1910.

Sarah Cheny *Read* Randall BRIGHAM (1824–1909)

Sarah was born October 25, 1824, in Brattleboro, Vermont, one of three daughters of Henry Read and his wife Mary Liscom. Nothing is known of her childhood and early education.

She was twice married, first to a man named Randall, with whom she had two daughters, Hattie M. and Ellen E. Only Hattie lived to adulthood, and she later assumed the surname of her stepfather, Hubbard Brigham. Hubbard Hammond Brigham (b. 1819) and Sarah were married March 25, 1851. At the time of his marriage, Hubbard was described as a botanic physician. Hubbard, also previously married, had four children by his first wife, who had died the year before. Only two of these children, George and Fred, were still alive when Hubbard and Sarah were married. George was eleven and Fred probably an infant.

The Brighams settled in Fitchburg, Massachusetts, where Hubbard had moved in 1845. Hubbard enrolled in Worcester (MA) Medical College (Eclectic) and graduated with an MD degree in 1855. Two years later, in 1857, Sarah earned her medical degree from the Eclectic College of Medicine in Cincinnati. She had also attended Worcester Medical College for a period prior to this. Thereafter, the couple practiced medicine together in Fitchburg for many years. They are listed as practicing physicians in national and local directories. In the 1856 and 1857 editions of the *Fitchburg Almanac*, Hubbard is listed as an "Eclectic Physician and Surgeon," Sarah as an "Eclectic Physician and Midwife." Their offices were separate but adjacent, at 11 and 13 Pritchard Street. In the 1874 Fitchburg directory (192), they offer, "Lung and catarrhal diseases treated by inhalation. Female weakness and spinal difficulties treated by electricity. Office hours 8–10, 2–3." (This gives an idea of what were prevalent problems.) By 1880, the Fitchburg directory lists them simply as "M.D.," both located at 202 Main Street.

Sarah retired about 1890. She died at her home at 4 Brigham Park, on December 15, 1909, of "senile debility," and is buried at Laurel Hill Cemetery. She had been a regular attendant at the First Universalist Church. Hubbard had died the previous February. Remarkably, but perhaps typical of the times, his extensive obituary did not mention that his wife had practiced with him for more than thirty years: "He was for a time in partnership with Dr. Artemas Farwell, under the name of Brigham and Farwell, but most of the time that he practiced in Fitchburg he had no partner."

References: Obituary, *JAMA*, 1910, 54:309; W. I. T. Brigham, *The History of the Brigham Family* (New York, 1907); William A. Emerson, *Fitchburg, Massachusetts, Past and Present* (Fitchburg, 1887), 6; *Fitchburg Almanac*, 1856, 1857; *Fitchburg Directory*, 1876, 1885; Hubbard Brigham obituary, *Fitchburg Daily Sentinel*, February 22, 1909; Obituary, *Fitchburg Daily Sentinel*, December 16, 1909; Funeral announcement, *Fitchburg Daily Sentinel*, December 18, 1909; Fitchburg Historical Society, *Old records of the Town of Fitchburg* (Fitchburg, MA, 1913), 109; Fitchburg city directories, 1874–89; Polk, 1886, 1890, 1893, 1896, 1898, 1900.

Hannah W. *BRINTON* Carter (1827–1910)

Hannah Brinton was born February 27, 1827, probably in Salisbury, Lancaster County, Pennsylvania, where, according to the 1830 census, her family was then living. She was the seventh of eight children (six girls, two boys). Her mother, Ann Fawkes, died when Hannah was two and a half years old, and her father, Caleb, remarried and had four more children. Nothing is known of Hannah's childhood and early education.

Hannah, by then living in nearby Christiana, attended the Female Medical College of Pennsylvania in Philadelphia and, in 1857, when she was thirty, graduated with an MD degree. She returned to Christiana and established her practice. The 1864 edition of the *Progressive Annual* lists her as still an active practitioner in that town.

On March 15, 1866, then thirty-nine, she married Benjamin Carter. They had one son who, in turn, had two daughters. Whether Hannah practiced after her marriage has not been determined. She probably practiced medicine in Christiana for at least nine years (1857–66). Hannah died in 1910. Her grave is in Arroyo Grande Cemetery, San Luis Obispo County, California.

Note: Attempts to contact Hannah's granddaughter, Florence Carter Innocent, a resident of California, were unsuccessful. In a letter in the archives of the Female Medical College of Pennsylvania, now housed at Drexel University School of Medicine, Mrs. Innocent states that she knew nothing of her grandmother, who had died before she was born.

References: Janetta W. Schoonover, *The Brinton Genealogy* (Trenton, NJ, 1925); Florence Carter Innocent, letter dated August 12, 1952, and postcard dated September 29, 1952, in the archives at Drexel University College of Medicine, Philadelphia; US census, 1830, 1850.

Permilia R. *BRONSON* (1807–71)

Permilia Bronson was the first woman with a doctor's degree to practice medicine in Connecticut. She maintained her practice in northwestern Connecticut for at least ten, possibly twenty, years. Permilia (sometimes Pamilia) Bronson was born February 28, 1807, in Winchester, Litchfield County, Connecticut, the third of seven children (five girls, two boys) of Salmon and Mercy Whedon Bronson. John Boyd, in his *Annals of Winchester, Connecticut,* described her father as "industrious, frugal, honest, moral and steadfast. His religion was something more than a profession." No information about her childhood has been found.

The 1850 United States census lists Permilia R. Bronson, age forty-three, as living in Winchester, Litchfield County, northwest Connecticut, in what appears to be a small hotel or boarding house, with William Sanford denoted hotelkeeper. A fellow boarder, H. B. Steele, twenty-five, is described as a botanic physician, and is probably the H. B. Steele that Permilia listed as her preceptor when she was at medical school.

Permilia attended and graduated from Central Medical College in Rochester, New York, with an MD degree on February 18, 1852. Her graduation essay was entitled "Fever." She apparently returned to Winchester and practiced medicine there. An 1857–58 business directory lists an M. R. Bronson as an eclectic physician in Winchester and

Harvey B. Steele as a physician in West Winsted. The 1860 federal census records for Winchester reads: "Permilia R. Bronson, age 50, born in Connecticut, E[c]lectic M.D., with $2,000 real estate and $500 personal property." In the same household are two Sylvia Kimberlys, ages fifty-seven and nineteen, probably a housekeeper and her daughter. Permilia is also listed in the 1860 *New England Business Directory* as a physician in West Winsted, a village close by Winchester: "Miss P. R. Bronson (ecl.), W. Winsted."

Dr. Bronson is not found in the 1870 Winchester census, though H. B. Steele, now forty-two, is listed as a physician in West Winsted with $13,000 real estate and $16,000 in personal property. Steele is also listed as being there in the 1867 and 1868 *Connecticut Register*s, the 1874 and 1877 Butler medical directories, and the 1886 and 1890 Polk medical directories. He was a member of the Connecticut Eclectic Medical Society from 1868. Dr. Bronson died, unmarried, in 1871 at the age of sixty-four.

References: John Boyd, *Annals of Winchester, Connecticut* (Hartford, 1873); Butler, 1874, 1877; *Connecticut Register*, Hartford, 1867, 1868; *International Genealogical Index*; Polk, 1886, 1890; *New England Business Directory*, 1860, 1861; Winchester, CT, vital records; US census, 1850, 1860, 1870; A. D. Jones, *The Illustrated Commercial, Mechanical, Professional and Statistical Gazetteer and Business-Book of Connecticut, for 1857–58* (New Haven, 1857).

Caroline *BROWN* Winslow (1832–96)

Caroline Brown was born in Appledore, Kent, England, on November 19, 1832. Her father, Samuel Brown, moved his family to Utica, New York, in 1836, where he would live until his death in 1857. Caroline was not very healthy as a child and, in her late teens, went to the Glen Haven Water-Cure, then run by the Drs. Rachel Gleason (q.v.) and James Caleb Jackson, in nearby Cortland County. Here she came under the care and tutelage of Gleason and undertook the study of anatomy. In 1853, after three full courses, she graduated with honor and an MD degree from the Eclectic Medical Institute in Cincinnati. She set up in practice at 178 Race Street in Cincinnati. In October 1855, she enrolled at the Western College of Homoeopathic Medicine in Cleveland (later, Western College of Homoeopathy; still later, Homoeopathic Hospital College of Cleveland), where she received a second medical degree on February 28, 1856.

Dr. Brown returned to Utica, drawn partly by the needs of her aging parents and partly to assume responsibility for the infant child left by her recently deceased sister. Caroline practiced medicine in Utica for the next eight years. She liked to deal especially with surgical problems and, according to early biographer Egbert Cleave, "performed successfully several important and difficult operations." She is listed in Utica directories as a physician in 1861–62 and 1863–64.

In April 1864, Dr. Brown went to Washington to help in the military hospitals, by then overflowing with Civil War sick and wounded. There she served as a regular visitor under the auspices of the New York agency not only as substitute mother and amanuensis but as physician as well. However, she had to use homoeopathic remedies covertly since they were proscribed by the "iniquitous ruling of the Surgeon-General" (Cleave). When the war was over, she went to Baltimore for eight months but then returned. She remained in Washington the rest of her life, practicing medicine until at least 1890. (She is listed in Butler 1877, Polk 1886, and 1890 medical directories.)

During the war she met Susan Edson (q.v.), another physician working in area hospitals as a nurse. After the war, the two were instrumental in starting a Homoeopathic Free Dispensary, a National Homoeopathic Hospital, as well as the Washington chapter of the American Institute of Homoeopathy. In 1866, she married Austin C. Winslow, a Washingtonian and "an artisan of good abilities, skill, and cultivation" (Cleave). It was said that Caroline herself had a philosophy of life that "was full of sunshine." She died at her home, 1 Grant Place, Washington, on December 7, 1896.

References: Butler, 1877; Cleave, 264; William H. King, *History of Homoeopathy and Its Institutions in America* (New York, 1905); Polk, 1886, 1890; Jane E. Schultz, *Women at the Front* (Chapel Hill, NC, 2004), 174.

Eliza A. BROWN (b. 1827)

Eliza Brown was already married and living in Morris, Illinois, with her two children when she went to the Eclectic College of Medicine in Cincinnati. She graduated with an MD degree in 1857. After finishing her education she moved farther south in Illinois to the larger community of Bloomington. The 1860 census lists her as a resident there, aged thirty-three, with two children: George, fourteen, and Clara, eleven. No husband is mentioned, so he had probably died, but no confirmation of this has been found. Eliza needed to support her children; this was probably her motivation for becoming a doctor. How long she practiced medicine has not been determined. It was at least until 1863. She is listed as a physician and paid the physician's Internal Revenue tax of $10 and $6.67 in 1862 and 1863, respectively.

References: US Internal Revenue Service tax assessment lists, 1862, 1863; US census, 1860.

Lucinda R. *Rowley* BROWN (1815–56)

Lucinda Rowley was born October 2, 1815, in Sharon, a village in the lower Mohawk River valley in eastern New York State. No information has been found regarding her background, parents, or early education. Probably in the early 1830s, she married Dr. Joseph Ransom Brown. They had two sons, William C. (b. ca. 1834) and Joseph R. (b. 1846 or 1848), both born in New York State.

Sometime before 1850, the family moved to Galveston, Texas, where Joseph practiced medicine until his death on September 5, 1854. In the meantime, Lucinda had matriculated at the Female Medical College of Pennsylvania and graduated with an MD degree in February 1854, seven months before her husband's death. After the death of her husband, she returned, presumably with at least her younger son, who would have been six or eight, to Gardnersville in her native Schoharie County. She probably practiced medicine here until her own premature death two years later (April 20, 1856) at forty-one.

Her younger son, Joseph R., who would have been eight or ten at the time of her death, later went to Albany Medical School, received an MD degree in 1868, and practiced medicine in Seward, a village of five hundred in Schoharie County for more than forty years. He is listed in Polk and AMA medical directories at least as late as 1912. Her grandson Joseph R. Brown Jr. wrote a letter in 1956 now at Drexel University School of Medicine, Philadelphia, giving the death dates and locations of his grandparents, adding that he was in possession of Lucinda's medical school diploma and some medical school lecture notes.

References: *American Medical Directory*, 1906, 1912; Joseph R. Brown Jr., letter dated April 5, 1956, Albany, NY, to the Woman's Medical College of Pennsylvania, Philadelphia.; Polk, 1886, 1890–1902; US census, 1850.

Chloe Annette *BUCKEL* (1833–1912)

Annette Buckel was born August 25, 1833, in the Western New York village of Warsaw. Her childhood was not a happy one. Her parents died before she was one year old. She went to live with grandparents who, in turn, died when she was four. For the next ten years she was the responsibility of two aunts, themselves initially aged fourteen and seventeen, who, it is said, made it clear to her that she was a burden to them. At fourteen, she set out on her own, teaching school in various towns in New York State and living in the homes of her students as partial payment for her teaching services.

At fifteen, she decided to become a physician. What influence Elizabeth Blackwell's (q.v.) recent matriculation at nearby Geneva Medical Institution may have had on her decision is not known. To finance the undertaking she gave up teaching and obtained more lucrative employment in a Connecticut burnishing factory, where she worked, it is said, with a Latin textbook propped up before her. She received her medical degree from the Female Medical College of Pennsylvania on February 28, 1858, and had a year of graduate training in New York at the Infirmary for Women and Children under Dr. Marie Zakrzewska (q.v.). She then moved to Chicago, where she set up practice and, with another woman, organized a dispensary for women and children similar to the one at which she trained in New York.

Then came the Civil War. As did many of these pre–Civil War woman doctors, Dr. Buckel served the army in a professional capacity, but as a nurse administrator, not as a doctor. In these roles they were referred to as "Miss" or "Mrs." In 1863, Buckel volunteered her services to Oliver P. Morton, governor of Indiana. Why Indiana and not Illinois is a question. In August 1863, the governor sent her to General Grant's Department of the Tennessee "to look after the condition and the wants of Indiana's sick and wounded soldiers" (Morton to Grant). In the course of her duties she set up half a dozen field hospitals but ultimately became responsible for selecting and recommending appointment of female nurses for the entire southwest area (Barnes).

Soon after that she became chief of nurses at Jefferson General Hospital in Jeffersonville, Indiana, where she would stay for the rest of the war. Joan M. Jensen, in her biography of Buckel in *Notable American Women* writes that Dr. Buckel seldom spoke of her wartime experiences in the years after.

After the war, Dr. Buckel practiced for a time in Evansville, Indiana. In September 1866, she became an assistant physician and soon thereafter resident physician at the New England Hospital for Women and Children in Boston, where she specialized in respiratory diseases. She is listed as a physician in Boston in the 1868 and 1871 editions of the *New England Business Directory*. A former student, writing in 1924 in the *Medical Woman's Journal*, "gratefully recall[ed] the valuable clinical teaching she gave to the hospital internes on this subject." From 1872 to 1875, because of poor health, she took a leave of absence, spent in Vienna and Paris in study and convalescence. Returning to Boston, she was appointed attending surgeon at the hospital but resigned two years later because of her health.

In 1877, she moved to Oakland, California, where she would live and practice for the subsequent twenty-nine years. She probably picked California because of its mild climate, and the Bay Area because her cousin, Washington Bartlett, was a prominent political figure in San Francisco (and later governor of California). She received a certificate of registration as a physician, dated November 10, 1877, was elected a member of the State Medical Society on April 17, 1878, and was soon appointed physician to the Pacific Dispensary for Women and Children (later San Francisco Children's Hospital).

Dr. Buckel was very much involved in other community activities, especially those involving child welfare and prevention of sickness. She served as trustee of homes for orphan and delinquent girls in 1901 and was active in organizing a commission to exclude milk from tuberculous cows from Oakland's milk supply (1904). She established a cooking school in her own home that led to the introduction of vocational training in Oakland public schools. By her will she left her estate in trust for the benefit of developmentally disabled children and, in 1914, a grant from this trust was used to establish a C. Annette Buckel Foundation Research Fellowship at Stanford for child psychology studies.

In the later 1890s, Dr. Buckel bought an acre and a half of land in the Piedmont Hills overlooking San Francisco Bay on which she built a log cabin retreat. Friends were welcome to come and use it, provided they replaced provisions and secured the door upon leaving. Later, she built a large house on the lot to which she and her friend and former patient, Charlotte Playter, retired a few years before her death. She died of a stroke August 17, 1912.

References: Medical Society of the State of California, *Transactions . . . during the Years 1877 and 1878,* 5; *Official Registry and Directory of Physicians and Surgeons in the State of California,* 13th ed. (San Francisco, 1901), 34; Letter from Morton to Grant, August 14, 1863, California Historical Society; Letter from acting surgeon general Joseph K. Barnes, December 23, 1863, California Historical Society; Obituary, *Ebell Society 1912–1913 Report* (Oakland, CA), 79–80; *Notable American Women,* 1:265–67; *American National Biography,* 3:853–54; Margaret E. Martin, "Dr. C. Annette Buckel, the 'Little Major,'" *California Historical Society Quarterly* 19 (1940): 74–76; Eliza M. Mosher, *Medical Woman's Journal,* 1924, 15–16 [biography of Buckel]; *New England Business Directory,* 1868, 1871; Obituary, *Oakland Tribune,* August 17, 1912; Woman's Medical College of Pennsylvania, *Transactions of the 38th Annual Meeting of the Alumnae Association, June 5 and 6, 1913* (Philadelphia, 1913), 378.

Alice *BUNKER* Stockham (1833–1912)

Alice Bunker, daughter of Slocum Bunker and Matilda F. Wood, both Quakers, was born November 8, 1833, in Cardington, Ohio, and later lived in Hastings, Michigan. When she was eighteen she met Emma R. Coe, a woman's suffrage activist said to be the first woman in the United States to study law. Mrs. Coe urged Alice to study medicine (this was in 1851). After education at nearby Olivet College, Alice attended and graduated in 1854 with an MD degree from Eclectic Medical Institute in Cincinnati. At EMI she was a classmate of Harriet Judd, later Sartain (q.v.). On August 11, 1857, Alice married Gabriel Henry Stockham of Cincinnati and had at least two children, a son, William Henry Stockham, born September 15, 1861, in Lafayette, Indiana, who became a prominent businessman in Birmingham, Alabama, and a daughter.

From 1854 until at least 1877, Dr. Stockham practiced medicine in Indiana. Sometime around 1872, she adopted the "Bloomer" costume; she also claimed that she never wore corsets. An active traveler, she visited various parts of the country giving parlor talks to mothers and daughters about physiology and hygiene, woman's suffrage, and sensible clothing. Probably in the late 1870s the family moved to Leavenworth, Kansas, and soon thereafter on to Chicago, where Alice went back to medical school, this time at the Chicago Homoeopathic Medical College, and received a second MD degree in 1882.

For the next twenty-five or thirty years she was far better known as an author and, in 1886, established and became president of the Stockham Publishing Company in Chicago, a firm that was to publish her several books as well as other "advanced" literature.

Her first and most famous book was *Tokology, a Book for Every Woman.* Published in 1883, this book on sex education went through many editions during the subsequent forty years, was issued in several languages, and is still in print today in some countries. Stockham advocated mutual fulfillment during the sexual act and the use of birth control, endorsed the practice of masturbation (at a time when a substantial subset of male physicians was making a living "treating" the "secret vice"), and favored complete abstinence from alcohol and tobacco.

Koradine, first published in 1893 as *The Koradine Letters,* was about a girl's awakening to womanhood. In 1896, *Karezza,* followed in the footsteps of John Humphrey Noyes's *Male Continence.* Wrote Stockham, "Copulation is more than a propagative act; it is a blending of body, soul, and spirit . . . [and if] the final propagative orgasm is entirely avoided . . . spiritual exhilaration increases . . . [and] all vestiges of the old idea of man's dominion over the woman" is gone. Here is embodied equality for women, birth control (a subject in the closet since passage of the 1872 Comstock Law), eugenics, and spirituality. In addition to these three works, were *Tolstoi, a Man of Peace* (1900), *The Lover's World, a Wheel of Life* (1903), and numerous pamphlets.

It is no surprise to find that Dr. Stockham was active in a variety of social causes—woman's suffrage, social reform, social purity—or that she established a school of philosophy at Williams Bay, Wisconsin, in 1900. She was also responsible for introducing "sloyd" into the curriculum of the Chicago Public Schools. Sloyd, derived from a Swedish word for skillful or crafty, was a program of manual training, especially woodworking, developed in Denmark in 1860.

It is not clear how active in later years Dr. Stockham was in clinical practice, but, having gone back to medical school in 1880, it seems likely that she was still in practice. She is listed in Polk directories as a practicing physician as late as 1898.

In 1905, Dr. Stockham joined the ranks of earlier writers who worked for sexual reform—Charles Knowlton, Frederick Hollick, Edward Bliss Foote, and Simon Mohler Landis, to mention a few—but, unlike them, she did not go to jail for it. In May of that year, she was indicted by a grand jury for misuse of the US mail. Post Office Inspector McAfee, Anthony Comstock's midwestern counterpart, had gathered the evidence. Stockham, of course, had written nothing different than she had been publishing for the past twenty years. But she summarized that material in a pamphlet—*The Wedding Night*—that caught McAfee's eye, a pamphlet that the government found so "indiscreet" that excerpts of it could not be placed even in such a matter-of-fact document as an indictment.

Though she was defended by Clarence Darrow, she was found guilty, fined $250, and her books on sexuality were banned. Neither the Alice B. Stockham Publishing Company nor Stockham's previous writings on marital sexuality survived the ruling. In 1909, only four years after the court case, attorney and free-speech activist Theodore Schroeder noted that neither Stockham's writings nor any like them were anywhere to be had in the United States.

After the trial, Stockham and her daughter moved to Alhambra, California, near Los Angeles, where she continued to practice "mental healing," but her career in sexual teaching was over. She died December 3, 1912. Wrote historian Beryl Satter in 1999, "The idea that women and men were not only equally sexual but equally able to direct and control their sexuality was unacceptable to the jittery mainstream of the early 1900s."

Bibliography: *Tokology, a Book for Every Woman*, 1st ed. (Chicago: Sanitary Publishing Co. 1883); *The Koradine Letters* (Chicago, 1895); *Karezza:*

Ethics of Marriage (Chicago, 1896); *Tolstoi, a Man of Peace* (Chicago, 1900); *The Lover's World* (Chicago, 1903); *Boy Lover, and Other Essays* (Chicago, ca. 1904); many pamphlets, including *Health Germs*, a paper read at Divine Science Congress, Chicago (1895?), and *The Wedding Night* (1905?).

References: Butler, 1874, 1877; Polk, 1886, 1890, 1893, 1896, 1898; Beryl Satter, *Each Mind a Kingdom* (Berkeley: University of California Press), 1999; *Sunday Record* (Chicago), May 21, 1905; *Who Was Who in America*, 1897–1942, 1189; s.v., "Alice Bunker Stockham," *Wikipedia*.

Frances BURRITT (b. ca. 1814–85)

Frances Burritt was born in Vermont about 1814. Her maiden name (and the names of her parents) is not known. Neither is anything known about her childhood and early education.

Sometime before 1833, Frances married Alexander Hamilton Burritt. Alexander was born April 17, 1805, in Troy, New York, and graduated with an MD degree from the College of Physician and Surgeons in New York in 1827. He practiced medicine as a Regular until 1833, when he turned to homoeopathy. In 1846, he became a member of the American Institute of Homoeopathy. His father, Ely Burritt, was a physician in Troy; his grandfather was a minister. Alexander and Frances had at least one child, a son named Amatus Robbins Burritt, born 1833 in Springfield, Illinois. Amatus became a physician (Western College of Homoeopathy, Cleveland, 1853) and practiced in Huntsville, Alabama.

In the later 1850s, Frances herself decided to become a doctor. She graduated from Cleveland's Western College of Homoeopathy in 1859. Sometime before this event the Burritts had moved to New Orleans, probably in the mid-1850s. The 1860 census shows Frances living in a household of three in New Orleans's Ward 3: J. T. Hill, age thirty-three, physician, born Canada, worth $800 in real estate and $1,000 in personal property; Frances Burritt, age forty-five, physician; W. Burk, age twenty-one, female, servant. Frances and Alexander were each listed in the 1866 directory as practicing homoeopathists. The listing for Frances reads, "Special attention given to diseases of women and children." Their offices were at different locations and, since it does not specify a residential address for Frances, one cannot tell whether Alexander and Frances were living together or apart, the latter case being the more likely.

By the time of the 1870 census, Frances had moved to Chicago, Ward 5, and was living with a family named Barnum. Mr. Barnum was a liquor broker and had a wife and a child. Frances is listed as a physician, so presumably she was still in practice. Alexander was still in New Orleans in 1870 and 1874. Though it is speculation, the evidence suggests that Frances went to medical school in anticipation of a divorce or separation and the need to support herself.

Alexander died in New Orleans October 9, 1877. Frances, who must have returned to New Orleans, died there on March 15, 1885.

Bibliography: "Hamamelis Virginiana," *American Homoeopathic Review*, August, 1858, 5.

References: American Institute of Homoeopathy, *Code of Medical Ethics, Constitution, By-Laws, and List of Members* (Boston, 1869); *New Orleans Directory*, 1860, 1870, 1874, 1880; Alexander's death notice, *New Orleans Daily Picayune*, October 10, 1877; Frances's death notice, *New Orleans Daily Picayune*, March 17, 1885; New Orleans Death Indices, 1877–95, 86:970; US census, 1860, 1870.

DeLavenna *BURROUGHS* (1826–94)

Born in Florence, Italy, August 11, 1826 (her tombstone says 1825), Miss Burroughs came to the United States prior to 1860. Nothing is known of her family background. According to her obituary, she settled first in Skaneateles, New York. However, when she matriculated at New England Female Medical College in 1858, she was listed as coming from Elmira, New York (possibly a patient or employee at the Gleason water-cure?). At medical school she held a Wade scholarship, an award made to non-Massachusetts residents. She received a medical degree from that institution in 1860 and settled in Lyons, Wayne County, New York, living successively in hotels run by Griffith C. Borradaile, William Smelt, and Lester J. Powell. Around 1877, she bought a house on William Street ("above the post office" and "near Canal Street").

Dr. Burroughs practiced medicine in Lyons as an Eclectic physician for twenty-five years. She died at her home of tuberculosis on September 11, 1894, having been an invalid for nine years and bedridden for five weeks. She is buried in Lyons Rural Cemetery. Records provide several variant spellings of her first name. In addition to DeLavenna, there is DeLavene (medical school catalogs), Delia (1867–68 Wayne County directory), DeLavone (1875 census), DeLavann (death certificate), Delavee (obituary and tombstone).

References: Map of Lyons, NY, *Atlas of Wayne Co., New York* (Philadelphia: Beers, 1874); *Gazetteer and Business Directory of Wayne County,*

N.Y. for 1867–8 (Syracuse, 1867); *Clyde, Lyons and Newark Directory for 1888* (Utica, NY, 1888), 69; Obituary, *Clyde Times*, September 13, 1894; *History of Wayne County* (Philadelphia, 1877); Polk, 1886; New York State census, 1865, 1875; US census, 1860; *Lyons and Clyde Directory for 1886–7*; *Lyons and Clyde Directory for 1891–92*; *Wayne County 1880 Directory*, 1880.

Lavinia Ann *Gates* BUSTEED (1820–95)

Lavinia Gates was born May 3, 1820, in Nova Scotia, the eldest child of O. Gates and his wife Lavinia McNeill. She had five brothers and three sisters. She belonged to the Church of England, which was a bit unusual for these early woman doctors, who were more apt to be Quakers or Methodists. Lavinia married George W. Busteed of Boston on December 12, 1843. Busteed's name appears in successive Boston directories as a commission merchant; later a real estate agent; later freestone; still later freestone, coal, iron, copper; and lastly a note broker. He was born in Ireland, was also an Anglican, and was sixteen years older than Lavinia. They had one child, Willard John, born July 7, 1846, who died a year later.

In 1858, Lavinia enrolled in the New England Female Medical College. She later transferred to Penn Medical University, an Eclectic medical school in Philadelphia, from which she received her MD in 1861. She was a resident of Boston at that time. Boston directories list her as a physician each year from 1862 through 1876 (except 1870; also 1871 and 1874 when there were no directories available). The Busteeds were at five different addresses in Boston during that period. She is not listed in the Butler medical directories for 1874 and 1877. According to the 1891 Nova Scotia census, both Busteeds were then residents of the province. Lavinia died in 1895.

References: Boston city directories, 1862–76; *New England Business Directory*, 1865, 1868; Nova Scotia census for 1891; Charles E. Slocum, *Of the Slocums, Slocumbs and Slocombs of America, Genealogical and Biographical* (Syracuse, NY, 1882), 510; US census, 1860.

Mary Ann T. *Denton* BUTTS (b. 1823)

Mary Ann Denton was born in 1823, in Georgia, probably in Hancock County. Her parents' names are not known, and no information has been found about her childhood and early education. On May 30, 1837, at the age of fourteen, perhaps fifteen, she married twenty-two-year-old Capt. Benjamin Kirby Butts. The *Macon Telegraph* reported,

"Married. In Sparta, at the house of R. S. Hardwick, Esq. on Tuesday last at 8 o'clock in the morning, by the Rev. Sereno Taylor, Capt. Benjamin K. Butts, to Miss Mary Ann T. Denton." The couple would have eight children, six of whom lived to adulthood. Only the eldest, David Lewis, was a boy.

Benjamin's father, Capt. James Butts, RS-VA, had migrated from Virginia to Georgia, where Benjamin was born, one of eight children of James and his wife, Sarah H. Simmons. James died in 1835. His will stipulated that the "balance" of his estate, including the slaves, be divided into eight equal parts, one part for each child. Since his wife was already dead, "balance" might suggest that land went to the eldest son. Since Benjamin's mother had eight children and was twenty-eight when Benjamin was born, it is highly unlikely that Benjamin was the eldest son. In any case, he and his family, by 1850 numbering six living children and twenty-nine slaves, moved west to Plantersville, Texas.

The family must have prospered. The 1860 census valued their real estate at $20,000 and personal property at $45,000. They had sixty slaves by 1860. In 1859 or 1860, Mary enrolled at New York Hygeio-Therapeutic College and, on March 29, 1861, received an MD degree. Three years later, in 1864, she subscribed $1,000 to her alma mater's college fund (*HOH*, 189).

Why did Dr. Butts want a medical education? All but two of her children had survived childhood, the youngest being then ten or twelve. She certainly did not need money (and practice in the Deep South was very difficult for women). Anticipation of wartime service seems an unlikely motivation: the firing on Fort Sumter was not until two weeks after she graduated from medical school. Could it have been that she would care for the sixty slaves? In the absence of hard evidence, one can only speculate.

Tragedy befell the family on June 27, 1862. The only son, 3rd Lt. David Lewis Butts was killed at the Battle of Gaines Mills, Cold Harbor, Virginia. He was twenty-four. What happened in Plantersville after the war is not known. Presumably, their sixty slaves were freed. In 1868, Capt. Benjamin Butts, then sixty-three, died. No information about the family subsequent to that time has been located. Did the five daughters find husbands? Did Mary, now presumably in economic straits, practice medicine to support herself?

References: *Herald of Health*, May 1864, 189; *Telegraph* (Macon, GA), June 13, 1837; US census, 1850, 1860.

C

Sarah C. CALDWELL (1834–91)

Nothing is known of Sarah's background, parents, or early education. It has not been possible to identify her positively in the census rolls, which list several hundred persons named Sarah Caldwell. She had married a man named William Caldwell, who had already died before Sarah went to medical school, possibly leaving her with children to support.

Sarah attended and graduated from Penn Medical University in 1859, at the age of twenty-five, and started practice in Philadelphia. Her name is listed in *Progressive Annuals* for 1863 and 1864 as a Philadelphia physician, as well as Philadelphia directories for 1861–68, 1870, 1876–80, 1881–87, 1889–93, and Polk medical directories for 1886, 1890, and 1893. All list her as a physician practicing in Philadelphia.

Unlike Hannah Longshore (q.v.) and Harriet Sartain (q.v.), each of whom had a large downtown practice and who moved either infrequently or within their own neighborhood, Sarah Caldwell moved at least ten times in the thirty-year period of her practice. Except for a few years in the early 1870s when she was located in central Philadelphia, her practice was in the outer neighborhoods, primarily in the northern part of the city: 1861–63, 1163 Passyunk Avenue (southeastern Philadelphia); 1864, 914 North Twentieth Street (north central); 1865–66, 954 North Sixteenth Street (north central); 1867–68, 925 Washington Avenue (south central); 1870, 706 Pine Street (downtown); 1876–80, 1103 Shackamaxon (northeastern); 1881–87, 2162 Franklin (north central); 1889–90, 816 Berks (north central); 1891, 911 Marshall (north central); 1892–93, 1124 Frankford Avenue (northeastern). It seems likely that her practice was a neighborhood one, among the less prosperous members of the community. The fact that she moved so often suggests she was searching for better practice.

Sarah died December 11, 1891. Her simple death notice in the *Philadelphia Inquirer* reads, "Sarah Caldwell, M.D., widow of William Caldwell," mentioning no children. It does include her professional status, which was often not the case in those days. The funeral was from the home, 1124 Frankford; she is buried in Mt. Moriah Cemetery in southwest Philadelphia.

References: *McElroy's Philadelphia City Directory*, 1861–68, 1870, 1876–87, 1889–93; Obituary, *Philadelphia Inquirer*, December 27, 1891; Polk, 1886, 1890, 1893; *Progressive Annual*, 1863, 1864; US census, 1860.

Elizabeth CALVIN

Nothing is known of Dr. Calvin's parents, background, childhood, or early education. She was a resident of Pennsylvania when she graduated from Penn Medical University in 1856. That she was already active in support of education for women is apparent from a letter she wrote at medical school to the editor of the periodical *Woman's Advocate*, which was accompanied by a manuscript of a paper on women's education written by Calvin three years earlier, which she hoped the editor would see fit to publish. She requested that her incognita be "strictly preserved."

Dr. Calvin is listed in the 1862, 1863, and 1864 *Progressive Annuals* as a physician practicing in Philadelphia. Her name is also found in Philadelphia directories, as a physician, from 1858 until 1864: at 923 North Sixth Street (1858 and 1859), 1302 Green (1860), 137 North Eighth (1861), 827 Race (1862), and 829 Race (1863 and 1864). Whether she married, died, or moved has not been determined. She is thought to have died before 1876.

References: Undated letter to Anne McDowell, editor of the *Woman's Advocate*, sold on eBay, May 2015, present location unknown; *McElroy's Philadelphia City Directory*, 1858–64; *Progressive Annual*, 1862, 1863, 1864.

Lydia S. CAMPBELL (b. ca. 1836)

Lydia Campbell was born in New York State about 1836. Nothing is known of her parents, background, or early education. On October 1, 1858, she graduated with an MD degree from New York Hygeio-Therapeutic College. Prior to that time she had married Elbert O. Campbell and was living in LaClaire, Iowa. Once a doctor, she and her husband moved forty miles west to the village of Tipton, where the following advertisement appeared on several occasions in the *Tipton Advertiser* during November 1858:

> Mrs. L. S. Campbell, Hydropathic physician, Would respectfully inform the citizens of Tipton and vicinity that she treats successfully all curable diseases *with strict adherence to hygienic principles*, being fully convinced that drugs are not only *unnecessary* in the treatment of disease, but *absolutely injurious*. Obstetrical Cases are also attended by her, special reference being had to the comfort and convenience of patients. Ladies wishing her services will do well to apply for advice at an early period. Residence at the corner of 7th and Linn Streets, formerly the house of Mr. Joseph Lee. Tipton, Oct. 30, 1858.

It seems likely that the residence was used to accommodate lying-in and other patients. The *Water-Cure Journal* for May 1859 says that Dr. Campbell is operating a water-cure for women (78). The 1860 census describes Mrs. Campbell as "doctress." Sometime before 1870, the couple moved to the smaller village of Onion Grove (now Clarence), a dozen miles to the north. There, Elbert established a variety store. The couple was still there in 1880. Though the fact that Mrs. Campbell is described in both the 1870 and 1880 census reports as "keeping house," it is not proof that she was no longer practicing medicine. However, no evidence has been found that she did continue to practice, either.

The Campbells must have had at least one child; its death is mentioned in Zina Warren's *Reminiscences of the Long Ago*. The child probably died in childhood since it does not appear in any census report. Warren's book, published in 1911, also mentions that Dr. L. S. Campbell is dead.

References: *Tipton (IA) Advertiser*, November 6, 1858; US census, 1860, 1870, 1880; *Water-Cure Journal*, May 1859; Zina Warren, *Reminiscences of the Long Ago* (Noblesville, IN, 1911).

Susan *Richards* CAPEN (1814–63)

Susan Richards was born October 29, 1814, in Sharon, Massachusetts, the daughter of Jeremiah and Susannah Hewins Richards. She was the fourth of eight children and the elder of two daughters. Two of her older brothers died prematurely, one at ten days, the other at three years. The names Capen and Hewins "go far back in Sharon history," according to the town historian. On October 12, 1837, almost twenty-three years old, Susan married Thomas Capen, a farmer. They had three children, Helen Frances (b. 1839), Artemas Alonzo (b. 1843), and Herbert Sylvester (b. 1845).

In 1857, now almost forty-three and her youngest child, Herbert Sylvester, almost twelve years old, Susan graduated from the New England Female Medical College in Boston, having been supported by a Massachusetts scholarship from 1854 on. She returned to Sharon, where she practiced medicine for the remaining six years of her life. Her name is found in the 1858 *Massachusetts Register* as one of two physicians in Sharon. (The 1860 *New England Business Directory*, however, places her in Charlestown.) In 1857, she served as treasurer of the New England Female Medical Society.

Susan died prematurely, of typhoid fever, at the age of forty-nine, on October 13, 1863. She lived almost her entire life in Sharon and practiced medicine there during her last six years. The listing of her death in Sharon, Massachusetts, Vital Statistics denotes her as a physician. Whether, and for how long, she may have been in Charlestown is not presently known. Thomas later married Rachel Hamden.

References: Charlestown, MA, directory, 1860; *Massachusetts Register,* 1858; *New England Business Directory,* 1860; Sharon, MA, directory, 1858; Sharon (MA) Vital Statistics.

Sarah Ann *CHADWICK* Clapp (1824–1908)

Sarah Chadwick was born July 17, 1824, in Windsor, Maine, the seventeenth of twenty children of Lot Chadwick and his wife Sarah. Nothing is known of her childhood and education. Sometime thereafter, the family moved to the frontier town of Lee Center, Illinois.

In 1856, then thirty-two, Sarah graduated from the medical school at Western Reserve in Cleveland. "An Essay on Contagion" was the title of her thesis. Among her classmates at medical school were Cordelia Greene (q.v.), Elizabeth Griselle (q.v.), and Marie Zakrzewska (q.v.). Both Zakrzewska and Chadwick received financial support for their medical education, Chadwick from the Female Medical Education Society of Cleveland. Chadwick and Zakrzewska were roommates at a Superior Road boarding house. In her autobiography, Zakrzewska says that she considered Chadwick a bit prudish. After medical school Sarah returned to Lee Center and presumably practiced medicine.

The principal information about Dr. Chadwick comes to us as a result of her Civil War service. Early in the war, when the western states were called upon to defend and hold the small southern Illinois town of Cairo, located crucially at the confluence of the Mississippi and Ohio Rivers, Dr. Chadwick volunteered to serve as a surgeon with the Seventh Illinois Volunteer Cavalry. Since women were not then given commissions in the army, she probably served as an unofficial assistant surgeon. However, according to historian Linda L. Goldstein, her services were so commended by the men of the Illinois Seventh that she was hired to continue in that role and served for a period of nine months.

After her wartime service, she returned to Lee Center, where she probably practiced medicine, at least for a while. She married a man named Clapp and may have given up the practice of medicine thereafter. Her name does not appear in the 1874 or 1877 Butler directories or the 1886 or 1890 Polk directories of practicing physicians.

In February 1892, then sixty-eight, she petitioned the US Pension Bureau, seeking recompense for her professional services rendered thirty years earlier. She supported her claim that she was indeed an army surgeon by presenting testimony from surviving members of the Illinois Seventh Volunteers to "show conclusively [that] she served successfully in the capacity indicated . . . but that owing to the refusal of the State medical examining board to examine for this service one of her sex, she could not be commissioned or paid. Testimony that the services were faithfully and intelligently rendered under trying circumstances and resulted in the saving of valuable lives is ample and apparently of a thoroughly reliable character." Three years later, in 1895, the bureau agreed to pay her a pension similar to that given surgeons of volunteer cavalry. It was not until 1906, when she was eighty-two, that the bureaucratic wheels rendered the first payment of $8.50, a sum less than most pensioners received. On appeal, Dr. Clapp was told that in order to receive the full $12.00 she would have to file again, but as an army nurse. Sarah died two years later, in Lee Center, on December 1, 1908.

References: Linda L. Goldstein, "Women Enter Medicine in the Western Reserve: The Graduation of the First Six Woman Doctors from Western Reserve College, 1852–1856," *Pan-American Medical Woman's Journal*, March 1952, 35–36; Jane E. Schultz, *Women at the Front* (Chapel Hill, NC, 2004), 194–95; US Fifty-Second Congress, 1st session, H.R. 1418, February 11, 1892, and US Fifty-Third Congress, 3rd session, H.R. 950, January 17, 1895, AGO Document File, Box 69, National Archives & Records Administration, Washington, DC; US Veteran's Administration, Sarah A. Clapp to Pension Commissioner Warner, September 9, 1907, and Pension Bureau to Clapp, October 18, 1907, Clapp pension file, #610330, Organization Index to pension files, Film Series T289, Pension Relating to 2,448 Army Nurses, Veterans Administration, RG 15, National Archives & Records Administration.

Elizabeth B. CHAMBERLIN

When and where Elizabeth Chamberlin was born is not known, nor is there any available information about her parents, background, or early education. When she graduated from New England Female Medical College in 1855, she was a resident of Boston and was thought to be a widow. At medical school she had been supported by a Massachusetts state scholarship in 1854–55. Various Boston directories list her as a physician in Boston in 1857, 1858, 1859, and 1860, first at La Grange Street (at #8, #1, and #4) and later at 273 Tremont, both addresses in downtown Boston. She was probably in Boston from the time of her graduation. The *Progressive Annuals* for 1862, 1863, and 1864 list someone named "Chamberlin" as a physician in Portland, New Hampshire, a village not found on the map. No Dr. Chamberlin is listed in the 1866 *New England Business Directory* in Portland, Maine, or Portsmouth, New Hampshire. Dr. Chamberlin is said to have died before 1876, but no confirmation of this has been found.

References: *Boston Almanac*, 1859, 1860; *Boston Directory*, 1857; *Massachusetts Register*, 1857, 1858; *New England Business Directory*, 1856, 1860.

Eunice S. CHOATE (b. ca. 1820)

Eunice Choate was born about 1820 in New York State. Her maiden name is unknown. The census of 1860 describes an Auburn, New York, family of four: Robert, age about forty-four, a traveling agent; Eunice, age about forty, MD; and two teenage daughters, Josie, eighteen, a music teacher, and Alice, fifteen.

An article by Choate in the *Water-Cure Journal* for September 1857, establishes that she was practicing medicine, at least as an accoucheur, before she went to medical school. In the article, she wrote that emphasis on a fruit diet and restriction of starchy foods during pregnancy would delay ossification of fetal bones and lead to an easier delivery, because the fetus would be more flexible. Once born, the baby should be fed generously on farinaceous foods to make up for the prior deficiency. Choate related the story of a woman who had borne two children with great discomfort and had had two miscarriages within the span of three years but who, on conversion to hydropathic principles, had a healthy child after an easy fifteen-minute labor. In advocating this dietary regimen, Choate was following the theories of Russell Trall, a leading hydropathist. (Trall's colleague, Joel Shew, thought the benefit came from the weight control resulting from the diet. Rachel Brooks Gleason [q.v.], on the contrary, thought it nonsense and said that eating less made women vomit more during pregnancy.)

On March 31, 1860, Choate received an MD degree from the New York Hygeio-Therapeutic College in New York. Graduating with her was an M. J. Choate, also from Auburn, about whom no information has been found. We know nothing of Eunice's whereabouts during the next three years. In the spring of 1863, she went to Wernersville, Pennsylvania, to take charge of a well-known water-cure establishment there, the Hygeian Home. According to an Auburn newspaper, she returned to Auburn in the summer of 1864. A newspaper advertisement (May 13, 1865) reads, "Lady Dr. Mrs. E. S. Choate, M.D., graduate of one of the best colleges in the land often cures when the best Old School doctors fail. . . . Obstetrics and diseases of her own sex a specialty. . . . Rooms 70 Genesee St."

Dr. Choate seems to have spent most of her professional life in Auburn. She is listed as a practicing hygienic physician, and later simply as physician, in city directories for 1865–56, 1867–68, 1868, 1869, 1870, 1871–72. She is also listed as a physician in the 1870–71 of the nearby city of Syracuse. The following advertisement appeared in the *Syracuse Daily Journal*, Tuesday, April 18, 1871: "Mrs. E. S. Choate, M.D., has taken rooms at no. 80 South Salina Street, having 18 years experience in treating all classes of diseases, uses electricity, magnetism and all nature's remedies. Cancers, tumors and catarrh successfully treated, and special attention given to female diseases, and has yet to lose her first patient in childbirth. Charges according to patient's means. The poor treated free."

In 1872, according to Weiss and Kemble's *The Great American Water-Cure Craze*, Dr. Choate was an attending physician at Dr. Trall's Philadelphia Hygienic Institute in Philadelphia. Consistent with this is the fact that her name appears as a physician in the Philadelphia city directory for 1875. In 1877, Dr. Choate reappears in the Auburn directory, is not listed for 1878–80, and is last listed in 1881–82. The 1884–85 Syracuse directory places her in Weedsport, a small community on the Erie Canal ten miles north of Auburn. When and where she died has yet to be established.

References: *Boyd's Auburn Directory*, 1865/66–1867/68, 1871–72; *Boyd's Daily Journal Syracuse City Directory*, 1871–72; *Boyd's Syracuse Directory*, 1884–85; *Auburn City Directory*, 1877–78; *Lamey's Auburn City Directory*, 1881–82; *Gopsill's Philadelphia City Directory*, 1875; *Auburn Daily Advertiser and Union*, April 20, 1863, August 23, 1863, August 30, 1864, May 13, 1865; *Syracuse Daily Journal*, April 18, 1871; US Internal Revenue Service tax assessment list, October 1864, June 1865; US census, 1850, 1860, 1870; *Water-Cure Journal*, September 1857; H. B. Weiss, *The Great American Water-Cure Craze* (Trenton, NJ, 1967), 190.

Betsey *Russell* CLARK (1821–89)

Betsey Russell was born July 6, 1821, in Mason, New Hampshire, the only child of Hubbard (or Hubert, or Hurbert) Russell and his wife Polly Woods. Nothing is known of her childhood or education. Sometime, probably in the early 1840s, she married Joel C. Clark, resident of Worcester, Massachusetts, a patternmaker by trade and a man fifteen years her senior. They had a son, Henry F. Clark, who became an Eclectic physician and established his own practice in Worcester.

Betsey attended Eclectic medical schools in Worcester and Boston. In 1861, she graduated from Penn Medical University in Philadelphia with an MD degree. She returned to Worcester and practiced medicine there for the next twenty-five years. She is listed as a physician in Worcester in the 1867 *Massachusetts Register and Business Directory* and in Worcester city directories as an Eclectic physician living first at 309 Main Street (1860–65), then at 7 Myrtle Street (1866–68), and later at 15 Myrtle Street (1872–86). (There were two other woman physicians in Worcester in the 1850s and 1860s, Mrs. Martin Goodwin and Mrs. S. W. Geralds. Neither was a doctor; both emphasized midwifery. Mrs. Geralds had attended lectures at Worcester Medical College and New England Female Medical College.) In the 1870 federal census Betsey is listed as "keeping house," but in the 1880 census as a "physician." Betsey died at her home, then at 173 Austin Street, May 30, 1889, of "paralysis and nervous prostration," at the age of sixty-eight.

References: William Lincoln, *History of Worcester, Massachusetts, from Its Earliest Settlement* (Worcester, 1862); *Massachusetts Register & Business Directory*, 1867; US census, 1870, 1880; *Worcester Almanac, Directory and Business Advertiser*, 1860–65; *Worcester Directory*, 1866–85; Obituary, *Worcester Daily Spy*, May 31, 1889.

Nancy Elizabeth *Talbot* CLARK Binney (1825–1901)

Nancy Talbot was born May 22, 1825, in Sharon, Massachusetts, the seventh of ten children—half of them boys, half girls—born to Josiah Talbot and his wife. Her Talbot ancestors came from England in the mid-seventeenth century. Several of her siblings had professional careers as ministers or teachers; a younger brother became a physician. Nancy went to Sharon Academy and, at age sixteen, was teaching school in South Dedham (now Norwood) where a brother and two sisters had preceded her. In 1845, at age twenty, she married a dentist, Champion W. Clark of Philadelphia. The couple moved to Baltimore and had a daughter in 1847, who died in the early part of 1848. Nancy herself was very sick at this time. Then, her husband developed typhoid fever and died on March 6, 1848, at twenty-seven. In due course, an older woman friend urged Nancy to go to medical school so she could help other women. She went to Western Reserve, a school that had not previously accepted any woman.

Why she made this choice is not known. Historian Frederick Waite suggests that Nancy may have been acquainted with the wife of the medical school's dean, John Delamater, who also came from Sharon. Records show that the medical school faculty had voiced opposition to the admission of women, but Drs. Delamater and Jared Potter Kirtland were faculty leaders, and they favored admitting women. They served as Nancy's preceptors. It is possible that Nancy intended to teach physiology and hygiene, not to practice medicine. In 1850, the Massachusetts legislature required that those subjects henceforth be taught in public schools. Waite quotes one of Nancy's teachers to the effect that was, indeed, Nancy's intention. She graduated with an MD degree on March 3, 1852.

Dr. Clark returned to Boston and set up her practice at 4 Bulfinch Place, just off Scollay Square, moving to nearby 49 Hancock Street the following year. She is listed as a physician in Boston directories each year from 1852 through 1871. In 1853, her second year of practice, Dr. Clark applied for membership in the Massachusetts Medical Society, was examined by its Board of Censors, and was found acceptable in every way. The board, however, was unwilling to take the responsibility of recommending a woman for membership. Under the Acts of Incorporation of the Society, which did not mention the possibility of a female candidate, the censors were obliged to examine and accept for membership all who could pass the examination or each, individually, would sustain a $400 fine. The membership at large turned down the application and indemnified the censors. It was not until 1881 that a woman was admitted to the society. In spite of her failure to breach the walls of organized medicine, she is said to have developed a good practice.

In 1854, Dr. Clark spent a year abroad training at the Paris and London hospitals, the only woman in Boston with such experience. A physician from Charleston, South Carolina, then studying in Paris on the wards of M. Dubois, described Nancy in the *Charleston Medical Journal*: "She is decidedly good looking, with large retreating blue eyes, dark hair, and a countenance which at once denotes intelligence and great resolution. Her bearing is certainly modest, yet when at the bedside of particular patients undergoing examination, and surrounded by medical students of the other sex, you can often notice the forced action of her lips restraining a smile, prompted evidently by feeling the ludicrousness of her situation." He further reports that she was always accompanied by her brother, a homoeopathic physician, that she spoke little French, and that the professor was at pains to explain things to her in English.

On the voyage over, Nancy met Amos Binney Jr. Amos, who had recently lost his wife and newborn child, was the eldest son of Dr. Amos Binney (1803–47), who never practiced medicine but was prominent in banking. On July 6, 1856, Nancy and Amos were married at West Church, in Boston. It was also the last year that Nancy is listed in Boston directories as a physician, so it would appear that she gave up practice after her second marriage. Instead, she raised six children: Amos, who graduated from Harvard and the Massachusetts Institute of Technology as a chemist and was later a businessman in Boston; two daughters who died while still young; two more daughters, each of whom had a good education, married, and lived in Philadelphia; and Harold, also an MIT graduate, who worked in the US Patent Office, later went to law school at New York University, and practiced law in New York City. During these years, Amos and Nancy lived with Amos's mother at 82 Beacon Street.

Nancy did return to practice for one year. In 1874, she opened an office and free dispensary for women on Charles Street in Boston, but the venture was short lived. In later years, the Binneys moved a lot. When first married, they lived in Roxbury. During the Civil War, Amos was a commissioned officer in the Paymaster's Department, becoming a Lieutenant Colonel, living in Baltimore and later Norfolk, Virginia. From 1867 to 1872, the Binneys lived in New York City, where Amos was in an unsuccessful banking venture with some colleagues. In 1872 they went back to Boston, but moved to Newport, Rhode Island, in 1877, where Amos died at fifty on March 11, 1880. Thereafter, Nancy lived in Newport, Boston, Philadelphia, and finally Haverford, probably to be near her daughters, where she died at seventy-six on July 26, 1901.

References: Boston city directories and almanacs, 1852–71; R. A. Kinloch, "Medical News from Paris," *Charleston Medical Journal* 10 (1855): 65, 159; Frederick C. Waite, "Dr. Nancy E. (Talbot) Clark," *New England Journal of Medicine* 205 (1931): 1195–98.

Emeline *Horton* CLEVELAND (1829–78)

Emeline Horton was born September 22, 1829, in Ashford, Connecticut, the fourth(?) of five daughters of Chauncey Horton and Amanda Chafee. Emeline was one of the eighty children in the seventh generation of Hortons in America. Earlier generations had graduates of Princeton and Yale. Along with many of their generation, Chauncey's family moved westward in the 1830s. In Chauncey's case, it was 1831, and the family settled in Stockbridge, Madison County, New York. An older sister described Emeline, then but two years old, occupying "a tiny chair which was fastened amid-ships of one of the large Conestoga wagons" in which they were traveling. (Forty-seven years later, Emeline would return to Stockbridge to visit her mother, arriving by New York Central Railroad in a Pullman car.) On the farm in Stockbridge, there were forty cows, and each girl had her chores. When older, Emeline was a milkmaid, performing morning and evening.

Father Chauncey set up a schoolroom in his corn barn, and, later, a tutor taught the Horton and neighboring family children in the house. On reaching maturity, Emeline taught in the local schools, and hoped to go to Mt. Holyoke, but in 1848 her father died, and the following year the teacher who had attracted her to Holyoke, Mary Lyon, died too. In the fall of 1850, she matriculated at Oberlin College. During the long winter vacations while she was there, she taught school, one year in Ashtabula, Ohio, and another, near Pittsburgh.

In the meantime, Giles Butler Cleveland, her Stockbridge neighbor who had just graduated from Hamilton College with a BA degree, began study at Oberlin Theological Seminary. Both Giles and Emeline graduated in August 1853 and on March 8, 1854, they were married in Stockbridge. He was ordained a Congregational minister in Arkport, New York. The couple planned to go abroad as missionaries, Emeline as a doctor. She matriculated at Female Medical College of Pennsylvania on October 1, 1853, supported at least in part by the Pennsylvania Ladies' Missionary Society. An apt medical student, she graduated in March 1855, joined her newly ordained husband in Arkport, in New York's Southern Tier, and practiced medicine there for a year.

In the spring of 1856, she was offered a position at her alma mater as demonstrator of anatomy. From the fall of that year until her death twenty-two years later, her career was at the Female Medical College of Pennsylvania. The following year she was made professor of anatomy, and Philadelphia became their home. Dr. Cleveland lectured in the school and saw patients at her home. Giles taught but was apparently soon disabled by some chronic disease. Their careers as missionaries were abandoned.

Shortly, some women of Philadelphia wished to establish a hospital for women and children. In anticipation of this, Emeline was sent abroad for further study. She entered the school of obstetrics at La Maternité in Paris on August 27, 1860, remaining until June 28, 1861, when she received five prizes, two of them "firsts," and an honorable mention for "clinical observation." She had to learn French along the way and undergo a public examination. She returned to Philadelphia to become resident physician at the newly chartered Woman's Hospital of Philadelphia. In 1860, she became professor of obstetrics, relinquishing the chair of anatomy.

During the Civil War Dr. Cleveland was an active volunteer surgeon. Shortly after the battle at Gettysburg, assisting surgeons on the field, she was described as "calm and strong, yet more than ever womanly." The observer told of "a poor fellow whose arm was shattered [and who shrank] fearfully, when, by the surgeon's direction, she was about to assist at an operation. But as soon as her hand, firm, yet tender, grasped his arm, he yielded and was quiet, feeling strangely satisfied and safe."

Back in Philadelphia, after six years at the new hospital, with her practice ever more demanding, she retired from her post as resident physician. She continued, however, to perform a substantial amount of gynecological surgery including, it is claimed, the first ovariotomy in the United States. Whether the claim is accurate or not, Dr. Cleveland was a pioneer among female surgeons. From 1872 to 1874, she was dean of the medical school.

In 1865, her only child, a son, Arthur, was born. An 1889 graduate of the University of Pennsylvania, he became an otolaryngologist in Philadelphia. Emeline contracted tuberculosis and was sick in her last years. She died at forty-nine on December 8, 1878, and is buried at Philadelphia's Fair Hill Cemetery. Her husband, the chronic partially paralyzed invalid, outlived her, remarried in June of 1880, and was still living in Belleville in northern New York State in 1893.

Tributes to Emeline invariably emphasize her "gracious womanhood," her "highly dignified bearing," her kindness to all. Described as a "tall, graceful figure . . . wholly devoid of pretension, she glided noiselessly into her Lecture Room. Quietly seating herself behind the lecture table, she began her lecture in a low, conversational tone, which was always distinct and dignified. Her sitting to lecture was characteristic." Kate Hurd-Mead summed her career: "Perhaps the greatest pioneer [woman] surgeon in America . . . she had rare native ability, a cool head, and a great deal of sympathy for suffering. She was a superior obstetrician and had an instinct for surgical cleanliness before the days of germ theories, hence her operative success was far above the average in the sixties and seventies." Much earlier in her career, another wrote of her in the *Herald of Health* that it was "a marvel that so much gentleness and sympathetic tenderness can be united to so much firmness and nerve."

Bibliography: Manuscript notes kept while studying in Paris, 1861, Archives of the Woman's Medical College of Pennsylvania, Drexel University College of Medicine, Philadelphia; *Introductory Lecture on Behalf of the Faculty to the Class of the Female Medical College of Pennsylvania, for the Session of 1858–59* (Philadelphia, 1858); *Valedictory Address to the Graduating Class of the Female Medical College of Pennsylvania, at the Eleventh Annual Commencement, March 14, 1863* (Philadelphia, 1863); *Valedictory Address to the Graduating Class of the Woman's Medical College*

of Pennsylvania at the Sixteenth Annual Commencement, March 14, 1868
(Philadelphia, 1868).

References: Rachel L. Bodley, "Tribute from the College Faculty," in
*Papers Read at the Memorial Hour Commemorative of the Late Prof. Eme-
line H. Cleveland, M.D. West Lecture Room of Woman's Medical College of
Pennsylvania, Philadelphia, Pa., Wednesday, March 12, 1879* (Philadel-
phia, 1879); Edmund J. Cleveland, *The Genealogy of the Cleveland and
Cleaveland Families* (Hartford, CT, 1899); Personal communication
from her great-grandson Arthur Cleveland, Riviera Beach, FL; *Herald
of Health*, September 1869, 108; Kate Hurd-Mead, *Medical Women of
America* (New York, 1933), 33; Howard A. Kelly, *Cyclopedia of American
Medical Biography* (Baltimore, 1912), 1:187–88; *Dictionary of American
Medical Biography* (Westport, CT, 1984), 140; Obituary, *Medical Record*,
1878, 14:499; Obituary, *Philadelphia Inquirer*, December 9, 1878; *Notable American Women*, 1:349–50; Adaline H. White, *The Hortons in America* (Seattle, 1929).

Abigail S. *COGSWELL* (1826–57)

Of her background, childhood, and education nothing is known. The
1859 census lists her as a twenty-four-year-old woman living in Scipio,
Cayuga County, New York, with the family of Josiah Letchworth, a
harness maker, and his wife Ann. There are three Letchworth children: Hannah, twenty; Charlotte, sixteen, and Isaiah, fourteen.
There is also a six-year-old named Hannah Cogswell. It might be reasonable to speculate that Abigail was the Letchworths' eldest child
and the younger Hannah her daughter. However, Abigail is referred
to as "Miss." In any case, she "was left dependent on herself early in
life" according to her obituary.

A member of the Society of Friends, she "was constantly aspir-
ing after an increase in intellectual treasure." She was interested
in science, so much so that her friends feared "that her talents,
designed for a nobler purpose, should be entirely devoted to the
pursuit of that knowledge which passeth away" (Friends' obituary,
37). She attended Nine Partners Boarding School, was trained as a
teacher, and taught for several years in a number of families belong-
ing to Scipio Monthly Meeting.

Later, "feeling herself called upon to instruct those of her own sex
in the rules which govern their physical being" and in poor health herself, she enrolled in 1853 at New York Hydropathic and Physiological
School (the not-yet-chartered predecessor of New York Hygeio-Therapeutic College). According to a report in the *Water-Cure Journal*, she

graduated in April 1854 but seems to have returned for another course the following year, after which she returned to Western New York to practice.

In the summer of 1856 she went to Hudson, Ohio, to care for her sick sister. While there, she wrote a long letter to the *Water-Cure Journal* in which she described various water-cures she had visited on a lecture tour made earlier that year. It gives some idea of her practice and of her personality. "From the 17th of Jan. up to June 10th, I have been traveling as a lecturer and for pleasure." During that time she talked with many people. Some of the water-cures were converts to hygienic living, others were not. Opinions of both were given in some detail. She especially liked an establishment in Bethlehem, Pennsylvania, run by Dr. A. Smith on "the strict principles of Hygiene, as taught in the Hydropathic College." Dr. Cogswell thought all other water-cures should send their cooks to this water-cure "to learn how to make bread. I can truthfully say, that in no house, public or private, did I ever eat better bread. Dyspepsia can't live long on *that fare.*" She was distressed that at many of the water-cures patients were being given medicine and not given much instruction in dietetics.

Her sister died, probably of tuberculosis. That fall Abigail joined the staff of the Cleveland Water-Cure run by Dr. Thomas Seelye. But she, too, was sick and died the following May 30 (1857) at the age of thirty-one, probably of tuberculosis. Her obituary in the *Water-Cure Journal* (July 1857, 14) said:

> Four years ago she came to us (the New York Hydropathic and Physiological School) in an exceedingly frail condition of health. . . . She had been seriously sick on several occasions, and had been repeatedly drugged nearly to death by the doctors. *Mercurial salivation* had made sad havoc with her vitality. . . . But by careful management she recovered a comfortable state of health. . . . The arduous and responsible position in the Cleveland Water-Cure . . . over-taxed her bodily powers. . . . It was impossible for Miss Cogswell to see suffering, and not sympathize with the sufferer. She could not witness error and ignorance, without striving with all her might to correct and enlighten. She was wholly consecrated to the work of her noble calling; and though her own career was short, she has been the means of leading thousands of her fellow-creatures into the ways of life and health.

In the *American Monitor,* the Society of Friends wrote that Dr. Cogswell was "called upon to instruct those of her own sex in the rules which govern their physical being" and that she labored not just for physical well-being of patients but also "their spiritual advancement."

References: *American Annual Monitor for 1858; or, Obituary of the Members of the Society of Friends in America, for the Year 1857* (New York, 1858), 36–38; US census, 1850; Letter from Dr. Cogswell published in the *Water-Cure Journal* 22 (1856): 61; Obituary, *Water-Cure Journal* 24 (1857): 14.

Elizabeth D. A. *Magnus* COHEN (1820–1921)

Elizabeth was born at 205 Hudson Street, in New York, on February 22, 1820. Much later in her life, Elizabeth claimed that her father was related to the Magnus family in Kent, England, one of whom was involved in the building of the *Great Eastern* steamship. The assumption that Magnus was her maiden surname is apparently incorrect. Her parents were David and Phebe Cohen. She was educated in New York and spent the early years of her marriage there. The exact date of her marriage to Dr. Aaron Cohen is not known, but it must have been in the early 1840s, since she already had five children when she went to medical school in 1854. Only one of the children lived to adulthood, and it was the death of her youngest son from measles that was one of factors motivating her to become a physician. At the time, she thought the physician could have done more to save him. "I knew later that I was wrong, but at the time it seemed as if the doctor could have saved him. And I determined to become a doctor myself, and to help mothers to keep their little ones well" (1920 interview). She was also encouraged in this by her husband, who went to New Orleans for surgical training when she went to medical school. How many of the children were still living in 1854 and whether they went with Elizabeth to Philadelphia when she enrolled at Penn Medical University or stayed in New York with grandparents is unknown. When she went to New Orleans after graduation at least some of the children went with her. Toward the end of her life she said, "I reared my family of five while practicing my professional duties, and the two duties never clashed." She and her husband had eighteen years together before his death, and they "never had a single disagreement."

In 1857, she graduated with an MD degree from Penn Medical University, an Eclectic, coeducational school in Philadelphia, not from the Female Medical College of Pennsylvania, as she remembered years later, when she was in her nineties. She recalled that she and her classmates at graduation received invitations to go to France to practice. With a family and a husband already in New Orleans, this seemed impractical. She described the trip to New Orleans to rejoin her husband: "I came down to New Orleans on the 'High Flyer,' a noted boat in those days, from St. Louis, and I can tell you that we had exciting times on the downward trip. There was gambling going on in the cabin and on deck, and there were races with other boats in the river, and altogether my trip down was a most memorable one" (*Daily Picayune*, 1913).

There were only thirteen physicians in New Orleans, then a city of more than 120,000. She was the city's first woman doctor. She set up practice in the French Quarter and worked there for thirty years. At first, she was registered as a midwife (in directories through 1868), was listed as a "doctress" in 1869 and, from the 1870s on, as a physician. The largest part of her practice was obstetrical. "In those days every physician had to register every case he treated, so if you consult the records in the Board of Health office . . . you will find that I had no mean practice" (ibid.). She delivered second genera-tions of her patients and "never lost a case in all my practice" (pre-sumably obstetrical). "People said I had a lucky hand in those days." She also practiced general medicine and surgery. She "never knew what it was to have a whole night's rest during thirty years. . . . We didn't have telephones, but messages came at all hours to my house in Baronne Street."

After the death of her one remaining son, then alone, she retired in 1887 and moved to the Julius Weiss Home for the Aged and Infirm. Here she would spend the remaining thirty-four years of her life. For many of them she ran the linen room, and in 1900 she presented the home with a fountain out front. In 1913, and again in 1920, on her one hundredth birthday, she was interviewed by a reporter from the local newspaper, interviews on which this sketch is largely based. Also on her one hundredth birthday, one of her nephews from New York, sixty-one-year-old E. P. Myerson, came to see her. Looking back over the years, she recalled yellow fever epidemics, working with Dr. Joseph Jones, and said that she never encountered any anti-Semitism. She spoke of a mysterious little wooden box under her table that con-tained information about titled relatives in Europe and other things that will make a good story for which "it will be time enough, though, when I die."

On her one hundredth birthday she told a reporter that she was "glad to see the girls of today getting an education. In my youth you had to fight for it. And it's the finest thing in the world—an education. And I believe in suffrage too—things will be better when women can vote, and can protect their own property and their own children." She died in the Touro Infirmary at the Weiss Home on May 28, 1921, more than 101 years old. Until a few months before her death, she had all of her faculties—mind, eyesight, and hearing. Her only complaint was lumbago. She left most of her property to the home.

References: Most of the information available for this biographical sketch came from two interviews given by Dr. Cohen when she was ninety-three and one hundred: *Daily Picayune* (New Orleans), January 26, 1913; *Times Picayune* (New Orleans), February 22, 1920, February 23, 1920, May 29, 1921.

Elizabeth *COLLINS* Jones (1834–96)

Elizabeth Collins was born in 1834 at the Lacey Collins homestead in Lower Buckingham, near Pineville, a village in Bucks County just north of Philadelphia. The homestead was situated on a four-hundred-acre tract granted the Lacey family by William Penn. Elizabeth's Lacey and Collins forbears were among the area's earliest settlers. On her mother's side, Elizabeth was descended from prominent Quaker preachers. The youngest of three children of Andrew Collins and Eleanor Simpson, she had a sister who died in early childhood and a brother, James, who also became a physician. Her mother died when she was an infant, and her father when she was fourteen.

Elizabeth attended local public schools, then went to Samuel Martin's boarding school in Kennett Square. Upon finishing, she taught school in Warwick Township but soon returned to school as a student herself at the Locust Street Institute for Young Ladies in Philadelphia (1850 and 1851). It was during this last period that she began the study of medicine with her cousin, Dr. Charles W. Smith of Pennsville, as her preceptor. She matriculated at the Female Medical College of Pennsylvania in 1853 and graduated in 1856. That same year she married Joseph L. Jones, a milk dealer. They had five children, three boys and two girls. The youngest child, Eleanor, became a physician.

She was listed in the 1864 *Progressive Annual* as a practicing physician in Philadelphia, but according to her obituary "she gave little attention to the practice of her profession after assuming household duties, but was always alive to the necessities and comfort of those around her, and was active in all charitable and benevolent works." Dr. Jones died in Philadelphia, October 31, 1896.

References: Obituary, *Philadelphia Inquirer*, November 3, 1896; US census, 1860; Woman's Medical College of Pennsylvania, *Report of the Proceedings of the Twenty-Second Annual Meeting of the Alumnae Association* (Philadelphia, 1893), 51–52.

Frances Sproat *COOKE* (1817–74)

Frances Cooke was born in 1817 or 1818 in Taunton, Massachusetts, the seventh of eight children (five girls, three boys) of Samuel F. Cook, Esq., and his wife Ann Nancy Padelford. Nancy was the daughter of the Hon. Seth Padelford, 1770 Yale graduate and judge of probate and, on her father's side, the granddaughter of Col. John Cooke, of Tiverton, Rhode Island.

As a young woman, Frances taught school in Taunton, where the 1850 census lists her as a schoolteacher living in a boarding house. She is mentioned in *School Chronicles* by Isaac W. Wilcox as a teacher.

When she was almost forty, she moved to Boston and enrolled in New England Female Medical College, where she was supported by a Massachusetts Commonwealth scholarship from 1854 to 1857. She graduated in 1857 with an MD degree. From that time until 1872 she practiced medicine in Boston and was on the faculty of her alma mater. An assistant instructor in 1857 and 1858, she became professor of physiology and hygiene on August 12, 1859, and professor of anatomy, physiology, and hygiene in 1866. She also lectured on physiology to students at Wheaton Female Seminary (Wheaton College after 1912) from 1859 to at least 1869. Dr. Cooke is listed as a physician in Boston in the 1860, 1865, 1868, and 1871 editions of the *New England Business Directory*.

In 1872, Dr. Cooke, along with two other faculty members, resigned from the faculty. Faculty and board minutes do not make clear the reason for this. It was probably because the trustees, without discussing the matter with the faculty, sought an agreement with the recently opened Massachusetts Homoeopathic Hospital that would allow the school's students to have clinical experience at the hospital, a privilege they had been denied at the Harvard-controlled Massachusetts General Hospital. The problem was that in that day Regulars, or allopaths, did not have professional relations with homoeopaths, and the faculty were Regulars. It was a moot point: two years later New England Female Medical College was assimilated by newly established Boston University. Contrary to the agreement, the medical school's name disappeared, and the school became homoeopathic. On September 29, 1874, Dr. Cooke died of carcinoma of the breast.

References: *Boston Almanacs*; Obituary, *Boston Evening Transcript*, September 1874; *New England Business Directory*, 1860, 1865, 1868, 1871; Massachusetts Death Records 1874, 267:206; US census, 1850; Frederick C. Waite, *History of the New England Female Medical College, 1848–1874* (Boston, 1950); Wheaton Female Seminary, *Chronological Catalogue of the Trustees, Principals, Teachers and Graduates of the Wheaton Female Seminary, Norton, Mass* (Boston, 1869); Isaac W. Wilcox, Article written for the *School Chronicles*, cited by the Taunton Public Library, original reference not located.

Maria Louisa *COOKE* Hooper (b. 1825)

Maria Louisa Cooke was born in July 1825, the youngest of three daughters of Caleb Cook (*sic*), a gunsmith, and his wife Lydia. Both Caleb and Lydia, as well as their children, were all born in Massachusetts. By 1850, the family had settled in Homer, Cortland County, in Central New York State. No information has been found about Maria's childhood or early education.

In 1856, then thirty-one and still single, Maria graduated from New England Female Medical College in Boston with an MD degree. It seems probable, however, that she was already a doctor of medicine when she matriculated at the Boston school. According to the February 1854 issue of the *Syracuse Medical & Surgical Journal,* "Miss Dr. M. Louisa Cooke, Homer, Cortland Co." is listed as having been a delegate to the fifth annual meeting of the New York Eclectic Medical Society held at Syracuse Medical College, January 10, 1854. (A fellow delegate was Miss Dr. D. A. Porter who graduated from Syracuse Medical College on February 16, 1854. It has not been possible to verify whether Miss Cooke was also a graduate that year, or merely a classmate.) The November issue of the journal reported that Dr. Cooke "commenced her course of lectures to the lady students," of whom there were seven so far. Soon after graduating from the Boston school, Dr. Cooke returned to Homer and started to practice her profession. The *Progressive Annuals* for 1863 and 1864 each list her as a physician practicing in Homer, as does the *Gazetteer and Business Directory of Cortland County* for 1869. In the 1870 census she is denoted as "physician."

Ten years later, now married to John W. Hooper, a local carriage maker with two grown children, Maria is listed as "keeping house." It was not uncommon at that time to so designate even women known to be practicing medicine, but, of course, she may have retired from practice after her marriage. (Note: The discovery that Maria married John Hooper was quite fortuitous. The 1880 census revealed that Lydia Cook, eighty-six, was the mother of Maria L. Hooper.)

Maria lived to be at least eighty-four and was still in Homer when she died. In the 1900 census, her older sister Lydia was living with her; her husband had probably died. In the 1910 census she is found living alone. As was often the case with these earlier woman physicians, it has not been possible to determine how much and for how long Maria practiced medicine in Homer. People got used to a woman doctor, if there was one, and no particular attention was given the matter. It is known that Maria maintained intellectual interests. In 1888, she graduated from Western New York's famous Chautauqua Institution, with a certificate from the literary and scientific circle. The date of Maria's death has not been found.

References: *Gazetteer and Business Directory of Cortland County, N.Y. for 1869* (Syracuse, NY: H. Child, 1869); *Progressive Annual,* 1863, 1864; *Syracuse Medical & Surgical Journal,* February 1854, 6; *Syracuse Medical & Surgical Journal,* November 1854, 312; US census, 1850, 1860, 1870, 1880, 1900, 1910.

Helen Caroline *COOKINGHAM* (b. 1835)

Caroline Cookingham, known as Carrie, was born November 25, 1835, in Clinton, Dutchess County, New York, the fourth of five children (four girls, one boy) of Daniel Cookingham and his wife, Margaret Crapser. She was christened the following year at St. Paul's Lutheran Church in Wurtemberg, Dutchess County, New York. Her forebears, then named Kuchenheim, had immigrated to America in the eighteenth century. Her father and older brother John were moderately prosperous farmers. (Daniel had $5,000 in real estate in 1850, and in 1860 $6,000 in real estate and $4,000 in personal property.) An older sister, Matilda, became a schoolteacher.

The 1860 census lists Caroline, then twenty-four, as a student of medicine. The following year, then a resident of nearby Staatsburg, she graduated from New York Hygeio-Therapeutic College with an MD degree. The *Progressive Annuals* for 1863 and 1864 list her as a physician in Staatsburg, New York. No further information about her has been found. Possibly she died. More likely, she married and she will be lost until her new identity is discovered.

References: *Progressive Annual,* 1863, 1864; US census, 1850, 1860.

Elizabeth *Bower* COOMBS Barnes (b. ca. 1832–1901)

Elizabeth Bower was born about 1832, in Clark County, Indiana, second of seven children and eldest daughter. Two younger brothers died in childhood, and a sister at twenty-one. Her grandfather, Adam Bower, was born at sea in 1754, while his parents were en route from Germany to America. He became a Dunkard preacher. Her father came to Indiana from North Carolina with his parents in 1806, became a well-established farmer, and was deacon in the Christian Church. Of Elizabeth's three surviving brothers, two, William and Abraham, became physicians. Elizabeth was educated at the seminary in Washington, Indiana.

She married a local farmer, Jesse Coombs, and had one child, who died. On December 8, 1853, her husband died. Elizabeth taught school for a couple of years and, in 1855, began the study of medicine in the office of Dr. Joseph Hostetler. She went to Eclectic College of Medicine in Cincinnati for the lectures, received her MD on May 23, 1857, and returned to Clark County to practice medicine.

On April 24, 1860, she married businessman John Clinton Barnes (b. 1835). He was the eldest of ten children, had an academy education, and had graduated from Scott's Commercial College in Indianapolis five years earlier. After his marriage, he too went off to Eclectic Medical Institute, the other Eclectic institution in Cincinnati, where he attended two lectures courses, one starting in November 1865, and the other following in January 1866. According to EMI records he did not receive an MD degree. That same year, the couple moved a hundred or so miles to the southwest into Douglas County, Illinois, where, a year later, John bought a farm three miles west of the village of Hindsboro. He farmed, and they both practiced medicine there for the next seventeen years. They are both listed in the 1874 and 1877 Butler directories as residents of nearly Arcola.

In the early 1880s, John gave up farming and the couple moved into the village of Hindsboro, where John ran a lumberyard and they both continued to practice medicine. Both are listed as practicing physicians in Polk medical directories for 1886, 1890, 1893, 1896, 1898, and 1900.

The Barneses were prosperous, prominent, and generous local citizens. They were members of the Christian Church. They had three children, Elmer B., who worked with his father in the lumber business, Calmer H., a school teacher, and Calmer's twin brother, Omer F., who became a physician, graduating from Kentucky School of Medicine in 1890. He returned to Hindsboro, where he practiced until about 1899, when he moved to Arcola. Elizabeth retired a little before 1900 and died November 9, 1901.

References: Butler, 1874, 1877; *County of Douglas, Illinois: Historical and Biographical* (Chicago, 1884), 524–26; John Gresham, *Historical and Biographical Record of Douglas County, Illinois* (Logansport, IN, June 1900), 285–86; *Portrait and Biographical Album of Coles County, Illinois* (Chicago, 1887), 426–29; Polk, 1886 et seq.

Sarah *Lamb* CUSHING (1818–1919)

Sarah Lamb was born in Pittstown, Rensselaer County, New York, on August 8, 1818, third child of Claudius Lamb and Betsy Hoag. She had two older brothers and a younger sister. She was four when her father died. Her mother died three years later, and she went to live with her Hoag grandparents until, at fourteen, she went to a Quaker boarding school near Albany. Later, in 1841, she graduated from Albany Academy. In 1846, on a visit to her brother in Portsmouth, Ohio, she met and married the Rev. David Cushing. Mr. Cushing had been pastor of the Presbyterian Church in Newark, New York, from 1837 to 1843, when he was dismissed. He moved to Portsmouth where, after a trial period, he became pastor of the Presbyterian Church there in March 1847. Because of poor health, he resigned this post on June 1, 1849. He died three weeks later. The Cushings had one child, a daughter named Martha Maria, who also died in 1849.

Now without husband or child, it is unclear what direction Sarah took, but a decade later, she graduated from Starling Medical School in Columbus, Ohio (1859). After being turned down for an internship at a Philadelphia hospital, she went for two years to the New York Infirmary for Women and Children, returned to Columbus for a year, and then moved to Lockport, New York, where she had Hoag relatives, to establish a practice that would continue for more than forty years. She was still listed under physicians and surgeons in the 1901 Niagara County directory.

Always interested in public affairs, Sarah supported women's suffrage and temperance movements. By the time of her one hundredth birthday, being by then housebound, she was sorry not to be able to enroll so that she might vote. She was then also the oldest resident of Lockport or Niagara County. She attributed her longevity in part to the fact that she avoided coffee, tea, and milk, but loved cocoa, meat, and potatoes.

In 1910, she established the Sarah Cushing Trust Fund with a $20,000 endowment. Half of the interest was to be paid to Sarah during her lifetime; the other half, and all of the interest after her death, was to benefit needy women patients at Lockport Hospital. By 1915, Sarah was ninety-seven, deaf and feeble, and had become unable to live alone. She moved to the home of Samuel Rising, where Mrs. Rising cared for her. When she died, at 101, her funeral was held at the First Presbyterian Church, though she had for many years attended Congregational services. She is buried in Cold Spring Cemetery, Lockport.

References: Biographical sketch dated September 1979 at the Lockport Public Library; *Niagara Falls Reporter*, August 26, 1908; *Lockport*

Union Sun and Journal, August 19, 1918; Obituary, *Lockport Union Sun and Journal*, March 12, 1919; *Roberts' Niagara County Directory for the Year 1901* (Lockport, NY), 1900–1901(?).

D

Maria J. *DENNETT* (1828–65)

Maria Dennett was born July 27, 1828, in Barnstable township, Massachusetts, the seventh child of fourteen (third of six daughters) of Oliver Dennett and his wife Eunice Seawards (or Seward). Nothing has been found regarding her childhood or early education. The 1850 census—she was then twenty-two—found her in New York, living with lumber merchant Erastus C. Sanderson and his family. In 1860, she was living in Philadelphia with the family of James Ruggles. Mr. Ruggles's daughter, Anna, and son, Augustus, as well as Maria, are all listed as medical students in the 1860 census.

At the age of thirty-two, she graduated from Penn Medical University (1861), where she had been a classmate of Anna M. Ruggles (q.v.), who may have been her cousin. Upon graduating, Maria and Anna went into practice together at 1540 Cherry Street in Philadelphia and are listed as physicians at that address in directories through 1865.

At the Yearly Meeting of Progressive Friends, Maria "presented the case of oppressed sewing-women of Philadelphia, reciting instances of trial and suffering that awakened the deepest sympathy. Her appeal for pecuniary aid on behalf of the class referred to met with a liberal response from many individuals." It would appear from this that Maria was a Quaker and that her practice was among the poor women of Philadelphia. Maria, then living at 1414 Ellsworth Street, died December 19, 1865, in Philadelphia at the age of thirty-seven. Her death certificate denoted her a physician. She is buried in Odd Fellows Cemetery.

References: *McElroy's Philadelphia City Directory*, 1863; *Proceedings of the Pennsylvania Yearly Meeting of Progressive Friends, Held at Longwood, Chester County, 1864* (New York, 1864), 10; US census, 1850, 1860.

Abigail Parthenia *DEWEY* Maurey Newhall (1822–67)

Abigail Dewey was born November 22, 1822, probably in Delta, Oneida County, New York, the third of four children of Josiah Dewey, a farmer, and his wife, Martha "Patty" Hitchcock. She had two older brothers and a younger sister. No information about her childhood or early education has been found. In 1850, she was living with her older brother Solomon.

In 1858, then thirty-six, she graduated from the New York Hygeio-Therapeutic College with an MD degree and returned to Oneida County and started to practice medicine. While in New York she met and married Jeremiah Maurey, a medical schoolmate from Sinking Spring, Bucks County, Pennsylvania. The marriage was short lived. Jeremiah apparently died. The 1860 census shows Abby, thirty-seven, and her mother, sixty-nine, living in North Bay, Oneida County, with the family of Abigail's older brother (Josiah) Davis Dewey, his wife, and three small children. Abby is described as "doctress," and her name is spelled Mory.

In the early 1860s, Josiah Dewey and his family moved west to Walworth in Wayne County, New York. Abigail must have gone with them because she soon married James Newhall, a reasonably prosperous farmer in Walworth ($5,000 in real estate, $2,000 in personal property, according to the 1870 census). No information has been found as to whether Abby practiced medicine in Walworth. Her days there were brief. She died December 16, 1867, at the age of forty-five. One might speculate that her first husband died of tuberculosis, infected her, and that she died from it, too. But that is no more than a possibility.

Abby is buried in a small, untended country cemetery near Walworth—the Freewill Cemetery. Her stone is tipped over, lying flat. Next to her is the grave of her successor, Mila, whom James Newhall married after Abby's death, and who died in 1882. And next to her is the eighteen-year-old daughter of Josiah Davis Dewey. That is all. Josiah and his clan moved to California. Newhall also moved, possibly to Michigan.

As was often the case, it is difficult to know how much or for how long Abby practiced her profession. The 1862, 1863, and 1864 *Progressive Annuals* describe her as a practicing physician in Delta, Oneida County, New York. The 1870 census describes her a "doctress." The Dewey family genealogy says she "was a doctor." So, she must have practiced in Oneida County, and possibly in Wayne County as well, albeit briefly.

References: Lewis M. Dewey, *Life of George Dewey . . . and Dewey Family history*, 2 vols. (Westfield, Massachusetts, 1898); *Progressive Annual*, 1862–64; US census, 1850, 1860, 1870; Walworth Center Cemetery (Freewill Cemetery), Walworth, NY.

Jane Elizabeth DOLLEY Laundon

Jane Dolley (her maiden name is unknown) was born in New York State about 1825 (census data vary from 1823 to 1818). Nothing has been found regarding her parents, background, childhood, or early education. In Elyria, Illinois, about 1846 or 1847 she married Paris Clark Dolley, MD (Eclectic Medical Institute, 1847). The couple had two children: Maria Estelle (b. October 14, 1850) and Paris (b. ca. 1854). Her husband Paris died of tuberculosis in September 1853, leaving Jane with two young children. Maria Estelle died in 1868 of tuberculosis at the age of eighteen. Paris Jr. died in 1872 aged nineteen.

After the death of her husband, Jane enrolled at Eclectic Medical Institute in Cincinnati and graduated with an MD degree on May 19, 1855. She returned to Elyria and started practice. Sometime before 1860 she married Thomas W. Laundon, a local merchant, born in England, who by the time of the 1870 census had $20,000 in real estate, and $10,000 in personal property. Jane bore two more children: Mary E. (b. ca. 1854) and Ernest T. (b. ca. 1856).

Though the 1870 and 1880 census reports give Jane's occupation as "keeping house," she almost certainly must have practiced medicine, at least for a while. Though her merchant husband, whom she married soon after the death of Paris, probably made it unnecessary from an income point of view, there is some evidence that she was professionally active. Her sister-in-law, Sarah Adamson Dolley, MD, a very active practitioner in Rochester, New York, sought Jane's professional care at the time of her own confinement (1856). Wrote Sarah's son, Charles Sumner Dolley, "My mother went to Elyria, for her confinement, to be under the care of her sister-in-law."

References: Charles Sumner Dolley, letter dated August 24, 1930, correspondence of Sarah Dolley, Dolley Papers, Edward G. Miner Library, Rochester, NY; Records of Ridgelawn Cemetery, Elyria, Ohio; US census, 1850, 1860, 1870, 1880.

Letitia (Lettice) *Hyde* DOUD (b. ca. 1815)

Little is known of the life and career of Dr. Doud. According to census records she was born about 1815 in North Carolina. While still a teenager, she married the Rev. Menzer Doud, a Methodist supply minister who was said to be "one of the most commanding and useful preachers of his age." Menzer, in poor health, was forced to retire from his post in Dansville, New York, "with his afflicted wife" to the home of his parents in Pittsford, NY, where he died April 27, 1834, leaving a nine-teen-year old widow and, according to one source, two small children.

It was not until seventeen years later that Lettice entered Roches-ter's Central Medical College. Following graduation in the spring of 1852, she set up practice in Rochester. An advertisement in the local *Rochester Daily Democrat*, which appeared from June through August 1852, read, "Mrs. L. A. Doud, MD, still renders medical and surgical aid to any who may desire it. She will receive into her family invalid ladies, and bestow upon them every medical and other attention req-uisite for a restoration to health. She will also take one or two Lady Students." This suggests that she may have been running some kind of nursing home prior to becoming a doctor. The 1860 census still records her as a physician in Rochester, living alone, and worth $75.

No subsequent record of her has been found unless she be the Lettice Doud recorded in the 1870 New York census as being sixty-five years old, born in Virginia, keeping house in Newark Valley, Tioga County, New York, worth $800.

References: F. W. Conable, *History of the Genesee Annual Conference of the Methodist Episcopal Church*, 2nd ed. (New York, 1885); O. L. Doud, *Doud and Allied Families* (Sun City, AZ, 1976); W. W. Dowd, *Henry Doude and His Descendants* (Portchester, NY, 1885); *Rochester City Directories*, 1853–54, 1855–56, 1857–58; *Rochester Daily Democrat*, June 23, 1852; US cen-sus, 1860.

Deborah *Smith* DRURY (1824–1915)

Deborah Smith was born January 1, 1824, and grew up in Andover, Massachusetts, the fifth of eight children, second of four daughters, of John and Abigail Bailey Smith. On May 7, 1846, in Andover's Christ Church, Deborah married Albert D. Drury of Farmington, Maine, described in the 1850 census as a "finisher." They had one son, Albert Jr. In later years, directories describe Albert Sr. as a "track layer" (1869–70) and a "railroad contractor" (1887).

In 1855, Deborah, her son no more than eight, attended New England Medical College for Women in Boston but later went to Penn Medical University, an Eclectic school in Philadelphia, from which she received an MD degree in 1857. Thereafter, she practiced medicine for thirty years—for the first few years in in the Boston suburb of Roxbury. She is listed as a physician in Roxbury in Boston directories for 1858 and 1860, in *Progressive Annuals* for 1863 and 1864, in the *Massachusetts Register* for 1867, and the *New England Business Directory* for 1868.

Sometime after the war the family moved to Haverhill, Massachusetts, where Dr. Drury practiced probably until the late 1880s. Living with them at the time of the 1870 census was a couple (the husband ran a "billiard saloon") and an unemployed couple (ages twenty-three and nineteen), as well as a sixteen-year-old servant. By the 1880s, Deborah and Albert had retired, moved back to Andover, and later to Salem, where they lived with son Albert and his wife. Dr. Drury lived to be ninety-one years old. She died August 22, 1915, at the Old Ladies Home in Haverhill.

References: Vital Records of Andover, Massachusetts to 1849, Topsfield, MA, 1912; Bailey family genealogy, typescript, Andover Historical Society, Andover, MA; Boston city directories, 1858, 1860; Butler, 1874, 1877; *Massachusetts Register and Business Directory*, 1859, 1867; *New England Business Directory*, 1860, 1868 1875; *New England Official Directory & Handbook*, 1878–79; *Progressive Annual*, 1863, 1864; US census, 1850, 1870, 1900, 1910.

E

Edith *Webster* EATON (1806–71)

Edee Webster, as she was known, was born December 9, 1806, in Wilton, Maine, the third of eight children, and second of six daughters, of Joseph Webster and his wife Ruth Butterfield. By his earlier wife, Betsey Walker, who probably died in childbirth, Joseph had three daughters and a son. So, over a period of nineteen years and with two wives, he had twelve children. Four of the girls did not survive to adulthood. Edee's older brother, Benjamin, wrote the following rhyme (in 1876) to explain the situation:

> My father was born in New Hampshire,
> In the town of Ware [Weare];
> There he found a wife
> And they were married there.
> When they had three daughters
> Then they moved to Maine
> And settled in the town of Milton
> When in 1800 they had a son.
> My father was a farmer
> And worked at clearing land;
> My mother was his second wife
> And I was her oldest son.

I had one half-brother
And he had three sisters older—
Which made quite a family
When we were all together.
My mother had six daughters,
And then she had a son.
And I was sixteen years of age
When my brother was born.
Then she had one daughter—
Although it was rather late;
She is all the sister that I have
Living in this state.
I have two more sisters more,
They both live out West;
And four have gone to Heaven,
If God their souls have blessed.

Edee grew up in Wilton. On March 28, 1826, she married Capt. Daniel Eaton, also of Wilton. They had eight children, five daughters and three sons. The family must have left Wilton in the mid-1830s, because their seventh child, Tappan Sargent, was born in Augusta, Maine, in 1838, and their last child, Edith A. R. Eaton, was born in Lowell, Massachusetts, in 1843. Captain Eaton died of tuberculosis in 1854.

By 1850, Edee was in Boston. Her husband may already have been an invalid, leaving Edee with at least two children to support. That year, she earned a certificate of proficiency in midwifery from the New England Female Medical College and is listed in the Boston directory as one of five midwives (out of a total of twelve) with this qualification. (The New England Female Medical College had been organized in 1848, but it was not until 1854 that it was granted a charter authorizing it to award doctor of medicine degrees.) From 1853 through 1858 Edee is listed in directories as a physician at 34 Albany. During the latter part of that period, she attended Worcester Medical Institution in Worcester, Massachusetts, and graduated with an MD degree on June 11, 1857. Thereafter, from 1859 through 1872 she is listed in the Boston directories as an MD physician, at 11 Common in Boston. She is also listed as a physician in Boston in 1856, 1860, 1865, 1868, and 1871 editions of the *New England Business Directory*. She died, in Boston, on November 25, 1871, of some kind of tumor, when she was just short of sixty-five. Dr. Eaton was one of the few woman physicians to have an obituary in the *Evening Transcript*. She practiced medicine, primarily midwifery, for twenty years.

References: *Boston Almanac*, 1851–75; Obituary, *Boston Evening Transcript*, November 25, 1871; Massachusetts Death Records, 1871, 240:194; *Massachusetts Register*, 1852, 1855; *New England Business Directory*, 1856, 1860, 1865, 1868, 1871; US census, 1860, 1870.

Susan Ann *EDSON* (1823–97)

Susan Edson was born January 4 (or June 24), 1823, youngest of four children and second daughter of John Joy Edson and Sarah Baker. Her father was a sergeant major in the War of 1812, an older brother was a physician, and her sister was a nurse. All sources agree she was born in Cayuga County, New York, but whether in Aurelius, Fleming (Cleave, 1873), or Auburn (*Lamb*, 1900 et seq.) seems to be in dispute.

After graduating from Western College of Homoeopathic Medicine (later Homoeopathic Hospital College of Cleveland) in March 1854, she practice for two years in Cleveland and then returned to Jefferson, Ashtabula County, Ohio, where most of her childhood had been spent, and developed "an extensive practice." (*Lamb* says she grew up in Auburn and returned to Auburn after medical school.)

With the start of the Civil War she gave up her practice and moved to Washington to serve in army hospitals. William H. King, in his history of homoeopathy, writes that she worked from August 1861 to March 1862 as a nurse at the hospital established in Columbia College on Meridian Hill, then moved to Hygeia Hospital at Fortress Monroe. She worked in hospitals during the entire war, usually as nurse, but sometimes as physician, as well. According to historian Jane Schultz, she went to New York in 1862 and established a training program for nurses with private support, the surgeon general having vetoed the idea. After the war she returned to practice, either in Auburn (*Lamb*), or in northeastern Ohio (King says Cleveland and Ashtabula; Cleave says Jefferson, Ohio).

In 1872, her own health somewhat compromised, she moved back to Washington, where she practiced as she was able to. Among her patients was the family of President Garfield, including the president himself. After Garfield was shot, on July 2, 1881, it is reported that Dr. Edson stayed at his bedside constantly, but for brief periods of sleep, until he died on September 19. For this service she was awarded $3,000 by Congress. Charles Roos, in his bibliography of presidential physicians, gives a somewhat different and more detailed report: Dr. Edson was Garfield's nurse until the president was moved to Elberon, leaving that place on September 8, returning for a visit on September 15. "Her presence at the end is doubtful. She is not included among those said to have been present in accounts in newspapers and medical journals, nor does she claim this in her own sketch 'The sickness and nursing of President Garfield.'"

In Washington, with Caroline B. Winslow (q.v.), whom she met during the war when they were working as nurses, she helped to organize the Free Homoeopathic Dispensary, the National Homoeopathic Hospital (of which her nephew, John Joy Edson, an attorney, was president 1889–95), and the Washington Chapter of the American Institute of Homoeopathy. One of the earliest woman to join the American Institute of Homoeopathy, she had become a life member in 1872, the same year as Eliza Pettingill (q.v.). Only Harriet Sartain (q.v.) in Philadelphia preceded them, becoming a lifetime member in 1871. Dr. Edson died, unmarried, in Washington on November 14, 1897.

References: American Institute of Homoeopathy, *Transactions,* 1898, 48; American Institute of Homoeopathy, *Transactions,* 1906, 883; W. R. Balch, *Life of President Garfield* (Philadelphia, 1881), 612–20 [includes Dr. Edson's description of her care of President Garfield]; John H. Brown, *Lamb's Biographical Dictionary of the United States* (Boston, 1900); Cleave, 135; William H. King, ed. *History of Homoeopathy and Its Institutions, in America* (New York, 1905), 1:321; Polk, 1886; Charles A. Roos, "Physicians to the Presidents, and Their Patients: A Bibliography," *Bulletin of the Medical Library Association* 49 (1961): 337; Jane E. Schultz, *Women at the Front* (Chapel Hill, NC, 2004).

Minna *ELLIGER* Piersol (1834–71)

Minna Elliger was born in Prussia about 1834, the eldest of six children (two girls, four boys) of George and Christeanna Elliger. The family immigrated to Pennsylvania in 1848, arriving in New York from Bremen. The youngest child was born in New York. George Elliger was a physician, and Minna's younger brother, Arthur, would later become one as well (MD, Jefferson, 1871). The timing of the family's emigration from Germany suggests that perhaps George had some involvement in the Revolution of 1848. When the 1850 US census was taken, the family was living in Allentown, and they were well off: George owned $8,000 in real estate and had domestic help.

On February 16, 1854, Minna, then a resident of Allentown, graduated from the Female Medical College of Pennsylvania. She had attended the sessions of 1851–52, 1852–53, and 1853–54 and submitted a thesis entitled "History of Chemistry." Sometime before 1860, she married Jeremiah M. Piersol, MD (b. 1826), who came from North Sewickley, Pennsylvania. The couple established their practices in central Philadelphia at 1110 Spring Garden Street and would live there the rest of their lives.

In 1860, their only child, George Piersol, who later became a well-known histologist, was four years old and the family had domestic help. McElroy's business directories for Philadelphia list Minna and Jeremiah as physicians in 1862, 1866, 1867, 1868, and 1870. Minna and Jeremiah each paid Civil War income taxes, $10 in 1862–63 and $6.67 in May 1863.

Minna died April 22, 1871, at the age of thirty-seven years. She is buried in Philadelphia's Laurel Hill Cemetery. On an 1857 passport application, she was described as age twenty-four, 5′4″ or 5′1/2″ (not clear), forehead full and broad, eyes dark hazel, nose medium, mouth large, chin oval, hair dark brown, complexion dark, face oval. She had become a US citizen by marriage. Jeremiah died April 27, 1882. As a retired physician he lived with his son and daughter-in-law at 1110 Spring Garden Street.

The great granddaughter of Minna Elliger Piersol, Anne Murray Morgan (b. 1925), attended Radcliffe College (graduated 1946) and was the first woman to be elected to the Harvard Alumni Association Council.

References: Anne Murray Morgan Papers 1890–1996, Schlesinger Library on the History of Women in America, Harvard University, Cambridge, MA; Internal Revenue Service tax rolls, 1862–63, May 1863; *McElroy's Philadelphia Business Directory*, 1862, 1866, 1867, 1868, 1870; Miscellaneous material on the Medical College of Pennsylvania, Drexel University School of Medicine, Philadelphia; New York passenger lists, 1820–1957, *Ancestry.com*, Provo, Utah, 2010; Passport application, Minna Piersol, November 7, 1857; US census 1850, 1860, 1870, 1880.

Hannah W. ELLIS (1807–65)

Hannah was born in 1806, probably in Philadelphia. No information has been found about her background, parents, childhood, or early education except that she was a Quaker. Sometime before 1831, she married a Philadelphia builder, Nathan W. Ellis. The couple had at least one child, William Penn Ellis, born December 4, 1831. William became a Philadelphia merchant.

In the early 1840s, Hannah became a midwife. She was said to have been practicing midwifery for at least a decade before she graduated, in 1853, from the Female Medical College of Pennsylvania, a member of the second class at that school. On the first faculty vote Hannah received only four white votes and three black votes, five white votes being required for a degree. The vote was reconsidered, and there were five white votes. Though she may have practiced general medicine after becoming a doctor, she probably continued to emphasize obstetrics. Her thesis at school had been "A Disquisition on Labor." She must have practiced for at least a few years in Philadelphia. She is listed in Philadelphia directories as a physician in 1854, 1855, and 1856, but not thereafter. She died July 16, 1865, with "softening of the brain" according to her death certificate, so she probably was not practicing medicine in her final years. However, she is listed in the *Progressive Annual* for 1864 as a practicing physician in Philadelphia.

Dr. Ellis was "amiable [and] intelligent . . . a fresh genial Quaker lady," according to a letter found in her medical school file, written by an unidentified person. She had been a member of the Green Street Monthly Meeting in Philadelphia. As were most Quakers, she was active in the antislavery movement. She attended the second and third antislavery conventions held in Philadelphia in 1838 and 1839. She was a supporter of the Northern Home for Friendless Children. Hannah and her husband are buried in Fairhill Friends Burying Ground in Germantown.

References: Anonymous, undated letter describing Ellis at the archives of the Woman's Medical College of Pennsylvania, Drexel University College of Medicine, Philadelphia; Obituary, *Friends Intelligencer*, July 1865, 22:331; *McElroy's Philadelphia Directory*, 1854–56; Pennsylvania, Church and town records, 1785–1915; Philadelphia, Death Certificate Index, 1803–1915; *Progressive Annual*, 1864.

Sarah Maria *Leonard* ELLIS (1828–1914)

Sarah Leonard was born August 10, 1828, in Barker, a small Quaker community in Western New York State. She was the last of five children (four girls, one boy) born to Joseph Leonard Jr. and his wife Margaret Hammar. The family migrated westward, settling in Troy, Michigan, just north of Detroit, before 1837. Sarah received her secondary schooling in Detroit.

On October 30, 1851, in Troy, twenty-three-year-old Sarah married Dr. John Ellis, a man twelve years her senior. Dr. Ellis had been married before, to Mary Coit, with whom he had three children, one of whom, Wilbur Dixon Ellis, lived to adulthood. Mary died October 15, 1850. John and Mary had a daughter and a son, but neither of them survived infancy. John himself was born in 1815 in Ashfield, Massachusetts, the youngest of his family. As a young man he learned dentistry, and, in 1840 and 1841, he traveled through the South on horseback as an itinerant dentist to pay for his medical schooling. Before and after this trip he attended, and in 1842, graduated from Berkshire Medical School in western Massachusetts. From there, he went to Albany Medical College and then to Chesterfield, Massachusetts, where he set up in practice and on June 29, 1843, married his first wife.

John and Mary moved to Grand Rapids, Michigan. While there, John became interested in homoeopathy, went to New York to attend lectures in the subject, and, on returning in 1846, set up an office in Detroit with a partner. The partner died of cholera in 1849 or 1850, and John's wife Mary died October 15, 1850. The following year he married Sarah Leonard. John lectured for six years at Western Homoeopathic College in Cleveland and was said to be an accomplished surgeon. Sarah and John lived in Detroit for ten years in a large four-story brick house where John had his office. During the later 1850s, Sarah attended and, in 1859, graduated from Western Homoeopathic College with an MD. Whether she practiced medicine with her husband in Detroit between 1859 and 1861 is not known.

The family moved to New York City in 1861 or 1862. Here, in 1863, Sarah was appointed chair of anatomy at New York Medical College for Women, a position she held for two years. Poor health and the requirement that she prepare her own cadavers for demonstration led to her relinquishing the position. She continued on the school's Board of Censors. In the fall of 1869, she and John traveled in Florida, and Sarah is reputed to have offered care to the women of Jacksonville. Toward the end of his life, John seems to have largely retired from medical practice and during his last fifteen years was involved in oil refining, by a process he had developed. With him in this endeavor were his son, Wilbur, and Sarah. In the 1880s, the Ellises took a year-long trip to Europe, Egypt, and the Holy Land. An account of the trip was published weekly in London's the *Dawn*. At home, they lived at the Chelsea, a new ten-story apartment block at 222 West Twenty-Third Street run as a co-op.

Sarah was described as a "very bright woman, well-educated. . . . She aided her husband greatly in his literary, medical and business pursuits." How active she was in medical practice after they moved to New York it has not been possible to determine. The 1870 census lists her as being "at home," and the 1880 census says she "keeps house." Sarah was an active supporter of Prohibition.

Sarah died on December 16, 1914, and is buried in Beldingville Cemetery, Ashfield, Franklin County, Massachusetts. John died at the Chelsea in December 1896. In addition to his medical and business

pursuits, he was a prolific author of religious tracts (*Address to the Clergy,
Skepticism and Divine Revelation*) that he sent gratis to, it is said, sixty
thousand American clergymen; *Deterioration of the Puritan Stock*; and two
medical books: *Avoidable Causes of Disease* and *Family Homoeopathy*. He
was said to have principles that were "fixed" and "inflexible" in religion, temperance, and medicine.

References: Cleave, 146; E. R. Ellis, *Biographical Sketches of Richard Ellis
the First Settler of Ashfield, Mass. and His Descendants* (Detroit, 1888);
Manning Leonard, *Memorial: Genealogical, Historical, and Biographical, of
Solomon Leonard, 1637, of Duxbury and Bridgewater, Mass. and Some of his
Descendants* (Southbridge, MA, n.d.); John's obituary, *New York Times,*
December 12, 1896; US census, 1870, 1880.

Susannah H. ELLIS

No information has been found about the birth, parents, background,
or childhood of Susannah Ellis. It was not possible to identify her in
census records and it is unknown whether Ellis is her maiden or married surname. Susannah graduated from Female Medical College of
Pennsylvania in December 1851, a member of the first class at that
school. She practiced medicine for at least a dozen years at five different locations, all in downtown Philadelphia, in an area just northeast
of present-day City Hall (306 1/2 Race, 1321 Vine, 231 N. 10th, 234
N. 12th, 147 N. 10th). She is listed in Philadelphia directories for the
last time in 1863. The *Progressive Annual* for 1864 lists her as a practicing physician in Philadelphia, but this publication is often a year or so
behind in its information. Whether Dr. Ellis married or died or moved
elsewhere after 1863 is not known. No marriage date, death date, census listing, or IRS tax roll listing has been found.

References: *McElroy's Philadelphia Directory*, 1854, 1855; *McElroy's Philadelphia City Directory*, 1858, 1860, 1861, 1863; *Progressive Annual*, 1864.

Sarah Ann *ENTRIKIN* (1819–88)

Sarah Entrikin (or Entriken) Fairchild was born January 16, 1819, in
East Marlboro Township, Pennsylvania. Nothing is known of her parents, background, childhood, or early education. The Entrikin clan, in
Chester County, was numerous, and one branch, that of Emmor and
his wife Susannah, moved to Ohio, where their son, Franklin, and his
son both became physicians.

Sarah graduated from Penn Medical University in 1854 with an
MD degree. She spent two additional years studying with a Dr. Thomas

in Philadelphia. From 1857 until 1882 she practiced homoeopathic medicine in neighboring West Chester. Of this, there is substantial documentation. The 1860 census enrolled her, in a fashion typical of the day, as a "doctress," noted that she had $700 in personal property and that she lived in a boarding house managed by Sarah Entrikin (age seventy-six), probably her mother. Local directories for 1857, 1870–71, and 1879–80 list her as a practicing physician. The tax assessment lists for 1863, 1864, and 1865 record her as paying $6.67 or $10 as a physician.

On January 16, 1880, seventy-five of her relatives and friends gave her a birthday party, organized by the reading circle, at which she was presented a medicine case. In June 1882, Sarah retired and moved to Juniata, Pennsylvania, to live with her brother Thomas. She died December 11, 1888, two days after suffering a stroke, while on a visit to a friend in Kane, Pennsylvania. A West Chester newspaper wrote, "Most of West Chester's citizen will remember Dr. Sarah A. Entriken [*sic*], who for several years practiced medicine in this place and was, we think, the first lady physician with a West Chester practice." The "several" years was actually twenty-five years.

References: *Boyd's West Chester Directory*, 1879–80; Robert E. Carlson, *Chester County (PA) Medical Practitioners to 1948* (West Chester, PA, 1986); *Chester County, Pa., Business Directory, 1870–71*; *Directory of the Borough of West Chester, for 1857*; Scrapbook with twenty-one newspaper clippings (source unidentified) regarding the Entrikin family, including four about Sarah Entrikin, MD, Chester County Historical Society; Dorothy I. Lansing, "Chester County in the 19th Century . . . a List of Practicing Physicians and Surgeons," 1977, typescript, Chester County Historical Society; Pennsylvania State census, 1865; US census, 1850, 1860; US Internal Revenue Service tax roll, Pennsylvania, 1863, 1864.

Susan *Maxson* ESTEE (1828–1914)

Susan Maxson was born March 3, 1828, in Petersburg, New York, a daughter of Daniel Maxson and Susan Armsbury Armstrong. No information has been found regarding her childhood or early education. On March 18, 1847, at the age of nineteen, she married the forty-four-year-old Rev. Azor Estee, longtime pastor of the local Seventh Day Baptist Church. Mr. Estee had been married before and had two sons; his first wife died in 1845. With Susan, he had two more sons, James Azor and Daniel.

In the late 1850s Susan attended lectures at the New York Hygeio-Therapeutic College and, on March 31, 1860, received an MD degree.

A notice in the 1863 *Herald of Health* reported that "Mrs. Susan M. Estee, M.D., is having excellent success in Quincy, Pa., in treating typhus fever, pneumonia, and diptheria [*sic*]."

On September 7, 1864, Azor died, leaving Susan with eleven- and fifteen-year-old boys. They moved to Alfred, New York, a community in the Southern Tier of Western New York, and another stronghold of the Seventh Day Baptists. Susan would remain there the rest of her life. She probably practiced medicine there, though the only supporting evidence is Susan's listing in the 1867 *New York State Business Directory* that year as a hydropathic physician. The 1870 census shows Susan as head of household, with sons James and Daniel and her seventy-eight-year-old mother-in-law living there. As late as 1891, she and son Daniel, who was principal of the local Academy, lived at 13 Academy Street. In her final years she lived with the family of Mark Sheppard, MD.

Susan died in Alfred, April 20, 1914. As her obituary put it, "As she had so greatly desired, her redeemed spirit went suddenly to her 'Father's House.'" She was described as "neighbor and friend . . . a cultured woman, a great reader, familiar with the Book of books, and a Christian, a wife and mother, of faith and faithfulness, goodness, gentleness, cordiality, strength of character, energy of purpose, and full of courage in the battle of life." But nowhere is mention made of her having gone to medical school or of practicing medicine.

References: Obituary, *Alfred Sun*, April 22, 1914; *Herald of Health*, February 1863, 92; *New York State Business Directory*, 1867; Corliss F. Randolph, *A History of the Seventh Day Baptists in West Virginia* (Plainfield, NJ, 1905).

Susan A. *Hamblen* EVERETT (1835–1914)

Susan Hamblen was born at Portland, Maine, in 1835, the second of seven (or eight) children of William Hamblen, a house carpenter (or mason), and his wife, Sarah Bartlett. Mr. Hamblen had $500 in personal property at the time of the 1860 census. Nothing is known of Susan's childhood or early education. In the 1860 census, Susan is listed as still living at home with her family, but as Susan Everett, so had married George H. Everett by that time. (Everett was probably the George Henry Everett who received an MD degree from the University of Pennsylvania several years later in 1869.) Susan graduated from Penn Medical University in Philadelphia in 1860.

The couple described themselves as "widely known lecturers and health teachers." They seem to have led an itinerant life, traveling from town to town, rather than maintaining a medical practice in one community. (This mobility may explain why they are not found in the 1870 or 1880 census.) During the month of April 1870, the *Herald of Health* reported, Mrs. Susan Everett, MD, "will lecture . . . in Canandaigua, Geneva, Waterloo, and Seneca Falls, N.Y." Her postal address was Syracuse, New York. In the August issue of the same periodical, readers were told that "Dr. Susan Everett has closed her season of lectures for the present, and will recreate until September, when she will open her fall campaign in New York and Massachusetts. She may be addressed during the summer at Aurora, Illinois." A year later, in November 1871, the following notice appeared in a Palmyra, New York, newspaper: "A lecture for the ladies. Mrs. Susan Everett, M.D., will give a Free Lecture at the Chapel of the Presbyterian Church, on Monday, Nov. 20th at half past 2 P.M. The lecture will be exclusively for the ladies and Mrs. Everett, who comes here with recommendations from far and near, is very anxious that the ladies of Palmyra will grant her their presence on this occasion. The subject of her lecture will be 'Intellectual and Physical Beauty of Woman as Modified by Health.'"

The Everetts are best remembered as authors of *Health Fragments; or, Steps toward a True Life: Embracing Health, Digestion, Disease and the Science of the Reproductive Organs.* . . . The book had two parts: the first, dealing with physiology, was by George; the second, embracing "dress, heredity, child-training, kitchen and dining-room ethics," was written by Susan. The book must have been popular, for it was published in six editions between 1874 and 1877. However, a reviewer for *Popular Science Monthly* was not impressed. Wrote he, "This book contains a few good things that have been said a hundred times before, and that are here scattered through a large amount of nonsense which might better been left unsaid."

The Everetts must have supported themselves either by accepting free-will offerings after lectures, possibly by providing consultations while they were in the towns where they lectured, and surely from the sale of their book, which was probably available at their lectures. The 1910 census lists Susan as a widow, boarding with a family named Hill, in Falmouth, Maine, supported by her "own income." She died March 1, 1914, in Falmouth, at the age of seventy-eight, with senile debility. Her death certificate said she was a doctor.

Bibliography: George H. Everett and Susan A. Everett, *Health Fragments; or, Steps toward a True Life: Embracing Health, Digestion, Disease and the Science of the Reproductive Organs.* . . . (New York, 1874; there were at least six editions by 1877).

References: Death certificate; George H. Everett and Susan A. Everett, *Health Fragments* (New York, 1874); *Herald of Health* 49 (1870): 191; *Herald of Health* 50 (1870): 94; *Palmyra Courier,* November 17, 1871; Book review, *Popular Science Monthly,* January 1876, 377; *Progressive Annual,* 1863; US census, 1860, 1910.

F

Laura Marion *Wheeler* FAIRCHILD Wheaton Plantz (1829–1923)

Laura Wheeler was born May 8, 1829, in Lyndon, Vermont, a village not far from St. Johnsbury in the Northeast Kingdom, the eldest of eleven children of Nelson Wheeler, village blacksmith and wagon maker, and his wife, Bersheba Moore. Years later, when she joined the Daughters of the American Revolution, Laura would establish descent from Benjamin Wheeler, a great-grandfather, and two other forebears who fought in the Revolutionary War. When Laura was ten, the family moved to Putney in southeastern Vermont. Laura attended nearby West Brattleboro Academy and then taught school for several years, in Dummerston, Saxton's River, and Putney, and then in Globe Village, Rhode Island. Later, she became principal of a young ladies' seminary in Jerseyville, Illinois, but soon returned to Putney because of poor health.

In 1853, at the age of twenty-four, she began the first of three marriages, this one to William Fairchild, a merchant in New Haven, Connecticut. Fairchild died two years later. Laura moved to Lowell, Massachusetts, where she worked in a mill and started to read medicine. In 1856, she enrolled in New England Female Medical College in Boston for at least one course of lectures, later transferring to Penn Medical University in Philadelphia, an Eclectic school that had separate classes for men and women, and from which she graduated with an MD degree in 1860.

She started practice in New York as resident physician and superintendent of an institution for the treatment of women and children at Ninety-First Street but left, shortly, to become superintendent of the Home for the Friendless on Thirtieth Street (where she was awarded $50 "for the superior sanitary condition" in which she maintained the home). She resigned this position to take charge of a corps of nurses being trained at Bellevue Hospital to serve in the army during the Civil War.

By the end of the war she had moved west to Rushford, Minnesota, where she set up in practice and where she met Col. William Wheaton, a civil engineer from Peoria, Illinois, who was in charge of building several railroads emanating from Chicago, among them the Chicago, Rock Island and Pacific. The couple soon moved to Kalamazoo, Michigan, where, in 1866, Laura's only child, a son, Walter, was born. Dr. Fairchild, now Dr. Wheaton, practiced medicine in Kalamazoo for eleven years, very successfully, it is said. She also participated in other community activities, especially the woman's suffrage movement.

Though her obituary reports that she was an ardent suffragist, this seems to be incorrect. Actually, she was opposed to giving women the right to vote. In 1870, she was on the lecture circuit in Michigan, Illinois, and Washington, DC, giving two different talks, "The True Woman" and "The Perils of the Hour," both of which received favorable comment in the press. "The Perils" was based on biblical sources and may have been the talk used when speaking in churches. In "The True Woman," of which a twenty-five page single-spaced legal-sized typescript exists among her papers, she contends that the woman's place is in the home, caring for children, supporting her husband, avoiding the base passions of politics that might sully her purity and allow that "the soft, persuasive words of love give place in the heated canvas to acts of chicanery and words that could emanate only from hearts full of corruption" (*Decatur [IL] Press*). The editor of the *Peoria Democrat* wrote that, "while we do not endorse the views presented, yet we must say, that it was one of the ablest lectures and as a literary effort, the best delivered in the city, on that side of the question." A writer for the *Freeport Bulletin* was even more enthusiastic: "Mrs. Dr. Wheaton's lecture on 'The True Woman,' was one of the most *womanly* lectures we have ever listened to. It was well written and *eloquently* delivered." Had Dr. Wheaton been on the other side of the issue, she might have been remembered along with Susan B. Anthony, Elizabeth Cady Stanton, and other leaders. She did apparently persuade the Illinois legislature in May 1870 to reverse its vote in favor of enfranchising women.

In 1875, Col. Wheaton's poor health led the couple to move to San Francisco, where he died on September 28 that year. Laura, after returning to Kalamazoo, later met and soon married (December 1876) sixty-five-year-old Tobias Avery Plantz, an attorney in Pomeroy, Ohio, former member of the Ohio Legislature, the US House of Representatives, then a County Court judge, and soon to be president of a local bank. Laura and her ten-year-old son moved to Pomeroy. After Judge Plantz died in 1887, Laura traveled in the southern and western states and, about 1891, moved back to Putney, where she built a large clapboard house on Depot Street in which she would live for more than thirty years. It is clear that she practiced medicine in Putney. Her license certificate from the Vermont State Medical Society, dated April 6, 1896, is among her papers, and her name appears in Polk medical directories for 1898, 1900, and 1902 and the AMA medical directories for 1906, 1909, 1912, and 1921. In 1918, she wrote, "I have just entered my 90th year and still do some office practice. I live alone and have just finished planning quite a large war garden."

In early 1900, when the wildly popular Admiral George Dewey, naval hero of the Spanish-American War, announced what turned out to be a brief candidacy for president of the United States, Dr. Plantz, who apparently had a good sense of humor, announced her own candidacy for vice president on the same ticket and, to her surprise, was besieged by members of the press. During the Putney years she was also active in the Congregational Church, the Woman's Relief Corps, the DAR, and the Order of the Eastern Star. On her ninetieth birthday, two of those organizations gave her a party at her home. In 1921, she moved to Columbus, Ohio, to live with her son, Walter, an accountant and banker, and where, on May 23, 1923, after a broken hip sustained in a fall on the stairs, she died at ninety-four. She is buried in Putney. On her tombstone is inscribed, "A dutiful child, an affectionate wife, a kind and loving mother, and a true friend."

In 1870, a newspaper editor described her as a person of "medium stature, very bright, but delicate, and modest in appearance, and when animated, earnestly, in her subject, exhibits much spirit, and mental power." Years later, her son wrote, "Mrs. Plantz was a lady of refinement and culture and maintained her mental faculties to the end of her long and useful life. She kept posted on the advancements in her profession; was interested in public affairs and news of the day. And her passing caused regret and grief to hundreds of widely scattered friends, to many of whom she had meant much more than one who had relieved only a physical pain."

References: *American Medical Directory*, 1906 et seq.; American Women's Hospitals. *Census of Women Physicians* (n.p., 1918), 104; John W. King, "Early Woman Physicians in Vermont," *Bulletin of the History of Medicine* 25 (1951): 429–41; Polk, 1886 et seq.; Putney Historical Society (Putney, VT) provided a clipping (1919) from the *Brattleboro Reformer* describing Dr. Plantz's ninetieth birthday party and a three-quarter-page typescript biographical entry from *People of Putney* (Putney, VT: Putney Historical Society, 1953); Joseph P. Smith, *History of the Republican Party in Ohio* (Chicago, 1898), 431–32 [information on Tobias Avery Plantz]; Frederick C. Waite, *History of the New England*

Female Medical College 1848–1874 (Boston, 1950); Plantz papers among those of her son, Walter G. Wheaton, at the Ohio Historical Society, Columbus: an obituary from an unidentified Brattleboro newspaper, her medical license from the Vermont State Medical Society, the typescript of her lecture "The True Woman" (1870), an advertisement for her 1870 lecture circuit accompanied by comments from the press, a biographical sketch by her son (1945), quotations from Decatur, Freeport, and Peoria newspapers accompanying a promotion for an 1870 lecture to be given by Wheaton in Kalamazoo.

Marion Augusta *FAIRCHILD* (1834–1923)

Augusta Fairchild was born June 7, 1834, in Newark, New Jersey, the youngest child in her family. When she was seven, her father died, followed shortly by her mother. She was raised by an older sister, under the guardianship of a paternal uncle, Dr. Stephen Fairchild, of Parsippany, New Jersey. At an early age she "showed a strong preference for the study of anatomy, physiology, materia medica and even pathology." Uncle Stephen, who had turned to homoeopathy, and who is said to have been the one who introduced that system into New Jersey, and his son, also a physician, were "amused and not a little pleased to observe the strong likings of the child, and they gave [her] much encouragement. . . . She was often permitted to visit both their hospital and private patients."

At thirteen, Augusta was sent to school in Philadelphia. Though she disliked both the place and the work, she finished and then, at seventeen, spent three years teaching school, which she didn't like either. At twenty, she developed "brain fever" from which she slowly recovered. When able to speak again, she is reputed to have told her nurse, "God has spared me, I mean now to live for a purpose." When the nurse asked her what she meant, she replied, "I mean to be a physician." At twenty-three, she enrolled at New York Hygeio-Therapeutic College and graduated with an MD degree in 1860.

For the first couple of years, she worked with Dr. Russell Trall at the Hygienic Institute associated with the college, caring for Trall's patients. It is difficult to trace with any precision the sequence of Dr. Fairchild's professional activities during the next ten years. Most of the time she seems to have been associated with a series of water-cure establishments and, later, with the hygienic homes into which water-cures evolved after the Civil War. Directories have her located in several places at once: three cities in Indiana: Milton (1861), Richmond (1863), Cambridge City (1863); and Dayton, Ohio (1862–64). Since all of these places are within a few miles of one another except Dayton, which is fifty miles to the east, but is the nearest large city to the other communities, and since the most definitive location was Cambridge City, it seems likely that she was most closely associated with that community. An advertisement in the January 1863 *Herald of Health* says that Dr. Fairchild was associated with Zachariah P. Glass, MD at Sunny-Side Water-Cure in Cambridge City.

The January 1864 issue of the *Herald of Health* reported that "Drs. Glass and Fairchild, late of Hygeian Home, have gone on an exploring tour to the West, with the view to establishing a Hygienic Institution at some convenient place, on a large scale. They will probably visit several places in Wisconsin and Minnesota, before locating. Dr. Fairchild will devote the winter to lecturing, for which purpose she is provided with anatomical and physiological drawings, especially adapted to 'Stereopticon' exhibitions which will render her lectures entertaining, as well as highly instructive." The pair settled on St. Anthony's Falls, in Minnesota where they established the Western Hygeian Home. The February issue of the *Herald* reported that Dr. Fairchild was, indeed, on the western lecture circuit, her purpose no doubt to convert new believers to reformed medicine and to drum up patrons for the home. The two would remain there for a year and a half.

Five months after a lecture tour into Iowa, Augusta described what it had been like. The piece, published in the *Herald*, though a bit long, gives an interesting description of the trials lecturers had to endure and what they hoped to accomplish, especially if they came from proselytizing schools like the Hygeio-Therapeutic one:

> [I have] travelled by stage-coach through a portion of Iowa during the winter, and in the thawy season. Three weeks ago I started on a stage journey of ninety miles, and having gone about twelve I found prospects looked very unlike my being able to go further, as the stage was crowded and the driver declared he could not take "that woman's big heavy trunk *this* trip." Now it was actually necessary that the "big heavy trunk" should go "this trip," for "that woman" was starting out lecturing, and could not possibly leave her pet apparatus, which works by magic—*lantern*. So I jumped from the stage, booked my name, trunk and all, for the very next trip, and started to walk to the place whence I came. . . . During the first seven miles I got along nicely—did not feel a hint at fatigue or tediousness—but then . . . I was *sloughed*.

The word is pronounced "slewed," and it describes sinking into mud like quicksand. It was up over the top of her boots, but she managed to extricate herself and, covered head to toe with mud, walk the other five miles back to where she had started, arriving after dark. Two days later, dried and brushed off, she started out again, traveled for two days and a night in a "lumber wagon" that could accommodate her trunk, and reached her destination. What made it all worthwhile were the receptions she and her message received: "Mothers cluster round and ask me questions in regard to health subjects, with such interest as testifies to their having lost all confidence in the doctors and their drugs. The mortality which attends the drug practice does not stupefy these noble, thinking, women into the belief that it is of God's will that men so traffic in human life. It rouses them to inquiry, and O that we had enough talkers of our school to visit every place and give the light that is so eagerly sought after" (*HOH*, June 1864).

Augusta found Minnesota too cold and left, intending to return to New York, but visited Hannibal, Missouri, along the way, to make a professional call, it was said. She remained there several months, built up a practice, and decided to stay in the West. It is unclear what she did between 1867 and 1872. She did spend two years in Chicago; that was too cold, as well. After 1872, she was either in Quincy, Illinois, or in Hannibal, Missouri, twenty miles downriver on the west bank of the Mississippi. Directories are confusing as to which community she was located in. It is possible that she lived in Hannibal and ran her Hygeian Home in Quincy.

In 1877, she established the Hygeian Home and Movement Cure at 537 Broadway on the northwest corner of Sixth Street in Quincy, where she offered "unequaled facilities for the treatment of chronic diseases." She may have operated a more modest establishment at her earlier Quincy location at 104 Eighth Street because, even there, she offered to send a circular upon application (*HOH*, January 1872). The newer building was perhaps the most elegant structure in the town, certainly the most sound. It had been built in 1837, for Joseph Bartlett, an Englishman who had retired rich to the West Indies, where his home was destroyed by a hurricane, along with much of his family. This new house was to be solid. Greek Revival in style, it had four enormous Ionic columns, cellar walls twenty feet high and four feet thick, sixteen-foot ceilings, and bricks made on the property, each one inspected twice before it was used. A garden in the rear extended through to the next street. The price to Dr. Fairchild was $10,152. (Years later the building would house the local telephone company and, more recently, the VFW.)

Dr. Fairchild's original partner was Dr. Thomas H. Trine, but after a year, her former colleague, Dr. Zachariah P. Glass, rejoined her. (Dr. Glass later moved to Hannibal, as did Augusta, and died in California, as did Augusta.) At the Hygeian Home the regimen sounds similar to that found at Our Home on the Hillside in Dansville, New York, and at the Clifton Springs (NY) Water Cure, except that it lacked the emphasis on religious observance. Temperance, vegetarianism, exercise, fresh air, and strict observance of the "Laws of Life" was the rule.

After fifteen years the home closed in 1892, and Dr. Fairchild retired to Hannibal where she practiced medicine for a number of years. She is listed as a practicing physician in either Hannibal or Quincy until 1890. She was licensed in Missouri in 1885. At some point she moved to Los Angeles where, on August 13, 1923, she died of carcinoma of the liver. According to her obituary in the *Journal of the American Medical Association,* she had been professor of gynecology at both Washington University School of Medicine and at St. Louis Medical College. However, her name is not found in the records of either institution. It is possible that she was a lecturer or demonstrator (these titles were not listed in the bulletins until the 1880s) or that her appointment was actually at the St. Louis Hygienic College of Physicians and Surgeons.

Bibliography: "Female Physicians," *Water-Cure Journal,* October 1861; *How to Be Well; or, Common-Sense Medical Hygiene* (New York: S. R. Wells & Co., 1879); *Woman and Health: A Mother's Hygienic Hand Book* (Quincy, IL, 1890).

References: Obituary, *JAMA* 81 (1923): 846; Butler, 1874, 1877; *Herald of Health,* January 1863, 4; *Herald of Health,* January 1864; *Herald of Health,* February 1864, 75; *Herald of Health,* June 1864, 234–35; *Herald of Health,* January 1872; *Herald of Health,* October 1881; *History of Adams County, Illinois* (Chicago: Murray, Williamson & Phelps, 1879); Carl Landrum, "House of 1837 Built to Last," from an unidentified Quincy, IL, newspaper dated February 20, 1966, at the Quincy Public Library; Polk, 1886 et seq.; *Progressive Annual,* 1862, 1863, 1864; *Quincy City Directory,* 1878–79, 1880–81, 1884–85; J. Annie Scripp, *Our Daily Bread, as Prepared for Us at Dr. Fairchild's Hygienic Home, Quincy, Ill.* (Detroit, 1879); Frances E. Willard, *A Woman of the Century* (Buffalo, NY, 1893), 283.

Eliza Wood *Burhans* FARNHAM Fitzpatrick (1815–64)

Eliza Burhans was born in Rensselaerwyck, New York, on November 17, 1815, the fourth of five children, and third of three daughters of Cornelius and Mary Wood Burhans. Her mother died when she was five, and, at six, Eliza moved west to Maple Spring (probably in Chautauqua County, New York) to live with adoptive parents. It is not clear whether the new parents were relatives. Later in life, Eliza wrote three fictionalized autobiographical books recounting this and other periods on her life. In one, she related that when she was eight, she told an elder who said she was not old enough to understand his thoughts, "When I am as old as you are, I shall know much more; for I shall read all the books I can get, and I shall talk with many wise people, and if you live in my part of the country you'll see what I think of now, for I shall be doing it then" (*My Early Days*). When asked what she wanted for her birthday she replied, "A book."

On July 12, 1839, then twenty-four, she married Thomas Jefferson Farnham, a lawyer eleven years her senior. They had three sons; the eldest died in infancy and the youngest in 1855, just before Eliza went to medical school. The surviving middle son, Charles H., became a magazine writer.

Both Eliza and her husband were social activists, and they seem to have spent a great deal of their ten years of married life apart. Before marriage, Thomas practiced law in Peoria, Illinois, but thereafter spent considerable time in Oregon, the Hawaiian Islands, and California, finally settling in San Francisco, where he practiced law from 1846 to 1848. He died there on September 13, 1848. Meanwhile, Eliza, always interested in the lot of the unfortunate, held a variety of interesting positions. From 1844 to 1848, she was matron of the female department of Sing Sing Prison in Ossining, New York. While there, she espoused using kindness in the treatment of her charges, an idea that received national attention. She edited *Rationale of Crime, and Its Appropriate Treatment* (1846). She was apparently forced out of this job because of her advanced ideas. It was during this period that she bore her other two sons. In 1848, she spent a year with Samuel Gridley Howe at Perkins Institute for the Blind in Boston.

Her husband made his second trip to California at this time and, for some legal services rendered was paid with a tract of land near the Santa Cruz Mission. He also built a schooner that plied the Sacramento River and San Francisco Bay transporting supplies to and gold from inland. Thomas died of intermittent fever in the fall of 1848. Following his death, Eliza moved to California to settle his estate, going from New York by the packet ship *Angelique,* around the Horn. In addition to her sons, she hoped to take with her a group of "intelligent, virtuous and efficient" young women who would find new homes and husbands from among the many men who had gone west in search of gold. The presence of the women, in turn, would have a domesticating influence on the frontier culture. Applicants had to be twenty-five years old, "bring from their clergyman, or some authority of the town where they reside, satisfactory testimonials of education, character, capacity, etc.," and contribute $250 to defray costs of the voyage. The project was recommended by, among others, James Cullen Bryant, Horace Greeley, and Henry Ward Beecher. Of the two hundred women who made inquiry, only three actually went, to Eliza's disappointment.

The trip was not a pleasant one. She later wrote that the captain was "brutal and cruel . . . [and the ship] carried bad water and insufficient fire." The nurse who cared for Eliza's two boys defected by marrying the steward. Eliza tried to hire a replacement in Valparaiso, and while she was ashore getting a passport for this person, the ship left with her boys aboard. A local clergyman gave Eliza clothes and money and, one month later she left aboard the *Louis Philippe*, landing in San Francisco forty-seven days later. Her boys had been cared for by a friend. After two months in San Francisco, where, she reported, "women are freaks," she had settled her husband's affairs and the family moved to the Santa Cruz property, El Rancho La Libertad. This would be their home for the next five years. It was in a beautiful area—redwoods and surf—but the house was a "forlorn habitation." There was "not a foot of floor, nor a pane of glass, nor a brick, nor anything in the shape of a stove." They lived in a tent, made the house habitable in ten days, and farmed it for five years. Help was scarce and costly, the crops were invaded by grasshoppers and mustard, and the trees she ordered were dead on arrival from delay and neglect. During this period her son Edward died (1855), and she had a short but stormy marriage to William Fitzpatrick. It was during these years that she wrote *California Indoors and Out* (1856), the book quoted here.

In 1856, Eliza returned to New York, where she soon enrolled in the New York Hygeio-Therapeutic College and graduated at age forty-three with an MD degree in 1858. We have no knowledge of her practicing medicine at this time. We do know that she was active in the women's rights movement and that she was a speaker at the 1858 Woman's Rights Convention. She returned to California and served as matron of the Stockton Insane Asylum (1859–62). During the Civil War she volunteered as a nurse, was active after Gettysburg, developed tuberculosis, and died on December 15, 1864. She is buried in the Hicksite Friends' Burying Ground in Milton-on-Hudson, New York.

Eliza was a doctor of medicine for only six years and may never have practiced. The definitive biographical sketch by Madeline B. Stern does not even mention her becoming a doctor. The biographical study in the *American National Biography* by Lori Ginsberg maintains that "she studied medicine" from 1856 until her death. Eliza's greater contributions were obviously in the realm of women's rights and other reforms.

Bibliography: *Life in Prairie Land* (New York, 1846); *California In-doors and Out* (New York, 1856); *My Early Days* (New York, 1859); *A Lecture on the Philosophy of Spiritual Growth: Delivered at Platt's Hall, May 18, 1862* (San Francisco: Valentine & Co., 1862); *Woman and Her Era* (New York, 1864); *The Ideal Attained* (New York, 1865).

References: Ann Braude, *Radical Spirits: Spiritualism and Women's Rights in Nineteenth-Century America* (Beacon Press, 1989); Samuel Burhans Jr., *Burhans Genealogy, 1660–1893* (New York, 1894), 194; *New York Times,* May 14, 1858; Obituary, *New York Times,* December 18, 1864; Obituary, *New York Tribune,* December 16, 1864, 4; *Notable American Women,* 1:598– 600; Madeline B. Stern, introduction to the 1972 facsimile of *California In-doors and Out,* vii–xlii; *Who Was Who,* historical volume; *American National Biography,* 7:722–23.

Wilhelmina (Willimanna) *FERGUSON*

Virtually nothing is known about Wilhelmina Ferguson except that she attended Penn Medical University, was a resident of Massachusetts at the time of graduation, when she received an MD degree in 1861. But the one thing that has been found is rather interesting. Four years after graduating, she signed on as a ship's surgeon on a freighter headed for Australia and, upon arrival, became the first female doctor of medicine in that country. Once there, she tried, on June 2, 1865, to register with the Medical Board of Victoria. The board claimed it lacked the power to register her and referred the issue to the Crown Law Department. The opinion of the Honorable Attorney General George Higinbotham was, "I think the Board are bound to give a certificate in this case." The opinion was signed July 30, 1865.

Dr. Ferguson's reception by the medical profession was less promising. Wrote the editor of the *Australian Medical Journal*:

> The applicant comes from America, where women insist on doing what is done for them in less advanced communities—and a woman who voluntarily devotes herself to a state in which the abandonment of the domestic qualification seems a necessity, is a being whom men do not love and with whom women can hardly sympathize. . . . But there is little fear in any British Community Medical Women will exist as a class. They will occasionally be imported like other curiosities and the people will wonder at them just as it wonders at dancing dogs, fat boys and bearded ladies, and in accordance with the demand for novelties they will perhaps be as successful in a material sense, but they are not likely to be included in the list of British institutions.

Whether Dr. Ferguson stayed and fought the battle or returned to the United States is not known. No further information about her career has been found. It was not until 1891 that the first two women graduated from an Australian medical school.

References: *Australian Medical Journal,* July 1865; I. Younger Ross, "The Advent of Women into Medicine," *Medical Journal of Australia,* May 30, 1953, 777.

Almira *FIFIELD* (1833–63)

Almira Fifield was born in 1833, somewhere in New Hampshire, the eldest daughter and second of five children of Thomas Fifield. Sometime before 1841, when her youngest sister was born, the family moved to Valparaiso, Indiana. The 1850 census of Porter County, Indiana describes a family consisting of Thomas, a forty-seven-year-old farmer, Susannah, his eighty-year-old mother, Thomas's developmentally disabled younger sister, and the five children, ages nine to twenty-two. Almira's mother had probably died. It must have been a religious family. Susannah, who received a small pension because she was the widow of a Revolutionary War soldier, gave ten dollars each year to support foreign missions. Almira herself had joined the Presbyterian Church at an early age.

In her youthful years Almira taught school, "and her impress has been left on many hearts and minds that are yet to tell her virtues to the world." In 1857, when she was twenty-four, "impelled by a sense of duty, though popular opinion and prejudice opposed," she entered New England Female Medical College, graduating in 1859. She was apparently already sick with what was probably tuberculosis ("the fatal disease that at last dried up the fountain of her life, was already fastened upon her," said her obituary).

When the war came, Almira had hoped to be assigned to the Ninth Indiana Regiment, but this did not happen, whether because of her health problem or some other reason is not known. She did have the support of Indiana's long-term congressional representative, Schuyler Colfax, who on December 19, 1861, wrote on her behalf to Dorothea Dix that Almira "was capable, zealous, worthy, robust and has withal a good knowledge of medicine" (quoted in Schultz, 126). In April 1862, she was sent by the Sanitary Commission in Chicago to an army hospital in Paducah, Kentucky, to work as a nurse but had to return home in July because of her health. Then, after spending three weeks at the newly opened Soldier's Hospital in Chicago (it is unclear whether as patient or nurse), she was sent back to Paducah, where she died March 8, 1863. She is buried in Valparaiso's Old City Cemetery.

References: Obituary from the *Chicago Tribune* reprinted in the *Valparaiso Republic*, March 1863; Jane E. Schultz, *Women at the Front* (Chapel Hill, 2004), 126; US census, 1850; Obituary, *Valparaiso (IN) Republic*, March 9, 1863.

Martha Jane *FLANDERS* (1823–98)

Martha Flanders was born in Concord, New Hampshire, January 15, 1823, to David and Martha Stark Flanders. She was one of their three daughters. When she was three years old, she attended the district school in Hopkinton, New Hampshire, and then went to Miss Susan Ella's "noted" school in Concord. After graduating from the New Hampton Seminary, she taught school in the West and South.

Returning to Concord, she began the study of medicine with Dr. Alpheus Morrill, "one of the first physicians to see that 'women needed the profession and the profession needed women.'" In 1861, she received an MD degree from New England Female Medical College in Boston and returned to Concord, where she practiced medicine for two years, in association with Dr. Morrill. In 1863, she moved to Lynn, Massachusetts—"that Quaker city of radical reformers"—where she remained and practiced homoeopathic medicine for the rest of her life. In the September 1869 issue of the *Herald of Health*, Dr. Flanders is described as a "singular example of rare professional skill, talent, and energy, united to the utmost feminine refinement, patience and sweetness . . . a true gentlewoman . . . yet of a manful courage and independence."

From 1879 to 1883 she lectured on diseases of children at Boston University School of Medicine (successor of New England Female Medical College). She was elected to membership in the American Institute of Homoeopathy and was a member of county and state homoeopathic medical societies. She retired in 1893 at seventy.

Whether Dr. Flanders or Dr. Breed (q.v.), each of whom came to Lynn in 1863, was the first woman doctor in that community, is not determined. Dr. Flanders was active in the community. Politically radical, she was described as being "a woman of very strong mind and conversant with all the topics of the day. She was greatly interested in governmental matters and an able adviser. [In 1861, she proposed arming blacks.] Her loss will be felt deeply by women all over the country." She was an early member of the North Shore Club and the Lynn Women's Club. She died, unmarried, in Lynn, November 1, 1898, having suffered from heart disease for several years. Obituary notices appeared in the Boston *Transcript* and New York *Tribune*, as well as local newspapers.

References: Obituary, American Institute of Homoeopathy, *Transactions*, 1899, 926; Obituary, *Boston Transcript*, November 3, 1898; *Herald of Health*, September 1869, 108; Lucinda M. Lummus, *Chronicles of the Lynn Women's Club* (Lynn, MA, 1914), 12; Lynn Historical Society, Obituary from an unknown source in Miscellaneous Scrapbook 2; H. H. Metcalf, *New Hampshire Women: A Collection of Portraits and Biographical Sketches* (Concord: New Hampshire Publishing Co., 1895); Obituary, *New York Tribune*, November 4, 1898.

Sophronia *FLETCHER* (1806–1906)

Sophronia Fletcher was born September 13, 1806, in Alstead, New Hampshire, the youngest of ten children (seven girls, three boys) of Peter Fletcher (1762–1843) and his wife Sarah Piper (d. 1848). Peter Fletcher was a private, at age sixteen, in the Cambridge, Massachusetts, Regiment of Guards in June 1778, and his father was one of the Committee of Safety at the time of the Battle of Lexington.

Sophronia was educated in New Hampshire at the Ladies' Seminary in Milford and at the Hancock Academy. She later taught in private schools in New Hampshire and New York. In 1845, at the age of thirty-nine, she decided to study medicine, after seeing the condition and needs of insane persons at South Boston. Her experience between that time and her graduation with an MD degree from New England Female Medical College nine years later in 1854 is not known. The 1853 *Boston Almanac* lists her as a practicing physician (but not an MD).

Upon graduation, she was appointed the first resident physician at Mt. Holyoke Seminary (later College), on "the recommendation of the Sanitary Committee to the Board of Trustees." The annual Mt. Holyoke catalog lists her as one of nineteen teachers (all female, all "Miss"). It is probable that she taught anatomy, physiology, and hygiene as well as serving as school physician. Sophronia was not popular with the girls at Holyoke. One of the students, Jerusha Usher, wrote of her, "She is to be physician and teacher of Physiology—looks weatherbeaten—don't know her principles—one of the girls had a slight sickness, and she gave her a mustard plaster, one sitzbath, two packs, two electric shocks, and what else I don't know. The girls don't give away as much as formerly to a slight illness, for if there was a toe ache Dr. F—— stands ready to be marshaled forward." Dr. Fletcher left this post in 1856 (to be followed by a male physician for four years and, thereafter, always by a woman physician, first Mary A. B. Homer [q.v.], and then Emily Norton Belden [q.v.]).

Whether Dr. Fletcher practiced office and house call medicine subsequently is not clear. It may have been primarily institutional, though the sources available suggest a wider practice. It is documented that she was for nine years "attendant physician" of the New England Moral Reform Association (i.e., "Society") and that her special interest was "educational and philanthropic work." Among her accomplishments was attaining passage by the Massachusetts State Legislature of a bill authorizing the appointment of women as physicians for females confined to state asylums and prisons. This was achieved with the help of Wendell Phillips, whose wife Dr. Fletcher had taken care of for several years.

Boston Almanacs list her as a practicing physician each year from 1856 to 1883. For 1859 and 1861 she is listed as a physician at 30 Eliot Street, Jamaica Plain. In the 1864 and 1867 *Boston Almanacs*, also under "female physician," her address is 250 Washington in downtown Boston, and at nearby 7 West Street in 1868 and 1869. So it seems likely that she was practicing in Boston during the 1860s. She is not listed in the 1874 or 1877 Butler medical directories or in the 1875 *Boston Almanac*. She is listed as being a physician in Claremont, New Hampshire, in 1878. In 1879, her name is again found in the *Boston Almanac* at 124 West Newton. From 1889, when she was eighty-three years old, she lived with her niece, Leonora Fletcher Lather, MD, in Cambridge, Massachusetts, and had probably given up practice. Her name does not appear in Polk medical directories for 1886, 1890, or 1893, or in the *Boston Almanacs* for 1881 or 1893.

After Sophronia was ninety, she remained active in her educational and philanthropic interests. She traveled extensively around the United States. At ninety-five, she traveled alone by trolley from Cambridge to Worcester. Her one infirmity seemed to be deafness, which she did not think could be helped by science and about which she did nothing. Devoted to her niece, her niece's grandson, and her niece's dog, she spent her final years happily, until July 17, 1906, when at ninety-nine years, ten months, and four days she succumbed to pneumonia, the last survivor of the 1854 class at the New England Female Medical College.

References: *Boston Almanac*, 1856–83; Obituary, *Boston Evening Transcript* 5 (July 19, 1906): 3; Cambridge, MA, city directories; Edwin H. Fletcher, *Fletcher Genealogy: An Account of the Descendants of Robert Fletcher, of Concord, Mass.* (Boston, 1871), 74; Massachusetts Vital Records, Cambridge, 1906, 26:267; Unidentified newspaper clipping, "Almost a Centenarian," 1905, Mt. Holyoke College Library archives, Health services records, 1841ff., RG 7.17 [the quotation of Jerusha Usher is found in a March 26, 1988, typed report from Librarian Edmonds to Dr. Carol Craig regarding seminary doctors]; Mt. Holyoke Female Seminary, *18th Annual Catalogue, 1854–55* (Northampton, 1855).

Amanda L. FOSTER Minor (b. 1827)

Amanda Foster was born in Vermont or New Hampshire (records vary) about 1827. Her maiden surname is not known and information about her parents, childhood, and early education is lacking. The 1850 census reports her as living in Woodstock, Vermont, and married to William Patterson Foster, a local farmer holding $1,500 in real estate. Two other Fosters, sixteen-year-old Charles and six-year-old Lois L. are in the household, but Charles, denoted a farmer, is too old to be the couple's child and was, perhaps, William's younger brother. By the time of the 1860 census, still in Woodstock, the couple have three children of their own: Ellen A., nine, Elsie M., seven, and Lydia C., five. Charles and Lois are no longer listed as part of the family. William and Amanda have either divorced, or, more likely, William died sometime between 1855 and 1858, and Amanda had become a physician, having received an MD degree from the New York Hygeio-Therapeutic College on March 29, 1859. She was listed as holding $500 in real estate and $900 in personal property.

Amanda returned to Woodstock after finishing medical school and must have practiced medicine to support her three small children. The following puff appeared in the May 1861 issue of *Water-Cure World*: "Mrs. A. L. Foster, M.D., Woodstock, Vt., is an earnest and true Hygienic or Water-Cure Physician, and we are happy to learn has a good run of practice with the best of success—as she well deserves." This, no doubt, in return for her having obtained several new subscribers for the periodical.

By 1862, she had married Levi Minor, a local farmer three years her junior. Levi had bought the farm of a Mr. Raymond about 1861 (Dana, 30). With Minor she had two more children, Lena M. and Allen L. Levi must have adopted the three Foster children: the 1870 census shows all five children with the Minor surname and living at home, and Amanda as "keeping house." She is not listed as a physician in Vermont directories for 1864, 1867, 1868, or 1870 (her fellow townswoman, Marenda Randall [q.v.] *is* listed as a physician in the 1864 W. W. Atwater Vermont directory), nor is she in the 1874 or 1877 Butler directories.

Probably Amanda did not practice medicine after her second marriage. She was raising five children and was soon running the farm, as well. By the time of the 1880 census, Levi had died and Amanda was head of the household, and she is listed in the census as a farmer. Aside from her youngest son, Allen, then fifteen and listed as a farm laborer, she had two adult farmhands and a domestic. How long Amanda lived after 1880 has not been determined.

References: Henry S. Dana, *History of Woodstock, Vermont* (Boston, 1889); *Progressive Annual*, 1863, 1864; US census, 1850, 1860, 1870, 1880; Vermont directories, 1864, 1867, 1868, 1870; *Water-Cure World*, Brattleboro, VT, May 1861, 37.

Almira L. *FOWLER* Ormsbee Breakspear (1826–99)

Almira Fowler was born March 24, 1826, in Cohocton, Steuben County, New York, to Horace Fowler and his wife. When she was nine years old, the family moved west, settling in Jackson, Michigan. According to Cleave, her early education was conducted by private teachers resident in the family. Later, she went to Jackson Seminary, of which the Rev. Marcus Harrison was principal. This was followed by two more years schooling in the "East."

Early in 1849, she began the study of medicine with Dr. J. W. Redfield as her preceptor, enrolled in the New England Female Medical College, and then transferred to the Female Medical College of Pennsylvania, from which she graduated with an MD degree in March 1853, with the school's second class. Cleave says that she attended three sessions, the middle one of which was in Boston as demonstrator of anatomy at the soon-to-be chartered New England Female Medical College. Following graduation, she was appointed demonstrator in anatomy and chemistry at her alma mater for the next year but declined subsequent offers there and at other schools. According to her *New York Times* obituary, she went next to New York, where she practiced a few years before settling, in 1858, in Orange Mountain, New Jersey, a village just west of Orange. She had bought some property there some years earlier and planned to oversee improvements to it.

According to Cleave, she did not intend to practice medicine, but circumstances soon led to her engaging again in her profession. At the end of six years, she had more than three hundred families for whom she cared. Her practice, a general one, continued to grow larger, and, by the late 1860s, she held daily office hours in the larger nearby community of Orange.

On October 18, 1871, she married J. Holden Ormsbee, a New York City merchant. She continued to practice and is listed in the 1874 and 1877 Butler medical directories as a homoeopathic physician practicing in Orange. Mr. Ormsbee died in 1876. Almira's name does not appear in the Polk medical directories from 1886 and thereafter.

She may have retired from practice. In 1884, she married Dr. Edward Breakspear of Birmingham, England. He died in 1899. Almira died at her home in West Orange, December 31, 1899.

In Cleave's biography, she is described as a woman of great self-control, "of possessing an unusual degree of sound judgment, equanimity of character, good taste, and great practical sympathy and kindness ... [and of being] passionately fond of children." In physical presence "she is of medium height; full, well-formed figure; has a wholesome, kindly face; is graceful in her movements, and accomplishes a vast amount of work by judicious planning."

References: Cleave, 464–65; Obituary, *New York Times,* January 3, 1900; Frederick C. Waite, *History of New England Female Medical College, 1848–1872* (Boston: Boston University School of Medicine, 1950).

Lydia *Folger* FOWLER (1822–79)

Lydia Folger Fowler, the second woman and first American woman to become a doctor of medicine, was born on Nantucket, May 5, 1822. She came of Quaker and Baptist forebears and was descended from Nantucket's ten original families, among them Folgers, Macys, Coffins, Swains, and Starbucks. A distant cousin of feminist and social reformer, Lucretia Coffin Mott, and niece of scientist, judge, and congressman Walter Folger Jr., both a generation senior to hers, Lydia belonged to that generation that, more than any of its predecessors, forsook Nantucket. For the century before 1840, Nantucket was the whaling capital of the world, prospering from the sale of whale oil, which provided the best artificial illumination then available. As sailing ships got larger, it became increasingly difficult for them to navigate the sand bars around Nantucket, and the industry began moving to New Bedford. After the successful drilling for oil in Western Pennsylvania by Drake in 1859, kerosene soon replaced whale oil as the preferred illuminant. Nantucket declined. A mass exodus ensued, especially of the talented.

The Folgers were not exempt from this economic disruption. Being the youngest of eleven children, Lydia's father, Gideon, had few prospects in Nantucket. He and all of his seven children who had survived to adulthood would leave the island, one by one. It was, perhaps, symbolic that nineteen-year-old brother Andrew, pursuing the calling of his ancestors, was lost at sea after falling from his ship's rigging. Josiah, the eldest, moved to New Orleans.

In addition to its failing economy, education did not have high priority on the island. As late as 1827, there was no free school. In that year, Sir Isaac Coffin, a sixth-generation descendant of Tristram

Coffin, who had joined the British navy in Boston in 1773 and had risen to the rank of admiral by 1817 (he had been made a baronet in 1804), decided to establish and endow a free Lancastrian school in Nantucket. (An important feature of this type of school was that older students helped teach younger students.) Seven years after the school opened, Lydia Folger, then thirteen, was listed as a student. Lydia was an "ardent" student. It was not long (1836) before she and her older sister Mary became assistants to the principal, Luther Robinson. This educational opportunity and the apparent recognition of teaching ability must have been a significant influence in Lydia's life. More than anything else, Lydia, as a physician, was a teacher throughout her life, whether as lecturer or professor at various medical schools, or giving public lectures to women on physiology, hygiene, and woman's problems, or as the prolific writer she became. Though she practiced medicine for several years in the 1850s, her principal contribution was as a teacher.

At age sixteen Lydia spent a year (1838–39) at Wheaton Seminary (later Wheaton College) on the mainland, an institution at which she would later (1842–44) teach. On September 19, 1844, she married Lorenzo Niles Fowler who, with his brother Orson Squire Fowler, was a well-known New York promoter of phrenology and a partner in the publishing house of Fowlers & Wells. Lorenzo was eleven years Lydia's senior. The Fowlers had three children: Amelia M. (1846), Lauretta L. (1850), and Jessie Allen (1856).

In 1847, Lydia published one of the several books she would write, *Familiar Lessons on Physiology,* "designed for the use of children and youth." During the later 1840s she and her husband were itinerant lecturers, she on human anatomy and physiology, Lorenzo on phrenology. Lydia's afternoon lectures to women were very popular, as attested by considerable newspaper coverage. Lorenzo's phrenological readings of heads, both private and public, predicting capabilities for future careers at ten dollars per examination, were lucrative.

In November 1849, with the help of her cousin, Lucretia Coffin Mott, Lydia enrolled in Central Medical College, an Eclectic institution then located in Syracuse, and the first school to admit women on a regular basis. In March 1850, because of factional disputes among the faculty, the prevailing group moved to Rochester, and, at the conclusion of the term on June 5, Lydia Fowler, alone among several woman matriculants, received the degree doctor of medicine, making her the second woman, after Elizabeth Blackwell, to do so. When the school moved to Rochester, it established a Female Department, and Mrs. Fowler, at age twenty-seven and already a well-known lecturer, was made principal of it, even though still a student herself. After graduation, she became also "demonstrator of anatomy to the female students." For the next year, 1851–52, she was appointed professor of midwifery and diseases of women and children, thus becoming the first woman to hold a professorship in an American medical school. Alas, Central Medical College was dissolved in October 1852 and absorbed by the rival faction at Syracuse Medical College, which Lydia did not join.

For the next eleven years Lydia practiced medicine in New York City and continued to lecture and to teach. In 1854, she advertised "a course of private medical lectures to females" to cost fourteen dollars, to last eight weeks, and given at the rooms of Metropolitan Medical College, a short-lived physio-medical school. She does not appear to have been on the faculty of this school. The lectures were offered over a period of several years. An auditor at one of Lydia's lectures wrote the following description:

> She was dressed in a very broadly striped silk, which was anything but a bloomer. Her hair was done up in a French twist with curls in front. Her face is pleasant, she has sunny blue eyes and a sweet mouth. She waved an elegantly embroidered handkerchief as she read her lecture. Quite a number of the little exhibited [babies] were present and contributed their full share to the festivities, at times almost drowning her voice, which is scarcely strong enough for a lecturer. (*NY Tribune*)

In 1862, Lydia held another formal teaching position as instructor in clinical midwifery at Russell Trall's famous New York Hygeio-Therapeutic College. In 1860, the Fowler brothers and Lydia had undertaken lecture tours in Britain, Lydia addressing the ladies on the "laws of life and health." Then came a trip to Italy, a period (1860–61) of medical study in Paris, and a three-month period in which she had charge of the obstetrical department of an unnamed London hospital.

Back in New York, she resumed practice. In 1863, the Fowler brothers withdrew from the publishing firm, and Lydia and Lorenzo moved to London, where they would be until Lydia's death sixteen years later. It appears that Lydia no longer practiced medicine but concentrated on lectures to women on physiology, hygiene, and diseases of women and children. She visited every large city in Britain and Ireland. In July 1863, she wrote from Dublin, "We have both been so busily employed, Mr. Fowler lecturing on the brain and myself lecturing on the body, constituting such a delightful harmony." But she rued the fact that "so many conservative contracted individuals would put stumbling blocks in [woman's] path, tie her hands and feet, shut her out from the temple of wisdom, and then proclaim her inefficiency and want of mental power." It was Dr. Fowler's hope that God might spare her life to labor for women. It was estimated that during her lifetime she had lectured to more than two hundred thousand women. She was also quite active in temperance work and in the women's rights movement. She served as secretary at several rights conventions. At the Seneca Falls convention, she befriended Elizabeth Cady Stanton, who would later list her as one of those to whom she dedicated *The History of Woman Suffrage* (1881).

Between 1865 and 1875 Lydia visited Turkey, Egypt, Palestine, and many places in Europe. She continued to write, including poetry and novels (see bibliography below), and to help her husband with his writing. In the words of medical historian Frederick C. Waite, "She was the intimate assistant of her husband in his editorial and literary work. Some of the works published under his name show in places her style of writing, which was direct and simple compared to the involved and pompous style of Mr. Fowler." Lydia died, at fifty-six, of pneumonia at her home in London on January 26, 1879.

Bibliography: *Familiar Lessons on Physiology* (New York, Fowlers & Wells, 1847; there were at least seven editions by 1860); *Familiar Lessons on Phrenology* (New York, 1847); *Familiar Lessons in Astronomy* (New York, 1848; three editions by 1870); "Introductory Address before the Class of Central Medical College, November 4, 1851," *Eclectic Journal of Medicine* 3 (1851); "Medical Progression," *Syracuse Medical and Surgical Journal* 6 (1854): 200–202; "Female Medical Education," *Journal of Medical Reform* 1 (1854): 43–45; "Suggestions to Female Medical Students," *Journal of Medical Reform* 1 (1854): 127–30; Letter from Mrs. Dr. Fowler, Paris, July 1861, to Dr. Trall, *Water-Cure Journal*, September 1861, 62–63; Letter from Mrs. Fowler, Dublin, May 18, 1863, *Herald of Health*, July 1863, 38; *Nora, the Lost and Redeemed* (London, 1863); *The Heart and Its Influences* (London, 1863); *The Pet of the Household and How to Save It* (London, 1865; published originally as a series of twelve pamphlets based on lectures pertaining to the rearing and diseases of children); "A Life-Leaf from My Note Book," *Herald of Health*, June 1868, 249–51; "A Sleigh Ride over the Alps," *Herald of Health*, September 1868, 124–28; "A Lesson for Parents," *Herald of Health*, November 1868, 193–97; "Pompeii and Its Baths," *Herald of Health*, May 1869, 217–21; "Shelley's Grave," *Herald of Health*, June 1869, 238–62; "The Nightingale; or, Instinct and Reason," *Herald of Health*, August 1869, 72–74; "At the Seaside of England," *Herald of Health*, October 1869, 166–70; *Poems: Heart Melodies* (London, 1870); *Woman and Her Destiny* (London, 1870); "Reminiscences of Sir James Y. Simpson," *Herald of Health* 50:106; "Robert Southey, the Poet Laureate and

His Grave," *Herald of Health* 50:210; "A Health Trip to the Orient," *Herald of Health*, October 1871, 155–60; "Hygiene," *Herald of Health*, November 1874, 201–2; "A Memorial to William Tweedie," *Herald of Health*, January 1875, 21–23; Unfinished manuscript of a temperance novel, 1879.

References: *Notable American Women 1607–1950*, 1:654–55; Phebe A. Hanaford, *Daughters of America* (Augusta, ME, ca. 1882); "Mrs. Lydia Folger Fowler," clipping from unidentified newspaper dated March 1, 1879, from the Nantucket Atheneum; *New York Tribune*, June 8, 1855; Marilyn Bailey Ogilvie, *Women in Science* (Cambridge, MA, 1986), 87–88; Edward A. Stackpole, "Lydia Folger Fowler: First American Born Woman with a Medical Degree," *Inquirer-Mirror* (Nantucket), 197?, from the Nantucket Historical Association; Madeleine B. Stern, "Lydia Folger Fowler, M.D. First American Woman Professor of Medicine," *New York State Journal of Medicine*, June 1977, 137–40; Zephorene L. Stickney, "Wheaton Graduate Becomes Doctor," *Wheaton College History Timeline*, n.d.; Frederick C. Waite, "Dr. Lydia Folger Fowler," *Annals of Medical History*, May 1932; Wheaton Female Seminary, *Chronological Catalogue of the Trustees, Principals, Teachers and Students of Wheaton Female Seminary, Norton, Mass.* (Boston, 1869).

Cecilia Pumpelly *Ricker* FREASE (1830–96)

Celia Ricker was born May 21, 1830, in Clermont County, Ohio, to Eben S. Ricker and Mary Pumpelly, both of whom had been born in Maine. Eben was nine years old when his family moved to Pleasant Hill in Clermont County, Ohio (1814). Eben taught school in his early days, at which he was apparently quite gifted. He later became a surveyor by profession and an active abolitionist. Though interested in politics, he declined public office. His religious views were liberal, and he belonged to no church. Farming and horticulture occupied much of his time, and his farm was a showplace.

Eben and Mary had two daughters, each of whom married a physician. The elder daughter, Cecilia, graduated February 3, 1855, from Eclectic Medical Institute in Cincinnati with an MD degree. On August 24, 1854, she had married fellow classmate Hiram Frease of Napoleon, a village in northwestern Ohio. Prior to this, in 1853, Hiram and Solomon Frease were operating a water-cure at Deardorff's Mills in Tuscarawas County, known as the Sugar Creek Falls Water-Cure, one of five water-cures in the state. After medical school, they moved to a new locale.

On May 1, 1855, the trio—Celia, Hiram, and Solomon—opened the Pittsburgh Water-Cure, notice of which may be found in 1855 issues of the *Water-Cure Journal*. It was located ten miles west of Pittsburgh, Pennsylvania, on the Ohio River, and one detrained at Haysville Station on the Pittsburgh, Ft. Wayne and Chicago Railroad. How long they remained here is undetermined, but Weiss and Kemble say they were there until 1860. However, in 1856, Solomon was listed as a staff member of the newly organized Clifton Springs Water-Cure at Clifton Springs, in Ontario County, New York.

No information has been found about the Freases' professional work in the subsequent thirty years. Hiram is listed in the first (1886) Polk medical directory as being in Locust Corner, Claremont County, Ohio (but not in the 1890 or 1893 Polk directories or the 1874 or 1877 Butler directories). This was the location of the Ricker homestead and was their home thereafter and probably for some years before. In the *History of Clermont and Brown Counties, Ohio*, the author writes, "Comparatively early in life he [Hiram] retired from professional life and located on a farm near Napoleon, Henry Co., Ohio, but spent most of his time after retirement with his family in Pierce township," which was the seat of his wife's family. The history goes on to say, "He made a great study of political affairs and understood politics better than the average citizen. He lectured in medical schools and colleges and made a special study of history. He was partly self-educated and was a man of a large fund of general knowledge, as well as knowledge along the special lines in which he was most interested . . . all held him in high esteem." (It sounds as if Hiram is a bit of a dilettante and as if the author hopes to sell him a copy of the book—not much meat here.) There is no mention of Celia being a physician in any of these sources. One might presume that neither husband nor wife practiced medicine after returning to the Ricker homestead at Locust Corners.

Hiram died on November 4, 1896. Celia lived until October 13, 1914, and died at the homestead. Solomon Frease, probably Hiram's brother, turned up in Rochester, New York, in 1885, having wintered in New York City where he was "investigating the latest medical research." He and a Dr. Stone operated the Rochester Sanitarium for chronic diseases, where they provided baths, including compressed air baths like those "conducted by Dr. von Liebig" in Germany. The enterprise was short lived, but Dr. Frease stayed on, practicing on Monroe Avenue in Rochester. He died January 25, 1892.

References: Polk, 1886; Clifton Springs Water-Cure, *Report of the Addresses and Sermon at the Dedication of the Clifton Springs Water-Cure Held July 25, 1856* (Rochester, NY, 1856); J. L. Rockey, *History of Clermont County, Ohio* (Philadelphia, 1880); *Water-Cure Journal*, 1855; Harry B. Weiss, *The Great American Water-Cure Craze* (Trenton, NJ, 1967), 184,

188, 193; Byron Williams, *History of Clermont and Brown Counties, Ohio* (Baltimore, MD, ca. 1987).

Martha Ann *FRENCH* (b. ca. 1832)

Nothing is yet known of Martha French's background, parents, or early education. When she matriculated at the Eclectic Medical Institute in Cincinnati, she was listed as a resident of North Clarendon, Vermont. French attended two terms at the institute, starting November 1853, and graduated with a medical degree on February 3, 1855. French returned for a third, postgraduate term. Her preceptor had been Nathan Bedortha, MD, proprietor of the Saratoga Springs Water-Cure, Saratoga Springs, New York.

In 1856 French became an assistant to Dr. Robert Hamilton, who headed the women's department at Bedortha's Saratoga Springs establishment. Two years later she was assistant to Dr. J. H. North at his Mt. Prospect Water-Cure in Binghamton, New York. Dr. French cannot be identified with certainty in the 1860 census. Nor is she listed in the 1862 or 1863 *Progressive Annual*. It is possible that she had died by then or, more likely, that she married and changed her name.

References: Eclectic Medical Institute of Cincinnati, Matriculation records, Lloyd Library and Museum, Cincinnati, http://www.lloydlibrary.org/EMI-1845-1939.pdf (accessed May 19, 2016); Harry B. Weiss, *The Great American Water-Cure Craze.*

Adeline *Johnson* FULLER (b. 1800)

Adeline Johnson was born March 8, 1800, in Cambridge, Massachusetts, the daughter of Edmond Johnson and his wife, Anna. Of her background, family, or early education nothing is known. On April 7, 1828, then twenty-eight, Adeline married seventy-one-year-old John Fuller, a widower and father of three grown children by his first wife. The new couple had three children: Edmund Johnson (1829), Adeline (1831), and Anna M. (1834). John died November 18, 1838, at eighty-one, leaving his widow with three children under the age of ten. How she managed financially is not known, but John appears to have left her reasonably well off. In the 1850 census she is listed as having $10,000. Cambridge city directories list Adeline as living at two different locations between 1850 and 1854.

In 1855, Adeline enrolled in the New England Female Medical College, then an unchartered school that awarded certificates in midwifery. In 1860, she graduated from Penn Medical University in

Philadelphia with an MD degree. Then sixty years old, she started practicing medicine in Cambridge forthwith. The 1861 Cambridge city directory lists "Mrs. Adeline J. Fuller, Eclectic physician, bds 39 Columbia." In 1862 and 1863, the entry reads, "Eclectic physician and nurse," and she is listed in the classified section under "nurses," suggesting, perhaps, that the doctoring business was not thriving. The 39 Columbia address was that of her son-in-law, daughter Adeline's husband, Wesley Ware, who, after 1867, is listed as an organ maker. There are no further listings in city directories after 1867. Dr. Fuller may have retired or died. For a brief period (1829–35) she had belonged to the First Evangelical Congregational Church of Cambridge.

References: Cambridge city directories, 1850, 1852, 1854, 1861, 1862, 1863, 1868; William H. Fuller, *Genealogy of Some Descendants of Thomas Fuller of Woburn* (New York, 1919); US census, 1850; Frederick C. Waite, *History of New England Female Medical College, 1848–1872* (Boston: Boston University School of Medicine, 1950).

Rebecca *Lewis* FUSSELL (1820–93)

Rebecca Lewis was born June 10, 1820, the second of five children (four girls, one boy) of John Lewis and his wife Esther Fussell. Son of a prosperous farmer, John was not healthy enough to operate the family farm. He died in 1824 of typhoid fever, leaving his widow with five children under the age of five. Rebecca was said to be a superior student and, later, a teacher. Little else is known of her childhood and education.

On January 20, 1838, at seventeen, Rebecca married Dr. Edwin Fussell, a man seven years her senior and her first cousin, and recent graduate of the University of Pennsylvania Medical School (1835). Between 1839 and 1849 the couple had five children, and fourteen years later, in 1863, a sixth (Edwin Neal). In 1843, the family moved to an area near Pendleton, Indiana, where there were other members of the Fussell and Lewis families living. They returned to Pennsylvania after five years. "In her own home she retained the habit learned in childhood . . . of having the current literature of the day read in the evenings to the gathered family circle."

In 1856, Edwin became dean of the Female Medical College of Pennsylvania, a post he would hold for a decade. The couple's Fussell grandfather, Bartholomew, had been one of the founders of the school. Rebecca, then in her middle thirties, enrolled in the school (her youngest child then seven) and graduated with an MD degree in 1858. She is listed as a practitioner in the *Progressive Annuals* for 1862–64 but not in directories thereafter. The fact that another baby had been born in 1863 may have been a reason for her leaving practice. Nancy P. Spears, archivist at the Friends' Historical Library at Swarthmore College, who is familiar with the Lewis papers there, reports that few of the many letters written by Rebecca mention anything about medical practice. Another source says that after graduation she "practiced with her husband in cases where her services could be of especial value." The 1863 annual report of the Woman's Hospital lists her as one of the twenty-four managers of that institution and her husband as a member of the Board of Trustees.

Rebecca's obituary records that "both she and her husband, in accordance with the traditions of their families, were earnest abolitionists, through all the years which called forth their devoted enthusiasm, and their active assistance in cases requiring the utmost heroism and the most dauntless courage." Edwin and Rebecca were among the founders of the Longwood Progressive Friends Meetinghouse in Kennett Square. This congregation held an annual meeting of "radicals and reformers" from 1855 until 1940, where many of the country's most famous abolitionist and civil rights speakers addressed them. The group was also an important stop on the Underground Railroad. Edwin died March 10, 1882, in Media, Pennsylvania; Rebecca, April 30, 1893. They are buried in Sandy Bank Graveyard in Media.

References: Obituary, *Friends' Intelligencer and Journal* (Philadelphia) 50 (May 13, 1893); Ellwood Harvey, "Edwin Fussell, M.D. 1813–1882," *Report of the Delaware County Medical Society*, 318ff.; Personal communication from Nancy Speers, archivist, Friends' Historical Library of Swarthmore College, February 7, 1989.

G

Anna Maria *Crane* GATCHELL (b. ca. 1821–85)

Anna Maria Crane was born about 1821, probably in Cincinnati where her father, Thurston Crane, was a prominent merchant, and her mother was Anna Owens. The scope of her early education and details of Anna's childhood are unknown. In 1843, Anna married Horatio Page Gatchell, about whom, in contrast to Anna, there is available a great deal of information. This biographical sketch will necessarily be primarily about Horatio, but that should give some idea of Anna's activities. The couple probably met while Horatio was a student at the Eclectic Medical Institute in Cincinnati in the early 1840s. They were married in 1843, had five sons, three of whom became physicians. The family lived in at least five different localities: Cincinnati, Painesville, and Ravenna, Ohio; Kenosha, Wisconsin; and Asheville, North Carolina.

The Gatchell family had immigrated to the mid-South, but Horatio's forebears had moved north to Maine, where he was born in Hallowell on February 12, 1814, graduated from Bowdoin in 1833, studied for the ministry, and was a preacher as late as 1840. Then twenty-six, he changed course and attended lectures at Louisville Medical College in 1840–41, and then moved to Cincinnati where he went to the Eclectic Medical Institute, from which he received an MD degree in 1842.

Horatio became professor of anatomy at Eclectic Medical Institute in 1849 and of physiology as well the following year. In the spring of 1851, he resigned this post and accepted the professorship of anatomy at Western College of Homoeopathic Medicine in Cleveland, where he became a homoeopath and a prominent practitioner in that community. It appears that he was also involved in a health resort of some kind in Painesville, a community on Lake Erie about thirty-five miles east of Cleveland. Knowledge of this venture comes from a letter Gatchell wrote: "When last year I wrote you from Painesville I was here as a visitor, now I write from under my own rooftop; then I was engaged in private practice in Cincinnati; now I am laying the foundations of an infirmary upon one of the most salubrious spots in the western country." Since medical school terms were then short—three or four months a year—it is likely that Painesville was his residence. In any case, Gatchell was described as "a tower of strength" at the school. In 1859, the medical school had changed its name to Western Homoeopathic College and that year his wife Anna, having attended lectures, graduated from it with an MD degree. The eldest of her five sons was fourteen years old at this time. The 1860 census places the family back in Ravenna, so they had apparently moved again.

After fourteen years in the Cleveland area, the family moved to Highwood, Lake County, Illinois, a town halfway between Chicago and Kenosha, Wisconsin (twenty-five miles each way). While here, Horatio was professor of physiology at Chicago's Hahnemann Medical College for five years, and he and Anna operated a health resort in Kenosha. The following advertisement appeared in the June 1870 issue of the *Herald of Health*: "Female Water Cure, Oak Grove Sanitarium, Kenosha, Wis. A Homoeopathic and Hydropathic Institute for the treatment of lady patients. Prof. H. P. Gatchell, consulting physician. Address Mrs. A. M. Gatchell, M.D. Drawer 46. Kenosha, Wis."

The conjunction of homoeopathy and hydropathy is noteworthy. Years earlier, while in Cincinnati, Horatio had edited (with J. H. Pulte) a short-lived popular journal designed to encourage the use of hydropathy in homoeopathic practice. While the Gatchells were in Kenosha, Horatio wrote a book entitled *Climate and Health of Kenosha, Wisconsin.*

The final move came in 1875 (another source says 1871, but both Horatio and Anna registered as physicians in Highland, Illinois, in 1877), when Horatio gave up active practice, moved to Asheville, and opened a sanitarium, said to be the first for the treatment of tuberculosis in North Carolina. He was joined by his son, Edwin, when he graduated from medical school in 1878. Here, Horatio wrote two more books: *Western North Carolina: Its Agricultural Resources, Mineral Wealth, Climate, Salubrity, and Scenery* and "Man and His Environments." The latter, which he considered his major life contribution, was destroyed in a fire that consumed his house in 1884. He also published an *Invalid's Guide* in 1880. The 1880 census places Anna and Horatio in Atlanta, so they may have retired there. Horatio died two years later at seventy-one of pneumonia and is buried in Asheville.

It has not been possible to determine whether Anna practiced medicine after graduation from medical school. Her name has not been found listed as a physician in any of the directories consulted. However, in each of the last three communities in which the family lived—Painesville, Kenosha, and Asheville—they had involvement with some kind of health institution, and it is likely she worked professionally at those institutions. Also, in 1877, when they lived in the Kenosha-Chicago area, she registered her license with the Illinois State Board of Health, as did her husband and one of her sons. There would not seem to be much point to doing this if she were not professionally active. Anna died after 1885, presumably in Asheville.

Bibliography: Mrs. H. P. Gatchell and J. S. Bradley. *Mrs. Bradley's Book of Cookery* (Cincinnati, 1853).

References: Illinois State Board of Health of Illinois, *Official Registry of Physicians and Midwives, 3rd Annual Report, 1880* (Springfield, IL, 1881); *Herald of Health,* June 1870, 41; William H. King, *History of Homoeopathy in America and Its Institutions* (New York: Lewis, 1905), 1:180, 3:16; *American Magazine Devoted to Homoeopathy & Hydropathy* 1, nos. 1–12 (1851–52).

Agnes Mitilda *GILKERSON* Smith (1838–81)

Agnes M. Gilkerson, who received an MD degree from Penn Medical University in Philadelphia in 1861, had a rather unusual career. While working in a Lowell, Massachusetts, textile mill and living in a boarding house, she met Hezekiah Bradley Smith, who had recently moved his factory to Lowell, where he made woodworking machinery of his own design. (Between 1849 and 1873, he received ten patents for these machines.) Hezekiah, a married man, met Agnes in 1854, made her his confidential secretary, sent her to finishing school, and, in 1859, to medical school in Philadelphia, where she lived with the family of Smith's Philadelphia sales manager. Agnes graduated in 1861.

That same year, Smith and Gilkerson were married in a civil ceremony in Lowell. Smith was still married to his first wife, who refused to give him a divorce. The two had lived apart since 1847, though Smith visited his wife periodically and fathered three sons with her. In 1861, Smith demanded, received, and burned all the letters he had sent her; opened a bank account for her; and gave her title to the Woodstock, Vermont, house in which she lived with her children. Both the bank account and the title were in his wife's maiden name. Hezekiah also cut out from the family Bible and burned all entries regarding his marriage and progeny. The sum of these acts he thought constituted divorce.

Smith and Gilkerson moved to Smithville (formerly Shreveville), New Jersey, where Smith continued the manufacture of woodworking machines. Gilkerson is said to have practiced medicine and sold remedies over the ensuing twenty years. After Dr. Gilkerson's death from cancer in 1881, her husband erected a canopied statue of her, made of Italian marble, in the yard of their home. Following the death of his mother, one of Hezekiah's sons destroyed the statue and threw it in the river.

Reference: s.v., "Hezekiah Bradley Smith," *Wikipedia*, https://en.wikipedia.org/wiki/Hezekiah_Bradley_Smith (accessed June 6, 2016).

Margaretta *Baldwin* GLEASON (1819–62)

Margaretta Baldwin was born in 1819 to Dr. William Baldwin, US Navy, and his wife. Nothing is known of her childhood. She was probably raised in Philadelphia. In 1844 she married Dr. Cloyes William Gleason (1821–1902), who received his MD degree that same year from the University of Pennsylvania and who was later professor of physiology at the Female Medical College of Pennsylvania. The Gleasons had four children: Eugene B. (1845), Horace B. (1847), Edward B. (1854), and Carrie H. (1857). The two older children died young.

In 1850–51, Margaretta matriculated at the Female Medical College of Pennsylvania, probably after the death of her two sons. The following year she changed to Syracuse Medical College (Eclectic), listing her husband as her preceptor. She graduated with an MD degree on March 6, 1851. While a medical student she wrote a letter entitled "Medical Education of Women" that was published in two installments in the *American Medical and Surgical Journal* (Syracuse, May and October 1851).

After graduation she returned to Philadelphia. Although her interest in the subject of educating woman doctors continued—she published another letter on the subject in 1854 (*Syracuse Medical and Surgical Journal*)—her name is not listed as a physician in the 1860 or 1861 Philadelphia directory or the 1862 *Progressive Annual.* She had two more children, Edward B. (1854) and Carrie H. (1857) and may have been fully occupied raising them. However, she was a member of the original 1858 Board of Lady Managers at the Woman's Hospital that opened in 1861, as were Emeline Cleveland, Rebecca Fussell, and Ann Preston. Margaretta died in Philadelphia on September 8, 1862, at age forty-three. She is buried at West Laurel Hill Cemetery in Bala Cynwyd, Pennsylvania. In 1865, Cloyes married Rebecca Nourse Hapgood.

Cloyes was a popular lecturer on physiology and hygiene, wrote *Everybody's Own Physician; or, How to Acquire and Preserve Health,* and was the first professor of physiology at Female Medical College of Pennsylvania. He had come from Barnet, in the Northeast Kingdom of Vermont and later in life bought an island there in the Connecticut River to which he retreated periodically. Edward Baldwin Gleason, son of Margaretta and Cloyes, graduated from the University of Pennsylvania (BS 1875, MD 1878), and he became clinical professor of otology at Medico-Chirurgical College in 1895 and professor in 1908. He wrote two books on otolaryngology subjects, and was visiting laryngologist at Philadelphia Hospital. He and his wife had one daughter, Helen B. (1897). His sister Carrie married J. W. Adamson and had a daughter, Mary.

Bibliography: "Medical Education of Women," *American Medical and Surgical Journal,* May 1851, 81–84, and October 1851, 189–91; Letter on the medical education of women, *Syracuse Medical and Surgical Journal,* 1854, 136–38, 167–69.

References: Obituary, *Public Ledger* (Philadelphia), September 9, 1962, 2; *Pioneer-Pacesetter-Innovator: The Story of the Medical College of Pennsylvania* (New York: Newcomen Society in North America, 1971).

Rachel Ingall *Brooks* GLEASON (1820–1905)

Rachel Brooks Gleason was the second child and eldest daughter among the four children of Reuben and Lucy Muzzy Brooks who survived to adulthood. Four more died in infancy. Rachel was born in Winhall, Vermont, November 27, 1820. Before she married Silas Orsemus Gleason, on July 3, 1844, she taught school. At the time of the marriage Silas had just graduated from Castleton Medical College.

From 1847 to 1850, the Gleasons were working at Glen Hill Water Cure on the western shore of Skaneateles Lake, one of the Finger Lakes in Western New York, a location about fifteen miles south of the village of Skaneateles. Situated on the lakeshore, at the bottom of a mountain that rose almost vertically a thousand feet and from which flowed a plentiful spring, it was a stunning site. Here the Gleasons were partners with Theodosia Gilbert, who kept the books; James Caleb Jackson, business manager; and Jackson's wife, Lucretia, matron. The Gleasons provided the medical care. Rachel, who was not yet a doctor, took care of the women.

During the winter months of this period, Orsemus lectured on hydropathy at the newly opened Central Medical College, an Eclectic school, in nearby Syracuse. He also persuaded the trustees to enroll women at the school (as nearby Geneva Medical Institution had recently done). Rachel matriculated, transferred the following year with the school when it moved to Rochester, and graduated with an MD degree on February 20, 1851, along with Sarah Adamson (later Dolley; q.v.), thereby becoming the third or fourth women to become doctors of medicine. (Rachel's diploma may be seen today, hanging on a wall at Arnot Ogden Hospital in Elmira, New York.)

When James Jackson, too, decided to become a doctor, the Gleasons sold out their share to the other partners for $500 and moved a few miles westward to the Forest City Water Cure on the east side of Cayuga Lake, just north of Ithaca. While they were there, Orsemus went to see a patient in Elmira. As Rachel later recalled it:

> My husband was called to Elmira to attend a patient, and on his return was not only enthusiastic over his success in treating a severe case of congestion of the lungs, with water only, but also that he had found just the place for our permanent Water-Cure home— a pretty town, accessible by railroad from every direction, a spring

of running water abundant for bathing purposes, delightful views, charming drives, pleasant walks on the hills and in the ravines, with the valley of the Chemung below us, was to be our home. Here in the midst of a wheat field with a rail fence about it was built our establishment. No vine or shrub or tree relieved the nakedness of our front yard; but the hills were grand and the valley beautiful, and on these we could feast our eyes till vines and trees could grow; and they have grown, till now we begin to cut away what was cultivated with so much care, that we may let in the sunshine and look out upon a charming landscape.

This became the Elmira Water Cure (later known as the Gleason Health Resort). By 1853, the Gleasons were reported to have fifty or seventy patients. After it had been open for five years, there were patients from fourteen states, two territories, and Canada. An observer said that "the establishment was cheap, clean and honest. Patients paid ten to twelve dollars per week, plus a charge for wood burned in the private rooms. Patients were expected to furnish 'for bathing purposes and comfort' one blanket, two cotton sheets, one old linen sheet, two coarse towels and table napkins."

The institution thrived. It became nationally famous and attracted many prominent citizens. Mark Twain called Rachel "the almost divine Mrs. Gleason" and called her to Buffalo to attend his wife who was doing poorly after the birth of their son. Many interns passed through the institution. One of Rachel's younger sisters, Zipporah, and her daughter, Adele, both became doctors and worked there.

The Gleasons retired in 1898 and moved to Buffalo to live with their daughter, who was then practicing there. Orsemus died the next year, Rachel on March 13, 1905. Both Gleasons were involved in community affairs. Rachel had been a popular lecturer on health topics during her active years and, like many of her female professional contemporaries, thought teaching patients about their bodies and physiology was important. She wrote a book, *Talks to My Patients*, that went through at least nine printings; it was well received from the first. Medical school classmate Sarah Adamson Dolley, practicing in Rochester, wrote of the book, "I have set it circulating among my patients." Caroline Winslow (q.v.), in Washington, DC, thought the book "will do everyone good for whom it was written."

Bibliography: "Notes of the Northwest," *Herald of Health* 47 (1869): 70–72; "Up the Mississippi," *Herald of Health* 47 (1869): 40–42; "Medical Education of Women," *Herald of Health* 50 (1870): 19–21; *Talks to My Patients* (New York, 1870; at least eight editions were published by 1895); "Woman's Dress," *Water-Cure Journal*, February 1851, 30–32, April 1851, 82–82, June 1851, 151–52.

References: Rachel Gleason Brooks, *This Is Your Inheritance: A History of the Chemung County, NY Branch of the Brooks Family* (Watkins Glen, NY, ca. 1963); Jane B. Donegan, *Hydropathic Highway to Health* (New York: Greenwood Press, 1986), 44–49; Evelyn Giammichele and Eva Taylor Giammichele, "Elmira Water Cure: Silas and Rachel Gleason and Their 'Tavern for the Sick,'" *Chemung Historical Journal*, December 1966, 1535–41; *Herald of Health* 50 (1870): 192 [Dolley quotation]; Frances E. Willard, *A Woman of the Century* (Buffalo, NY: C. W. Moulton, 1893), 322.

Ellen Hermans *GOODELL* Smith (1833–1905)

Ellen Goodell was born August 25, 1833, in Belchertown, a village in south central Massachusetts. She was the eldest of nine children of Ashbel Goodell and his wife Cynthia Tilson Newell. Ellen "acquired her elementary education in the common schools, and, after pursuing higher branches of study two terms at the Amherst Academy, taught school one term. Compelled by ill health to relinquish her labors in 1857 [then age twenty-four] she entered Dr. William T. Vail's Granite State Health Institute, at Hill, New Hampshire, an establishment that took pride that it was 'not a fashionable resort.'" Ellen became interested in the successful method practiced there of treating the sick and decided to become a teacher and a practitioner of the new school.

She remained at the Health Institute for two years as patient, student, and assistant. In 1859, she enrolled at the New York Hygeio-Therapeutic College (Dr. Vail was an alumnus), graduated with an MD degree in 1861, and returned to the Health Institute as matron and physician. In the fall of the following year, she went on the lecture circuit "again." This experience is well detailed in a communication published in October 1863 issue of the *Herald of Health*. The piece is of particular interest because it shows the economic importance of such tours in drumming up clientele for the institution the speaker represented, not to mention the missionary fervor speakers felt in promoting health truths as they saw them. Wrote Dr. Goodell, "I am preparing to start out on another lecturing tour, and I think I need some charts to illustrate my lectures to ladies. I find that they are much more interested in lectures if they can *see*, as well as hear what we are talking about." Lectures were usually given in churches; on this particular circuit, Ellen spent three months in Vermont's Lamoille and Orange Counties as well as stopping at several towns in New Hampshire.

She wrote that she had "never spent seven months more pleasantly, than while engaged in heralding the gospel of health to drug-cursed communities. . . . I met with excellent success, especially in view of the fact, that health reform had scarcely been heard of in many places, and the idea of curing sick people without 'something to take,' or raising up a patient without 'stimulants' was to many people simply absurd." Though "opposition met me everywhere . . . our glorious cause is progressing."

In 1864, Ellen left New Hampshire and became resident physician at Dr. Trall's sanitarium in New York City. She would have similar posts at three other institutions during the decade that followed: Westboro, Massachusetts, St. Paul, Minnesota, and Philadelphia. While in New York, she was in charge of the Swedish movement cure and Turkish bath departments. After two years she went to Dr. J. H. Hero's Willow-Park Water-Cure in Westboro, where she was medical director, responsible again for the movement cure and Turkish baths.

In 1868, Ellen joined Thomas W. Deering, MD, at the Hygienic & Movement Institute in St. Paul, Minnesota. He was surgeon and physician, she was physician. While in St. Paul she met and on April 16, 1871, married Dr. John Brown Smith of Northfield, Minnesota, a man four years her junior, with whom she had one child seven years later when she was forty-five—Lindsey Goodell Smith, who became an actor. Husband John, Canadian born, came to the United States at seventeen, served in the Civil War in the Tenth Minnesota, and must have been a trifle eccentric. Though he had also acquired a medical degree, it is not clear that he ever practiced medicine. One of his principal occupations was in developing a shorthand system, but he was also an author, a tax evader, and, some say, an anarchist. In 1879–80, he spent almost a year in Belchertown jail for refusing to pay a $2 poll tax (because he was not a citizen), being finally released when a friend paid the tax and accrued costs ($5.62).

After leaving St. Paul in 1871, Ellen became resident physician at Dr. Trall's Philadelphia establishment, a post she held for three years. While there, she introduced parlor lectures for ladies. She returned to Belchertown for the birth of her son on August 24, 1874. There she remained, practicing medicine and active on the lecture circuit until retiring at fifty in 1883. In retirement, she wrote two books, *The Fat of the Land and How to Live on It* and *The Art of Living*. During her last six years, she was one of the editors of the popular *New York Health Magazine*. She also helped out as an assistant at her brother Lafayette's seed business.

In the spring of 1905, then seventy-two, she had a fall from which she never recovered—slight improvement and then relapse—suggesting a subdural hematoma, rendering her helpless and leading to her being taken to a sanitarium in Brooklyn, New York. Cheerful and courageous, she died November 13, 1905. Her funeral was at the home of her brother, Wesley Melancthon, merchant and postmaster of Dwight, Massachusetts. She is buried in Dwight Cemetery. Said her obituary, "She strove to teach people how by right living to prevent sickness as well as to cure. Unselfish to a fault, of a genial, cheerful nature . . . she had the faculty of imparting much of her cheerfulness and optimism to others. Her life was devoted to the uplifting of humanity without regard to mere self-interest and all who knew her became her lasting friends."

Bibliography: ALS, Belchertown, January 1, 1850, to her cousin Angelo Goodell, New York City; "Lecturing Reminiscences," *Herald of Health*, October 1863, 154–56; *Fat of the Land and How to Live on It* (Amherst, MA: Carpenter & Morehouse, 1896); *The Art of Living* (Amherst, MA: Author, 1903).

References: Obituary, *Amherst Record*, November 1905; Three-page manuscript biographical sketch of E. G. Smith at the Jones Library, Amherst, MA; Advertisement for the Hygienic & Movement Institute, St. Paul, MN, in *Herald of Health*, December 1868, 42; *Water-Cure World*, Brattleboro, VT, June 1860 and May 1861; "John Brown Smith," *Wikipedia*; George E. Williams, *A Genealogy of the Descendants of Robert Goodale/Goodell of Salem, Mass.* (West Hartford, CT: Author, 1984).

Anna *Eames* GOULDING (1799–1866)

Anna Eames was born March 20, 1799, in Ashland, Massachusetts, the third of five children and second of four daughters of Jesse Eames and his wife Anna Lovering. On June 2, 1824, she married John Goulding. He died ten years later, September 14, 1834. In 1852, Anna enrolled in what was then known as the Boston Female Medical College (later the New England Female Medical College) and presumably earned a certificate in midwifery. In 1855 and 1857, she is denoted an early manager of the New England Female Medical College and the Female Medical Society in the Boston directory for that year. She was a resident of Boston when she graduated with an MD degree in 1860 from Penn Medical University in Philadelphia, at the age of sixty-one. The 1860 census lists her as a resident of Ward 8, Boston and as owning $800 in real estate. Boston directories list her as a physician each year from 1861 through 1869 but not thereafter. She died with pneumonia on November 6 or 7, 1866, at 39 Eliot Street, Boston.

References: Boston city directory, 1861–69; Moses Eames, *Of One Branch of the Descendants of the Thomas Eames' Family, Who Came from England about 1630, and First Settled at Dedham, Mass., in 1640* (Watertown, NY, 1887), 12; US census, 1860; Waite, *History of the New England Female Medical College 1848–1874.*

Cordelia Agnes *GREENE* (1831–1905)

Cordelia Greene was born July 5, 1831, and grew up in Lyons, in Western New York, the eldest of five children of Jabez and Phila Cook Greene. Her parents were raised as Quakers but became Presbyterians. Jabez was a school trustee in Lyons, and during his tenure he introduced the graded system. In her youth Cordelia obtained a teacher's certificate. In the late 1840s, the family moved farther west in New York State, first to Pike and, in 1849, to Castile, where Jabez started a water-cure.

There are conflicting data about what Cordelia was doing at this time. Most sources say that she attended the Female Medical College of Pennsylvania and graduated in 1853. However, the published catalog of graduates of the school does not list her name. Another source says that she worked for six years at the Cleveland Water Cure Establishment, in charge of the female department (*WCJ,* January 1856, May 1856). In either case, she attended Western Reserve Medical School and received an MD degree in 1856. For the next six years she was back in Western New York on the staff at Henry Foster's Clifton Springs Water-Cure. In 1863, on the death of her father, she took charge of the water-cure in Castile, New York. Under her management, it was to become nationally known.

Greene's first patient at Castile, Mrs. M. H. Rossiter, had followed her from Clifton Springs. She later recalled the time: Patients were awakened at 6 a.m. and went to the bathroom to receive either "a pail dash or a dripping sheet." One "stood a little way from the nurse and she threw half of the [warm] water over your chest and limbs, then you turned and the other half was thrown over your back." This was repeated with a cold dash. "It almost took your breath away . . . [but] you felt fine afterwards." Then a cold dripping sheet was thrown over you, followed by a wet rub and then a dry rub. It was "exhilarating."

Early in her life, Cordelia experienced a religious conversion and remained devout thereafter. Prayer was an important feature of treatment at Castile. She was also active in temperance circles and the political equality movement. Susan B. Anthony and Frances E. Willard were both friends and patients. She became a member of the New York State Medical Society and the American Medical Association.

She wrote three books: *Build Well,* published in 1885; *The Castile Sanitarium Cook Book,* 1902; and *The Art of Keeping Well,* published posthumously in 1906. She was also instrumental in building a library for the village, contributing land across the street from the sanitarium and providing a $12,000 endowment and $500 with which to buy books. Though never married, she adopted six children, four of whom lived to adulthood, and two of whom became physicians. Dr. Greene died in New York City, January 28, 1905, following surgery at Presbyterian Hospital. Her ashes are buried under a marked boulder in Grace Cemetery. After her death, her niece, Mary Theresa Greene, MD, took over management of the sanitarium. It continued in operation until 1957, when it was sold, to be used as a nursing home.

Bibliography: *Build Well* (Boston: D. Lothrop, 1885); *The Castile Sanitarium Cook Book* (Castile, NY: Fred Norris, 1902); *The Art of Keeping Well* (New York: Dodd, Mead & Co., 1906).

References: *American National Biography,* 9:522–23; Elizabeth Gordon, *The Story of the Life and Work of Cordelia A. Greene, M.D.* (Castile, NY: Castilian, 1925); Edward Greene, "Recollections of Early Days at the Water Cure with Dr. Cordelia Greene," *Historical Wyoming,* April 1958; Douglas Morgan, "Castile Landmark Sold, January 1957, Arcade, N.Y.," *Historical Wyoming,* January 1957; Obituary, *New York Times,* January 29, 1905; "Miss C. A. Greene in Charge of Female Department at Cleveland Water-Cure Establishment Run by T. T. Seelye, M.D.," *Water-Cure Journal,* January 1856; "Cordelia Greene Now a Graduate of Western Reserve Who Has Practiced the Water-Cure for Six Years at Cleveland Water Cure Establishment," *Water-Cure Journal,* May 1856.

M. Adelaide *GRENNAN* (b. ca. 1821–96)

Adelaide Grennan was born about 1821. Nothing is known of her early life and education. She received a medical degree from Penn Medical University in 1861. At that time she was listed as living in Walton, Kentucky, a community just south of Cincinnati. The title of her medical school thesis was "The Agency of Electricity in Reproduction."

According to the *Progressive Annual* of 1862, she was still in Philadelphia. That same publication in 1864 places her in Pawlet, a hamlet in southwestern Vermont not far from Manchester. She must have soon moved to St. Louis, where she would live and practice medicine the rest of her life. Though not listed in either of the Butler medical directories (1874, 1877), she is listed in Hoyne (1881) and Polk

(1886) at 1725 Washington Avenue, St. Louis, and at 1210 Washington Avenue (Polk, 1890). She is not in the 1893 Polk but is found in the 1896 Polk at 2645 Pine Street. At the time of her death, she was living at 2736 Olive Street.

In 1896, she was run down by a trolley while returning from a dramatic recital at the Young Men's Hebrew Association. Said her obituary, "She was highly cultured, conversant with ancient and modern languages and interested in a number of movements for the uplifting of her sex. She was a charter member . . . of the Equal Suffrage Association, which was organized in St. Louis in 1864, and which, its members assert, was the first woman's suffrage association." Adelaide never married and, at the time of her death, had no known relatives.

References: Harold J. Abrahams, *Extinct Medical Schools of Nineteenth Century Philadelphia* (Philadelphia: University of Pennsylvania Press, 1966), 222; T. S. Hoyne, *Hoyne's Annual Directory of Homoeopathic Physicians, 1881* 1, no. 9 (Chicago, 1881): 18; Polk, 1886, 1890, 1896; *Progressive Annual*, 1862, 1863, 1864; Obituary from an unidentified St. Louis newspaper at the Missouri Historical Society, St. Louis.

Maria Jane *GRIER* (1832–65)

Maria Jane Grier was born November 9, 1832, in Chester County, Pennsylvania, the second of eight children (two girls, six boys) of Joseph F. Grier and his wife, Margaret Graham. Nothing is known of her childhood or early education. Sometime between 1845 and 1850 the family moved to Lewisburg, Pennsylvania, where Maria's father practiced medicine. In 1853, when she was twenty, Maria matriculated at Penn Medical University in Philadelphia and the following year graduated with an MD degree. She returned to Lewisburg and presumably practiced medicine, although the 1860 census denotes no occupation for her, and no definite information on the subject has been found. Maria died in Lewisburg twelve years after her graduation, on December 7, 1865, probably of tuberculosis.

References: Personal communication from Joanne Kramer, Union County Public Library, Lewisburg, PA; US census, 1850, 1860.

Elizabeth *GRISELLE* (1830–1910)

Elizabeth practiced in Salem, a small Quaker community in eastern Ohio, and, for a short period, in San Francisco. She was born October 31, 1830, near New Garden, Columbiana County, Ohio, a village about ten miles south of Salem, the second of six daughters of Charles and Mary H. Griselle. Her early life was spent in their country home, attending school there, with an occasional year in Salem. Later she went to Delaware, Ohio, to pursue her studies preparatory to the study of medicine.

Though her obituary and two standard histories of Columbiana County say she graduated from the Female Medical College of Pennsylvania, this is incorrect. She received her MD degree from the medical school at Western Reserve in Cleveland in 1856. She is not listed in the catalog of the Female Medical College. Perhaps the graduate clinical training she had as an assistant physician at Woman's Hospital in Philadelphia, an institution associated with the Female Medical College of Pennsylvania, is what was being referred to. She returned to Cleveland and started practice.

After practicing in Cleveland for eight years, she returned to Salem. In Cleveland she is said to have had trouble with asthma. In Salem, she "soon found that she had a good practice among the best families in the town and country." About 1877, she went to San Francisco where she was "in private practice in hospital work." She is listed in the 1878 and 1879 San Francisco directories as a physician. In the early 1880s, she returned to Salem and continued her practice there; the 1886 Polk directory lists her there. Except for an occasional winter trip to Florida, she remained in Salem thereafter, gradually slowing down in the early 1890s.

> Earlier in her life she was an active and devoted member of the Episcopal church, but on account of advancing years she relinquished all the strenuous duties of life, which she never evaded when younger, but always remained hopeful, cheerful, and sympathetic when needed among the sick. She was often asked her reason for studying medicine and stated that it was her belief in the refinement and modesty of women and the example of the Blackwell sisters that induced her to adopt the profession that required at the same time great courage and self-denial. (Obituary)

In *Women of Cleveland*, Mrs. Ingham describes Dr. Griselle as

> an elegant woman, tall, stately, belonging to the Society of Friends [who] attracted my admiration when a young girl here in 1855, because she drove so splendid a horse and had a unique profession; she was a doctor. . . . Not a Quaker as to the cut of her garb; she wore lovely grays and lavenders and had breezy ways—one of the most delightful ladies ever at home in Cleveland; but she did not long remain under the chilling influence of our lake winds. She returned to her home in Salem, O., became a member of the County and State

Medical Associations, and when for her own health's sake she practiced some years on the Pacific Coast, she joined a similar Society for California. There is a bit of romance in Miss Griselle's early life, which determined the direction of her future effort. Tenderly attached to a young physician, her fiancé, he suddenly died, and the strongest tribute of affection she could pay was to take up his life work: to pursue it until the close of her own career. She graduated at Cleveland and Philadelphia, guided here by H. A. Ackley and Elisha Sterling, M.D. Across the continent she was very successful, and in Salem is greatly beloved and sought for. Her specialty is the ills to which her own sex is subjected. Womanly, true, unselfish, she wears a crown invisible.

Dr. Griselle, "one of the most prominent physicians in this part of the country," died at her home on August 23, 1910. She had been in decline for a year prior to this. She is buried at Grand View Cemetery.

References: Cemetery inscriptions, Columbiana Co., OH, at the Stark County Public Library, Canton, OH; *History of Columbiana County Ohio* (Philadelphia: D. W. Ensign, 1879), 47; George D. Hunt, *History of Salem and the Immediate Vicinity, Columbiana County, Ohio* (Salem: Author, 1898), 151; Mrs. W. A. Ingham, *Women of Cleveland and Their Work, Philanthropic, Educational, Literary, Medical and Artistic* (Cleveland: Author, 1893), 316–17; Polk, 1886; Obituary, *Salem News*, August 24, 1910; San Francisco city directories, 1878, 1879.

Maria Maxwell *Tooker* GROSS (1833–99)

Maria Tooker was born March 28, 1833, in Elmira, New York, the only daughter of the Reverend Manly Tooker and his wife Roxanna Farwell. She had two brothers. Her father was an itinerant Methodist minister who served at least twenty different communities in Central and Western New York during the forty years before the Civil War. Manly, the eldest of eight children, recalled in 1849, "It is twenty-nine years this morning since I mounted the horse my father gave me, for the itinerant work. I left my father, as I suppose, in the closet, and my mother at the door, in tears."

After elementary education, Maria attended and graduated from Canandaigua Female Seminary in 1851. Sometime thereafter, while on a visit to Henry Foster's nearby Clifton Springs Water Cure (org. 1850), she met James Eldredge Gross, a native of Maine and then resident physician at the cure. He had attended the medical school at Bowdoin in 1847 but transferred to Hahnemann Medical College in Philadelphia, where he graduated in 1850. The couple was married in Vienna, New York, by Maria's father on February 8, 1853.

Late the next year, the couple moved to southern Wisconsin where, with three partners (including an ex-governor and two real estate speculators), they built, just south of Madison, a four-story, steam-heated water-cure hotel amid a fifty-acre oak grove overlooking a lake, and named it the Lakeside Water-Cure. The building could house eighty patients and had a large two-story wing on the back that contained the baths. Board and treatment was twelve dollars a week. The 1850s were the height of the water-cure craze, and many were built but few survived. (Those that did, like James Jackson's Home on the Hillside and Henry Foster's Clifton Springs Water-Cure, both in Western New York, usually had a religious component and a leader with a strong personality.) Lakeside was not an exception. By 1858, having seen five successive resident physicians, it closed.

The Grosses had long since moved on to Cleveland, where Maria enrolled at the Western Homoeopathic College, from which she graduated with an MD degree in the spring of 1859. Meanwhile, husband James was associated with a Dr. Strong at the Forest City Water-Cure in the eastern part of the city. In 1859, Dr. Strong sold out to Dr. Thomas T. Seelye, who combined Forest City with his own Cleveland Water-Cure and the Grosses moved on, joining with Dr. Charles M. (or E.) Seeley to manage Glen Forest Water-Cure in nearly Yellow Springs, Ohio.

The Glen Forest Water-Cure was already quite well known. Started around 1850 by Dr. Abner Cheney, it was bought by Dr. Ehrmann, a homoeopathic physician in Cincinnati, who leased it to Thomas and Mary Gove Nichols, who planned to open "a School of Health; a School of Progress; a School of Life" to be called Memnonia. But their liberal ideas of social reform and their advocacy of free love led to considerable opposition from the local citizenry, and especially from Horace Mann, president of nearby Antioch College. In early 1857, Memnonia disbanded, the Nicholses converted to Roman Catholicism and left Yellow Springs.

At Yellow Springs, the rates were seven to ten dollars a week for room, board, and treatment. "The female department is under the direction of Mrs. Gross, who has a very large experience in the treatment of diseases peculiar to her own sex," said a promotion. While they were here, James published a monthly newsletter, and for the first New Year's issue (1860), Maria's father wrote a poem, the last stanza of which read:

> Come soon, and be healed, ye sick and ye lame
> And add a few gems to the crown of our fame;
> Yet we say, *not to us, not to us*, the glory be given,
> But to sov'reign *Hygiene, Hydropathy*, and *Heaven!*"

The Grosses stayed here for three years until November 1862, when the cure burned to the ground and they moved on to their fifth, and last, water-cure. This was in Richmond, Indiana, where they bought the building that had housed Green Mount Seminary, remodeled it, renamed it the Green Mount Health Club, and were in business for five years, until that structure burned down in 1867. In its heyday, Maria is said to have cared for as many as one hundred patients at a time, which suggests that though many of the patrons probably had organic illness such as tuberculosis or gynecological problems, many too were tired, neglected (some perhaps merely spoiled) housewives who sought attention, care, and a sympathetic ear.

After 1867, the Grosses moved to Chicago, where James went into business as a pharmacist and, with a partner, as principals in the publishing house of Gross & Delbridge. Maria set up in practice, emphasizing care of women and children, and was soon very successful. Her name appears consistently in medical directories of the period. On January 5, 1898, she registered as a physician, as the law then required. The biographical sketch of her in Cleave says:

> She is a member of the American Institute of Homoeopathy, and possesses one of the best libraries in the West, which is fully supplied with the periodicals of both schools of medicine. The reputation she enjoys for attainments and skill is such as to place her in the front rank of gynecologists, and her tact and success in the treatment of children are equally characteristic of her pre-eminent abilities as a physician. With all her professional reputation, she impresses those around her with the fact that they are in the presence not only of a lady of great personal charms, but of refinement and culture. . . . She attributes her success chiefly to a happy faculty for diagnosing diseases, and a cheery hopefulness and sympathetic "way" that characterizes her in the sick room.

(Cleave tends to be fulsome and somewhat promotional in his biographies, but this one seems a bit more substantive than many.)

Maria's younger brother, Robert Newton Tooker, MD (1841–1902), also a homoeopath, and professor of diseases of children in Chicago Homoeopathic College, dedicated his textbook, *Diseases of Children and Their Homoeopathic Treatment*, to his sister, "who was among the first of her sex to demonstrate woman's fitness for the study and practice of medicine, and whose advice and counsel have been of great value to the writer in critical cases, this work is affectionately dedicated by her brother, the author." The Grosses had three children, each of whom married and had children, four altogether. Maria died August 1, 1899. Husband James lived twelve more years.

References: Cleave, 462; Ronald L. Numbers, *Wisconsin Medicine Historical Perspectives* (Madison: University of Wisconsin Press, 1981), 55; Manly Tooker, *Poems and Jottings of Itinerancy in Western New York* (Rochester, NY: R. Darrow, 1860); Robert N. Tooker, *Diseases of Children and Their Homoeopathic Treatment* (Chicago: Gross & Delbridge, 1895); John H. Treat, *The Treat Family* (Salem, MA: Salem Press, 1893), 330; *Water-Cure Journal*, March 14, 1859, 2; *Water-Cure Journal*, March 24, 1859, 3; Jeffrey M. Wehmeyer, "The Yellow Springs Water Cure," *Ohio Academy of Medical History*, May 7, 2011; Harry B. Weiss, *The Great American Water-Cure Craze* (Trenton, NJ: Past Times Press, 1967).

Emily M. *Smith* GUTHRIE (b. ca. 1829)

According to the 1850 US census, Emily Smith was born in New York State about 1829. No information has been found regarding her parents, background, childhood, or early education. On October 24, 1848, then nineteen, she married George Guthrie in Rockton, Illinois. Ten years later, on April 13, 1858, still a resident of Rockton, she graduated from New York Hygeio-Therapeutic College with an MD degree. Neither of the Guthries is found in the 1860, 1870, or 1880 census. Nor has any other information about them been located.

References: Illinois Marriages to 1850; US census, 1850.

H

Lucinda Susannah *Capen* HALL (1815–90)

Lucinda Capen Hall was the first woman doctor to practice in New Hampshire. She was born July 13, 1815, on a farm near Stewartstown, on the Connecticut River in northern New Hampshire where the Canadian, Vermont, and New Hampshire borders meet. She was the fifth of nine children, fourth of six daughters (one was her twin) of Ebenezer and Abigail Carter Capen. When she was ten, the family returned to Concord, New Hampshire, from whence they had come in 1806. It was here that Lucinda received a common school education.

At eighteen, on July 4, 1833, she married her neighbor Robert Hall, at the North Congregational Church. The Rev. Nathaniel Bouton performed the ceremony. (Thirty-three years later, Mr. Bouton's son would marry the Halls' daughter, and much of the information here available came from the son of that couple, Tilton Clark Hall Bouton.) The newly married couple lived for two years in Loudon, just east of

Concord. They moved back to Concord, where they lived for the next seven years and where their two children were born, Ann Louesa, on June 21, 1834, and Tilton Clark, on July 7, 1839. At this time, Robert was making his living as a maker and purveyor of patent medicines.

About 1842, though the medicine business was doing well, Robert decided he wanted to learn more about the diseases he was treating, and he became an assistant to Dr. Lemuel Paige (1807–57), a physician in South Weare, a village a dozen miles southwest of Concord and to which the Halls moved. By 1847, Robert was sufficiently proficient to be a pharmacist in Concord. In the meantime, Lucinda took to reading the medical books in the doctor's library and, as one thing led to another, decided she wanted to become a doctor. There were then no medical schools to which a woman could go, so she enrolled in the Boston Female Medical College, an unchartered precursor of New England Female Medical College, from which she received a certificate of proficiency in midwifery. Instruction started November 1, 1848; while at the school, Lucinda lived with her maternal uncle, Dr. Thomas Carter, in East Boston. The course completed, she returned to Concord and practiced midwifery. She was long the only certified midwife in the state.

While this was going on, Worcester Medical Institution had been established in 1846, and, partly under the urging of Lucinda's uncle, it was persuaded to accept women in 1852. Lucinda was one of the first three matriculants and, with three years practical clinical experience and her midwifery certificate, was able to receive her MD degree after one lecture course, given June 23, 1852. This was the first MD awarded to a woman by a school in New England. While at the school she advertised her services as midwife to the local community. Her husband had matriculated with her but, having no prior credentials, was required to take three lecture courses.

Encouraged to do so by her Worcester professor of surgery, Walter Burnham (MD, University of Vermont, 1829), who lived and practiced in Lowell, Massachusetts, the Halls moved to Lowell, 120 Merrimac Street, and both went into practice. Lucinda is listed as an MD in Lowell directories for 1855, 1856, and 1857. But misfortune was to befall the couple. On October 11, 1856, their seventeen-year-old son was killed by accidental discharge of his gun while hunting near Concord. On January 2, 1857, less than three months later, their daughter Ann died. Ann had married at sixteen, moved to Ohio, where she and her husband contracted cholera; he died. She returned to Concord and in 1856 married the Rev. Mr. Bouton's son, had a baby, but died two months later, January 2, 1857, as not long after did young Mr. Bouton, also. The grandparents raised the child, who, in due course, became a minister. He is the source for much of what is known about the grandparents.

The devastated parents left Lowell and returned to Concord in 1857, bought a small house on Birchdale Springs Road, and continued to practice medicine. According to their grandson, Lucinda was more enthusiastic about their work than was Robert. Her practice was mostly obstetrics and diseases of women. She continued to see some of her old patients in Lowell and even in Boston.

In 1866, the Halls bought land across the road from their house, where were located the Birchdale mineral springs, and built a sanitarium. This was not a water-cure but a home for convalescents and chronic cases—a large, three-storied, cupolaed structure that could accommodate fifty patients. It opened in 1867 and soon became a popular temperance health resort. The Halls sold the hotel and several outbuildings in 1877 but continued to live in the house until 1892. Early Sunday afternoon, July 27, 1885, the hotel and all the outbuildings burned to the ground within an hour's time, a loss of $20,000 as well as most of the guests' belongings.

Earlier, Lucinda had developed respiratory disease with hemorrhages in 1866, so her practice was limited thereafter, but although afflicted she continued to accept obstetrical cases, in Boston and Lowell as well as in Concord. She also visited former sanitarium patients. After 1876, she saw only old patients but continued active practice until shortly before her death at seventy-five of a cerebrovascular accident, on August 27, 1890. Her husband, Robert, died in 1902, at ninety-one. They are buried in Millville Cemetery, three miles west of the State House.

Various sources attest to the "high regard in which she [Lucinda] was held in the community, both professionally and personally" and report the enthusiasm she showed for her work. Robert was similarly respected.

References: Grace P. Amsden, *A Capital for New Hampshire* (Concord, 1961); Obituary, *Concord Daily Monitor*, January 10 (or 12), 1902 [quotes extensively from an interview with Dr. Hall some years earlier by a reporter from the *Boston Globe*]; Obituary, *Concord Evening Monitor*, August 28, 1890; Frederick C. Waite, "Dr. Lucinda Susannah (Capen) Hall," *New England Journal of Medicine* 210 (1934): 644–47.

Susan Emily *HALL* Barry (1826–1912)

Susan Hall, one of the earliest to volunteer as a nurse during the Civil War, was born in Minisink, Orange County, New York, on March 19,

1826, the eighth of ten children (seven girls, three boys) of Lewis Hall and his wife Mary Cory. The Halls were natives of Orange County where Mr. Hall farmed. Each of them had ancestors who fought in the Revolution. In 1844, the family migrated one hundred miles westward to Tompkins County, on New York's Southern Tier, and settled in Ulysses. By the middle 1850s, seven of Susan's eight surviving siblings were married and gone, her younger brother Gilbert was at college at Louisiana State, mother Mary had died, and her father was too infirm to run the farm, which was sold. Susan had been doing missionary work among the Choctaw Indians with her friend Harriet Dada. Then almost thirty years old, she followed her eldest brother, Jonathan, and her sister Eliza Jane (q.v.) into the medical profession. She enrolled at New York Hygeio-Therapeutic College, where Eliza Jane had studied a few years earlier and graduated with an MD degree on March 29, 1859. The 1860 census found her living in Rosamund, Christian County, in central Illinois, with her next-older sibling, Hannah Rosamund Hawley.

At the start of the Civil War, Dr. Elizabeth Blackwell, recognizing that there would be a need for nursing (as the military authorities apparently did not) called for a mass meeting to be held at Cooper Union in New York City on April 24, 1861. At the meeting, attended by four thousand, women were urged to enroll as nurses under the aegis of the newly organized Ladies' Central Relief Association of New York, whose purpose was to care for soldiers in the Union army. It was the hope of the organizers to expand the group into a National Sanitary Commission. President Lincoln, at first, thought the women would be a "fifth wheel" but later, on June 13, relented. Susan, and Harriet Dada, volunteered at once, underwent examination, took a two-month course in wound dressing and general nursing at Bellevue Hospital.

On Sunday, July 21, 1861, the Battle of Bull Run took place. News of the disaster reached New York the next day. At noon, Susan and Harriet received orders. At 6 p.m. they were on a train to Washington, where they reported to Dorothea Dix, who was in charge of all nurses. She directed them to Alexandria, Virginia. They arrived next evening and went to work in an old seminary building turned hospital, caring for casualties from Bull Run. For the next four years the two women would labor, usually together, in many different hospitals, with poor food, little rest, and no furlough. After a couple of weeks at Seminary Hospital, Harriet found time to write letters in which she described the situation, later related by Brockett and Vaughan (1867): "There they lay, the wounded, some on beds, many on mattresses spread upon the floor, covered with blood from their wounds, and the dust of that burning summer battle-field, many of them still in their uniforms" (432).

In her later memoir Harriet Dada related that "we had wounds to dress with water every hour; faces, hands, and feet to wash, beds to arrange, food and water to distribute, medicines to give, and, in fact, everything to do for the sick and wounded." The hospital, of course, was in Virginia, and Southern whites did not visit the patients; blacks did, bringing gifts and moral support. Among the clergy, only the local Roman Catholic priest came. The nurses played an important role as chaplains in addition to their other duties. "No soldiers were detailed as attendants for the first few weeks, and even the most menial duties fell upon these ladies. Sometimes a contraband was assigned them as assistant, but he soon tired of steady employment and left. They had little sleep and food and that was neither tempting nor sufficient. . . . A busy month passed thus, and then the numbers in the hospital began to decrease, many of the convalescent being sent North, or having fur-loughs, till only the worst cases remained" (Brockett, 432–33). Soon, however, soldiers with typhus began to arrive at the hospital. Miss Dada further relates:

> It is well known that from the first there was opposition to having female nurses in the hospitals. Surgeon-General Finley was always opposed to them, and many others under him felt the same. This subjected us to more or less annoyance. One of the surgeons in this new hospital [in Alexandria, to which they had just moved] said to one of the ladies: "A lady ceases to be a lady when she becomes a nurse." In March 1862, Hall and Dada moved to still a third hospital, just opened in a couple of large residences, one with eighty-two beds, the other with sixty-one beds, with Dada in charge of one, and Hall the other. Both were filled with soldiers with measles, mostly from the Fifth Michigan. (Raus, 16)

Early in April 1862, Miss Dada and Dr. Hall were ordered to Winchester in northern Virginia, to care for those wounded in the recent battle in which Stonewall Jackson was defeated. They worked at three different hospitals, staying the longest at the third and only there getting to know the patients. On May 22 they were sent to nearby Strasburg, but the rebels returned and the nurses had soon to retreat to Winchester with their patients. Even there, however, they were soon prisoners in their hospital with a rebel guard surrounding it. This was the only time in the war in which they were directly involved in hostilities.

The two women had arrived in Winchester two weeks after the battle.

> We found everything very much unsettled in the Union Hotel hospital. Nothing was ready for the comfort of the wounded as they were brought in from the battlefield. On Monday, after the battle, thirty-seven had died in this hospital. For days they laid on the floor. The Confederate women brought things for their wounded, but passed ours by. . . . In the ward to which I was assigned were eight who had been severely wounded, and the nurses had been bathing all their wounds from one basin of water, which set on a table in the center of the room. . . . Why the surgeon had not instructed them to do differently, I never knew. (Raus, 18)

Susan, in spite of hardships, apparently was doing well. In June 1862, her twenty-two-year-old nephew, Henry H. Hall, a Union soldier posted in Winchester, was surprised to encounter his aunt at the Union Hotel hospital. Writing to his fifteen-year-old brother back home in New York State, he related that "she is looking very well I think in consideration of the arduous duties she has to perform." In August, the two nurses were reassigned to Armory Square Hospital in Washington to care for the wounded from the second battle at Bull Run. After the battle at Antietam in September, Hall and Dada were separated, with Susan going to Antietam. In November, the two were working together again, having moved to Harper's Ferry, where the medical director of the Twelfth Army Corps had opened a hospital.

> The next day the sick and wounded from the regimental hospitals were brought in. They had suffered for lack of care . . . many of them had long been ill, and want of cleanliness and vermin had helped to reduce them to extreme emaciation. Their filthy clothes were replaced by clean ones, and burned or thrown into the river, their heads shaven, and their revolting appearance removed. But many a youth whom sickness and suffering had given the appearance of old age, succumbed to disease and suffering, and joined the long procession to the tomb. These were sad days, the men were dying rapidly. (Brockett, 435)

In the late spring of 1863, Hall and Dada were at Acquia Creek caring for the wounded from the battle of Chancellorsville, and by July 8 they had moved to Gettysburg: "Miss Dada at the hospital of the Twelfth Army Corps, at a little distance from the town, and Miss Hall at that of the First Army Corps, which was within the town. The hospital of the Twelfth Army Corps was a farmhouse. The house and barns were filled with wounded, and tents were all around, crowded with sufferers, among whom were many rebel prisoners, who were almost overwhelmed with astonishment and gratitude to find that northern ladies would extend to them the same care as to the soldiers of their own army" (Brockett, 436).

In December of that year, the two women were ordered to Murfreesboro, Tennessee, a city by then in shambles as a result of the war.

> Two Seminaries, and a College, large blocks of stores, and a hotel, had been taken for hospitals, and were now filled with sick and wounded men. A year had passed since the awful battle of Stone River . . . but the hospitals had never been empty. When they arrived, they reported to the medical director, who "did not care whether they stayed or not, [but] if they remained wished them to attend exclusively to the preparation of the Special Diet." They received only discouraging words from all they met. They found shelter for the night at the house of a rebel woman, and were next day assigned—Miss Hall to No. 1 Hospital, Miss Dada to No. 3.

The surgeon at No. 1 Hospital told them the chaplain thought "they had better not remain." They were coldly received "and it was evident that the Surgeons and chaplains were very comfortable, and desired no outside interference." The ladies saw that they were needed and stayed. Some of the patients had been recently wounded at Lookout Mountain, others remained from Chickamauga. When a doctor they had known at Gettysburg visited in January, he told the medical director that he knew two of the ladies (Hall and Dada) from before. The director's response: "We have no ladies here! A hospital is no place for a lady. We have some women here, who are cooks" (Brockett, 436–37).

Finally, in May 1864, the two were sent to Chattanooga, where their reception and working conditions were better. Patient outcomes were dreadful, however. In one of the hospitals, "not a large one, and containing but seven hundred beds, there were two hundred sixty-one deaths in the month of June, and there were from five to twenty daily." November brought many new patients, wounded in Sherman's advance on Atlanta. In March, the following spring, came many soldiers with measles. One of them, who would die a few days after his arrival, said, "You are the *God-blessedest* woman I ever saw." Of fifty-three deaths on one of the wards, thirty-seven were from measles (Brockett, 438).

It had been four long years of constant work, no respite, and often lack of respect and cooperation from the surgeons. It is not clear how much help Susan's medical training was to her. Harriet Dada, who would go to medical school after the war (MD, 1868, Medical College and Hospital for Women) and who would practice medicine as a homoeopath in Syracuse for thirty years, seemed quite as qualified as Susan in their nursing role. Medicine was primitive: surgeons amputated, sometimes with ether or whiskey, and prescribed morphine for pain. Nurses bathed, fed, and consoled. Most patients died from infection. The importance of asepsis was yet to be recognized. The bathing was probably one of the most important therapeutic modalities, though it usually first came after an infection was established.

The end of the war found Dr. Hall's health permanently impaired. She left Chattanooga and spent the winter at Our Home on the Hillside, Dr. James Jackson's increasingly well-known water-cure in Dansville, New York, seeking rest and recovery. The following year, in Homer, New York, she married Robert E. Barry of Chicago. Barry had been a soldier in the Chicago Board of Trade Light Artillery Battery. Susan had cared for him after he was shot. Barry, born in England, had immigrated in 1857, and was a bookkeeper by profession. The couple moved to San Francisco and, in 1869, had a child who died at birth. From 1867, Robert worked as a bookkeeper for Moss & Beadle and later for T. H. Hatch & Company. Apparently unable to continue this work because of his drinking problem, he worked as a traveling salesman from 1874 until 1879. In 1875, he had a stroke while in Virginia City, Nevada. Susan took him home and nursed him. After 1879, he is listed in directories as bookkeeper, but it is not certain that he was able to work. Though he had recovered from his war wounds, he suffered from "battle fatigue" or what is today called "posttraumatic stress syndrome" and was alcoholic as well. In her pension application Susan stated that "Robert had a defective memory . . . his nervous system was shattered . . . he suffered intensely with his neuralgia."

The couple lived at 21 Prospect Place from 1872 until 1898. Robert probably went to the Sawtelle Veteran's Home in Los Angeles at that time. Susan is listed as a resident of the Alms House in 1895 and 1896, and she probably moved to Pasadena after this time. She is not listed as a physician in any directory consulted: Butler, Polk, or San Francisco directories. It seems almost certain that she never practiced medicine after her Civil War nursing career. That contention is supported by family tradition. Robert died in 1906 at the Veteran's Home. Susan died in Pasadena on March 15, 1912. She is buried at Rosedale Cemetery, Los Angeles, in a plot owned by the local Women's Relief Corps of Stanton Post, GAR, of which Susan was a member. Her tombstone says, "Susan E. H. Barry, US Army Nurse," nothing more.

References: L. P. Brockett, *Woman's Work in the Civil War* (Philadelphia, 1867), 431–39; Clifford Hall, "Descendancy Narrative of Lewis (Robert) Hall," typescript [Hall is a grandnephew of Susan Hall Barry]; Henry H. Hall, ALS, Winchester, VA, June 11, 1862, to Thomas Fisher Hall, Spencer, NY, transcribed by Clifford Hall; San Francisco directory, 1867–99; Rosamund Hawley, Biographical sketch of her sister Susan Barry, *Marinette Eagle-Star*, March 8, 1918; Edmund J. Raus Jr., *Ministering Angel: The Reminiscences of Harriet A. Dada, a Union Army Nurse in the Civil War* (Gettysburg, PA, 2004); Obituary, *San Jose Mercury News*, March 17, 1912; Obituary of Harriet Dada Evans, *Syracuse Herald*, September 2, 1909; US census, 1850; Frances E. Willard, *A Woman of the Century: Fourteen Hundred-Seventy Biographical Sketches* (Buffalo, NY, 1893).

Mary Elizabeth *Baum* HANCHETT (1826–89)

Mary Baum was born February 10, 1826, in Minden, Montgomery County, New York, the fourth of ten children (second daughter) of the Rev. John Philip Baum, a Methodist minister, and his wife, Magdelena Elwood. A younger brother, Adam Clarke Baum (1832–88), was a physician, Civil War surgeon, banker, businessman, travel agent for the West Shore Railroad, and in the Castoria business. A son, Stephen A. Douglas Hanchett (1860–88), was a physician (MD, Long Island College Hospital School of Medicine, 1882) but died prematurely, and a grandson, Charles Hanchett Hitchcock (1896–?), became an internist in Syracuse (BS, Amherst, 1917; MD, Johns Hopkins, 1921). A nephew, L. Frank Baum, was author of the Oz books.

Mary attended Albany Academy, graduated in 1848, returned to the Syracuse area, and soon attended Syracuse Medical College, an Eclectic school, from which she received an MD degree on March 17, 1852. According to her obituary, she also attended medical lectures while at the academy in Albany. While at medical school she met and married a fellow student, Sylvanus Dyer Hanchett (1828–1912), who was a year ahead of her. They had nine children, six of whom died before the age of five.

The couple moved to Chittenango, New York, in 1852, and together practiced medicine for the next four decades. In 1871, they built a large brick house on the Main Street, where they lived until their deaths, after which the house continued for many years as the home of physicians. (By 1989, it had become a law office.) An interesting insight regarding the attitude of the public toward woman doctors appears in Mary's obituary. Writing of the success of her practice, it said, "She has been of much value to her husband in his professional work."

An active member of the Methodist Church, she was for many years secretary of its Woman's Foreign Missionary Society. It was while giving a paper at a meeting of this group at her house, a year before she died, that she had the first symptoms of the cerebro-vascular disease that would cause her death at sixty-three a year later, on July 19,

1889. That was a bad year for the family. Her doctor brother and a younger sister both died, and her twenty-eight year-old son died, just six months out of medical school.

Bibliography: "Woman: Her Sphere and Influence," *American Medical and Surgical Journal*, April 1851, 77–78; "Medical Reform," *American Medical and Surgical Journal*, December 1851, 238.

References: Frank J. Baum, "Baum Genealogy," typescript (1958), Syracuse Public Library; "Dr. Hanchett," *Madison County Times*, April 14, 1876; Obituary, *Madison County Times*, July 26, 1889; Marriage notice, *Syracuse Medical Journal*, December 1851, 249; Personal communication from Richard F. Sullivan, Chittenango Village Historian, March 13, 1989.

Sarah Gates *Farnsworth* HARRINGTON (1816–99)

Sarah Farnsworth was born December 3, 1816, in Worcester County, Massachusetts, the daughter of a Mr. Farnsworth (given name unknown) and Mina Gates. Nothing is known of her childhood, education, or how many siblings she had. In 1838, she married Maverick Wilder Harrington, a maker of chairs. Over the next twenty years they had six children: Frances Amelia (b. 1839), Maverick Irving (b. 1842), Stillman Benjamin (b. 1844), Sarah L. (b. 1848), Asa Nelson (b. 1852), and Ezra (b. 1859). Sometime between 1850, when they were living in Westminster, a village west of Worcester, Massachusetts, and 1852, when Asa was born, the family moved west into New York State. The 1860 census shows them living in Florence, a hamlet in Oneida County, north of Oneida Lake.

In the late 1850s, Sarah attended the New York Hygeio-Therapeutic College and graduated from that school on May 29, 1859, with an MD degree. The exact date of baby Ezra's birth that year is not known, but presumably Sarah was carrying him during the three months she was at medical school. By 1862, the family had moved to Oswego, thirty miles to the west of Florence, and then a thriving port on Lake Ontario, with a canal connecting it to the Erie Canal. An 1862 Oswego city directory lists Sarah as a physician there and her husband as a chair maker, living at 152 East Second Street. The *Herald of Health* for February 1863 reported that Dr. Harrington was "practicing successfully in Oswego." The IRS tax roll for May 7, 1863, showed Dr. Harrington paid a ten-dollar tax as a practicing physician. The month before this, the same journal published the following advertisement:

> Mrs. Dr. S. G. F. Harrington, Hygienic Physician, would invite the citizens of Oswego, who wish to get well when sick without having their systems filled with poisonous drugs, to curse them for a lifetime—and those who would learn how to live so as not to be sick—to give her a call. She is ready at all times to attend cases of midwifery, and all female diseases, feeling confident that her thorough knowledge, long experience, and excellent success in this branch of medical science, justify her in warranting satisfaction to all who need her assistance. She treats most successfully those terrible and much dreaded diseases, Diptheria [*sic*], Scarlatina [*sic*], Croup, Measles, Worms, and all diseases with which children are afflicted. Baths given at her residence whenever desired. Office and residence, 152 East Second Street. Consultation free.

Oswego was apparently not a success. The 1870 census found the family in Newburgh, Ohio. By 1880, Maverick and Sarah had settled in Meridian, Michigan, a suburb of Lansing, where they would spend the rest of their lives. In Meridian, Maverick is no longer denoted a chair maker in census records but a farmer. Two of his sons, thirty-one-year-old Benjamin and twenty-eight-year-old Nelson, both single and living at home, were farm laborers, presumably on the family farm. Sarah probably continued to practice medicine in Newburgh and Meridian, although no evidence to document this assumption has been found. In none of the census entries is Sarah listed as a physician, although it was then common practice for women physicians to be listed simply as "keeping house," especially if their husbands were physicians. Her name is not found in the 1874 and 1877 Butler medical directories or the 1886 Polk medical directory. However, she was denoted a physician on her death certificate and in the Michigan Deaths and Burials Index 1867–1995. Maverick died in 1889. Sarah died in Meridian, March 17, 1899, at eighty-two and is buried at Glendale Cemetery, Okemos, Ingham County, Michigan.

References: *Herald of Health* 1 (January 1863): 3; *Herald of Health* 35 (February 1863): 92; Oswego city directory, 1862; US census, 1850, 1860, 1870, 1880; US Internal Revenue Service tax roll, Oswego, NY, May 7, 1863; Sandra Moore, "Sarah Gates *Farnsworth* Harrington," August 21, 2012 (https://www.findagrave.com/cgi-bin/fg.cgi?page=gr&GRid=95705007).

Fidelia Rachel *HARRIS* Reid (1826–1903)

Fidelia Harris, or Rachel, as she was usually known, was born April 26, 1826, in Portland, Chautauqua County, in Western New York, the fourth of nine children, who, remarkably for the time, all lived to grow up. Her parents, Ebenezer Harris and Rachel Baldwin, first cousins, had come from Halifax, Vermont, and were pioneers in the Western New York area.

Rachel was educated in public and private schools and in the village academy. At the age of fourteen, she started teaching school and, as was the custom, "boarded around." She gained a reputation for managing unruly pupils without applying the rod. According to Cleave, "At seventeen she underwent a severe and painful operation on her neck to relieve a troublesome disfigurement caused by a frightful burn received in infancy." This experience influenced her to become a physician. She continued to teach to earn the money for medical school and in 1854 began her studies under a tutor. During the winter of 1855–56, she read medicine and practiced with Dr. Orrin Davis, then of Attica, New York, as her preceptor. Dr. Davis had been professor of obstetrics at Central Medical College. Rachel attended formal lectures at Eclectic College of Medicine in Cincinnati and received an MD degree in 1857.

Moving to Beaver Dam, Wisconsin, she set up practice and remained for ten years. On Sunday evening, July 1, 1860, at her father's house in Fredonia, New York, she married Hiram A. Reid. Reid, orphaned in infancy, had learned the printing trade, attended college with the aid of a Congregational parish in Boston, and somewhere along the line qualified as a clergyman. The young couple (she was thirty-four and he a mere twenty-six) returned to Beaver Dam.

In May 1861, a few weeks after the firing on Fort Sumter, Rachel, with the approval of the governor and other state officials, organized a group of army nurses "ready to go to any point for service at a day's notice." Later, in September 1861, she was called to St. Louis by Dorothea Dix, then national superintendent of volunteer women nurses, and became, it was said, the first woman in the West to be mustered into the army hospital service.

There, she helped to establish, under the auspices of the government officers and the Sanitary Commission, "the Fifth, the Fourth Street, and the Marine Hospitals. The *Progressive Annuals* for 1862, 1863, and 1864 all locate her at St. Louis Army Hospital. She also acted for a time as agent of the Sanitary Commission in visiting and distributing supplies to the Ironton, Pilot Knob, and Victoria Hospitals; and for a month had charge of the Post Hospital at Sulphur Springs" (Cleave). In June 1862, "with broken health, through labors in caring for the sick and wounded from the battle of Pittsburg Landing, she was compelled to return home."

In 1869, the Reids moved to Nebraska City, apparently in search of better health. Rachel had still not resumed full practice. Rachel taught black freedmen, aged five to fifty, in a mission school supported by the city school board and the Episcopal Church. Hiram did newspaper work. In 1874, a scourge of grasshoppers destroyed almost everything, and the couple moved to Des Moines, where they would remain for the next nine years. For one of those years Rachel was special lecturer to "lady students" at Drake University and lecturer on diseases of children at the medical school. Hiram attended lectures at the medical school and, in 1883, received an MD degree.

In 1883, the Reids moved to California in company with former governor Samuel Merrill and his family, patients of Dr. Rachel. In California, the couple continued an active life. Hiram became principal editor of the *Pasadena Standard* and wrote a history of Pasadena. Both Reids were active in temperance work and in keeping Pasadena a "dry" community. When Rachel was over sixty-five, she and Hiram climbed nearly to the top of Precipicio Peak "over craggy peaks, and along spaces thickly strewn with sharp angular fragments of rocks and through thorny chapparal."

Though not listed in either Butler directory (1874, 1877) or the first Polk directory (1886), both Hiram's and Rachel's names are found regularly in the six Polk directories (1890–1902) as active practitioners. Rachel was probably the more active of the two. Rachel often lectured to women "on physiological and hygienic matters of special concern to them." Though they had no children, later in life they adopted the widowed Olive Douglas and, upon her premature death, assumed responsibility for raising her two small daughters, Verna and Helen. After watching a parade on New Year's Day, Rachel developed pneumonia. She died at seventy-three, on January 7, 1903. Later, two years to the day, Hiram married the widow Magoon.

References: Thomas L. Bradford, "Homoeopathy in Wisconsin," in *History of Homoeopathy and Its Institutions in America*, W. H. King (New York: Lewis Publishing Co., 1905); Cleave, 394; 40th wedding anniversary, *Pasadena Daily News*, June 30, 1900, and July 3, 1900; Obituary, *Pasadena Daily News*, January 8, 1903; Hiram A. Reid, *History of Pasadena* (Pasadena: Pasadena History Co., 1895).

Lucy Amelia *Brown* HARRIS (1818–59)

Lucy Brown, was born December 16, 1818, and raised in North Stonington, Connecticut, the fifth of eight children of Christopher Brown and his wife Charlotte Pendleton. Nothing is known of her early education. On April 3, 1838, when she was nineteen, Lucy married Benjamin Niles Harris Jr. (b. 1808), eldest son of a Baptist clergyman. The couple lived in North Stonington until the early 1840s, when they moved to Boston, and then on to Rockport, Massachusetts, in the late 1840s, and finally, in the early 1850s, to Waterville, Maine. Benjamin and Lucy had seven children, three girls and four boys. The second boy, Charles Franklin, born in 1847, died the following year. Two other children, the eldest, Mary Ann Brown Harris, and the youngest, Benjamin Franklin Harris, died in 1864.

After the family moved to Waterville and the death of infant son Charles Franklin (1848), Lucy decided to go to medical school, enrolling at New England Female Medical College in Boston. She graduated with an MD degree in 1854. The Brown genealogy states that Lucy practiced medicine in Boston, Rockport, and Waterville. If this is correct, she must have been practicing medicine before becoming a doctor. (Neither the Waterville Public Library nor the Waterville Historical Society were able to provide any information about Lucy as a local physician during the 1850s, partly because the local newspaper, the *Waterville Mail*, did not go back to that time.) Lucy probably practiced medicine in Waterville from 1854 to 1859. She died July 26, 1859, at the age of forty.

References: Cyrus H. Brown, *Brown Genealogy*, vol. 1 (Boston: Everett Press Co., 1907), 108; Vital Records of North Stonington, New London County, Connecticut, book 1, p. 178.

Mary Ann *HARRIS* Butler (1813–1906)

Mary Ann Harris was born October 30, 1813, in Troy, a village in southwest New Hampshire, near Keene. Her parents were Luke Harris, a Troy entrepreneur, and his wife, Polly Whitney. Mary Ann attended either the academy or the medical school in Worcester, Massachusetts (which is not clear), and later went to the New England Female Medical College in Boston, graduating with an MD degree in 1859.

She apparently stayed in Boston for a while; her name appears in Boston directories for 1859, 1860, and 1861, and she is denoted a doctor of medicine. She moved to North Abington, Massachusetts, for the next three years. Abington was a small community south of Boston where, during the Civil War, half of the boots used by men in the Union army were made. After this brief period, she moved back to her native Troy, either because of poor health (as was claimed) or because her practice was not thriving. In Troy, she practiced, at least in summer, for the next few years.

In 1869, then fifty-six, she married Jabez Butler, a sash and blind maker who had five probably grown children by his first wife, who had died. It is said that Dr. Butler gave up practice after marriage. The family moved to south central Vermont, where they lived for at least twenty years either in Plymouth Union or North Shrewsbury. Subsequent knowledge of Dr. Butler depends on Walton directories. She is listed as a physician in Plymouth Union from 1877 to 1883, moved to nearby North Shrewsbury in 1884 (Child's directory) but is not listed in Walton directories as a physician there until 1888–92, then back to Plymouth Union in 1894 and 1895. Since she listed herself as a physician, it is presumed that she was in practice during these years. The original town clockworks in her native Troy were the gift of Dr. Butler. The clock was razed in 1938 because the steeple had rotted. Dr. Butler died at the home of Marshall Adams in Marlborough, New Hampshire, on May 27, 1906, and is buried in Troy. She was ninety-two and a half years old.

References: Charles A. Bemis, *History of the Town of Marlborough, Cheshire County, N.H.* (Boston: G. H. Ellis, 1881), 434–35; Hamilton Child, *Gazetteer & Business Directory of Windsor County, Vermont* (Syracuse, 1884); Obituary, *Keene Evening Sentinel* (New Hampshire), May 28, 1906; John W. King, "Early Women Physicians in Vermont," *Bulletin of the History of Medicine* 25 (1951): 429–41; M. T. Stone, *Historical Sketch of the Town of Troy, New Hampshire, and Her Inhabitants . . . 1764–1897* (Keene, NH: Sentinel Printing Co., 1897), 277–78; Boston city directories, 1859, 1860, 1861; *Walton's Vermont Register.*

Rachel *Hamlin* HARRIS (1833–89)

Rachel Hamlin was born in Washington, Pennsylvania, in 1833. Information about her parents, childhood, and education has not been found. On February 17, 1854, in Warren, Iowa, she married Ephraim Harris. Harris was born in 1827 at Harrisville, Butler County, Pennsylvania. As a young man he had apprenticeships with two different physicians in Pennsylvania and practiced medicine there for a year before moving to Farmington, Iowa, where he practiced for a year before moving in March 1855 to Grinnell, Iowa, which became the permanent home of the couple. In 1856, he graduated from New York Medical College with an MD degree. At the same time Rachel attended and graduated from New York Hygeio-Therapeutic College.

Both Ephraim and Rachel practiced medicine in Grinnell for the rest of their lives. Ephraim as listed in Polk directories for 1886,

1890, and 1896; Rachel is listed in 1886. The United States census rolls for 1860, 1870, and 1880 record only Ephraim as a physician; Rachel, as was often then the case with women physicians, was listed as "keeping house." *The History of Poweshiek County* (1880) states that Rachel was a practicing physician. In 1870, Rachel received a second medical degree from Chicago's Hahnemann Medical College and Hospital.

The couple raised four sons: Luther C., Willard H., Arthur J., and Clinton Ephraim. Arthur became a physician (Bennett, MD, 1887) as did Clinton (Rush, MD, 1899). Willard was a pharmacist. Rachel died in 1899 at the age of sixty-six.

References: *The History of Poweshiek County Iowa: A History of the County, Its Cities, Towns, Etc.* (Des Moines: Union History Co., 1880); Polk, 1886, 1890, 1896; US census, 1860, 1870, 1880.

Sophia *Roper* HARRIS (1822–1916)

Sophia Roper was born May 14, 1822. She graduated from Worcester Medical College (Eclectic), Worcester, Massachusetts, with an MD degree in 1853 at age thirty-one. Since she is known to have lived and practiced medicine in Worcester from 1886 on, it is likely that she started practice there after graduating from medical school, but this is not documented.

Sometime prior to 1853, she married Gideon Harris, a cotton manufacturer. According to the 1900 and 1910 US census reports, Dr. Harris had two children, neither of whom were then living. They are not listed as part of the family in the 1870 census. Whether they had died by then or grown up and left home is not known.

Polk, AMA, and local directories list her as a physician at 76 Summer Street, Worcester from 1886 to 1906. She is not listed in Butler directories for 1874 and 1877. Husband Gideon had probably died before 1900; he is not listed in that census. About 1906, Sophia moved to 530 Park Avenue in Worcester. She died there of bronchopneumonia on March 23, 1916, at ninety-three years. She probably practiced medicine in Worcester from 1853 to 1906. A 1906 real estate record, probably made at the time of her husband's death or when the house was sold, valued the house at 76 Summer Street at $2,900, recorded a lot size of 14,806 feet, and attributed to her $4,100 in personal property.

References: *American Medical Directory*, Chicago, 1906; Massachusetts Vital Records; Polk, 1886 et seq.; US census, 1870, 1900, 1910; Worcester real estate record, 1906; Worcester city directories.

Amelia A. *HASTINGS* (1825–78?)

Amelia Hastings was born in Maine in 1825. She had at least one sibling, a sister, Clara, two years her senior. She probably grew up in Maine because she was still a resident of that state when she matriculated at Penn Medical University in Philadelphia. After receiving an MD degree in 1857, she moved to Baltimore to establish a medical practice there. The 1860 census and the 1863 and 1866 IRS tax rolls all place her in Baltimore and list her as "doctor" or "physician." An 1863 Baltimore city directory characterizes her as offering "homoeopathic medicines, etc."

In 1866, she moved to Springfield, Illinois. Local directories list her as a physician in 1866, 1868, and 1869. By 1870, she had moved to Quincy, Illinois, where she was living with the family of Charles and Lydia Clowes. It is not clear whether she practiced medicine in Quincy. No further information about her has been found. The death, on November 24, 1878, of an Amelia Hastings was recorded in Cook County. Whether it is the same person described here is uncertain.

References: Baltimore city directory, 1860; Springfield, IL, city directory, 1866, 1868, 1869; US census, 1869, 1870; US Internal Revenue Service tax rolls, May 1863, April 1866.

Esther Jane *Hill* HAWKS (1833–1906)

Esther Hill was born on August 4, 1833, in Hooksett, New Hampshire, the fifth of eight children of Parmensas Hill and Jane Kimball. Both of her grandfathers served in the Revolutionary War army. She attended public schools in Hooksett, Suncook, and Exeter; high school in Manchester; and the academy in Kingston, New Hampshire, and later taught in schools at Kingston, Merrimack, and Thornton's Ferry.

In October 1854, she and John Milton Hawks, MD, of Manchester, a man seven years her senior, were married. The young couple went on an extended wedding trip to Florida, sailing from New York to Tampa. They spent the winter in Manatee, and Esther taught in a local Methodist school. In the spring, they returned to Manchester by way of New Orleans; a Mississippi River boat to St. Louis; and rail to Manchester by way of Indianapolis, Terre Haute, and Niagara Falls. Esther had studied her husband's medical books by then and was able to give public lectures on physiology in Vicksburg and St. Louis, along the way. This added to the couple's meager funds but made Milton unhappy. Once home, Esther set up as a housekeeper and student in her husband's office, clerking in his drug store and visiting his patients. She enrolled at New England Female Medical College in Boston and graduated with an MD degree in 1857. For the next five years she practiced medicine in Manchester.

Just what motivated Esther to become a doctor is not clearly stated in her diary. She may have recognized that Milton's bent for reform would always stand in the way of his attention to full-time practice. Her temperament was certainly one that needed to be contributing. Milton was not happy with her becoming a physician. In later years he is quoted as saying, "I wish Ette had never seen a medical book, or heard a lecture. It is not a business man-like worker that a husband needs. It is a loving woman." They had no children, a matter of great regret to Esther. On May 1, 1864, she wrote in her diary, "What can be sadder than to pass through life with nothing to love. To live through the long weary months and years with an ever increasing yearning in the heart for some object dearer than all the world besides, on which to lavish the strong pure heart love. The mother love—dearer than all others! I have longed for this, prayed for it with all the passionate entreaty of a desolate nature. Why am I denied[?]"

In the summer of 1861, Esther went to Washington, hoping to serve the army as a doctor but was, of course, turned down. Then she applied for work as a nurse, again unsuccessfully. According to reports, Dorothea Dix thought her too attractive to serve. So, after caring for casualties from the first battle at Bull Run, Esther returned to Manchester and took over the practice of her husband. Milton, in addition to being a physician, was an abolitionist and social reformer at heart, and had gone to Haiti, where for six months he looked after freed slaves who had moved there.

In the fall of 1862, Milton was appointed surgeon in charge of the First General Hospital for Blacks at Beaufort, South Carolina. Esther joined him there and became a schoolteacher for blacks, adults and children, from Beaufort and the adjacent Sea Islands, an area in Union hands. Union women were then allowed in the Southern area only in the role of teacher, but Esther did practice medicine as well, caring mainly for black Union soldiers. She thought the military officials in Washington did not care about the black regiments. She later recalled a twenty-one-year-old black ex-slave, Charlie Reason, as "noble looking" and "uncomplaining" even after an arm was amputated. "The majesty and mistery [*sic*] of death stole over his face, fading the eager look from his giant mournful eyes, and clinging close to my hand, with a whispered 'pray with me,' he sank into unconsciousness" and died.

During the 1862–65 period, Esther often assisted her husband in surgery; when he was absent, she was in charge of the hospital. Life must have been difficult during those years. In her diary, Esther describes the bad behavior of Union soldiers, a corrupt quartermaster, and fighting off rats, among other unpleasantries. After the war, the couple moved to Port Orange, Florida, where Milton ran the Florida Land and Lumber Company, a nonprofit organization that built homes for freedmen (and others). By 1870, the organization was out of money and Esther returned to New England.

Now thirty-seven, she went into practice in Lynn with her medical school classmate, Lizzie Breed Welch. In 1874, she visited her husband, still in Florida and, after returning home, established her own office at 81 Broad Street, in Lynn, where she stayed for ten years until buying a house at 16 Newhall Street. There she would live and practice for the remaining twenty-two years of her life and where she died on May 6, 1906. She is listed as a practicing physician regularly until 1902.

Esther's community activities were legion. She was a member of the New England Hospital Medical Society, an honorary member of the New Hampshire Association of Military Surgeons, and a member of the Society for the Prevention of Tuberculosis. She was a founder and for many years an officer of Associated Charities of Lynn, a patron of Boys' Club, of Day Nursery, and of Reading and Rest Rooms. She was active in the woman's suffrage movement, worked forty years in the Woman Suffrage Club (of Lynn) formed in 1877, and was an officer in the Equal Rights Club. Add to these membership in the Civic League, the Lynn Woman's Club, the Lynn Historical Society, and the Houghton Horticultural Society. She served for six years (1889–95) as a member of the Lynn School Board. John Milton Hawks died in Florida, where he grew oranges, practiced medicine, and was considered a local patriarch.

Bibliography: *A Woman Doctor's Civil War, Esther Hill Hawks' Diary* (Columbia: University of South Carolina Press, 1984).

References: "Biographical Sketch of Esther Hill Hawks," undated two-page typescript at the Lynn Historical Society; Obituary, *Boston Medical and Surgical Journal* 154 (1906): 594–95; William R. Cutter, *Genealogical and Personal Memoirs Relating to the Families of Boston and Eastern Massachusetts* (New York: Lewis Publishing Co., 1908), 1:359–62; Lynn Historical Society, Register, 1907, 40–44; Jane E. Schultz, *Women at the Front* (Chapel Hill: University of North Carolina Press, 2004); Glenna R. Schroeder-Lein, *The Encyclopedia of Civil War Medicine* (Armonk, NY: M. E. Sharpe, 2008), 126–27.

Susan N. *HAYHURST* (1820–1909)

Susan was born December 25, 1820, at Attleboro (now Langhorne), Pennsylvania, the second of ten children. Her father was a teacher and a leader in the local Quaker community. At sixteen, she also became a teacher, apparently a very effective one. Katharine A. Williamson, chairman of the 1909 necrology committee for the Woman's Medical College of Pennsylvania, wrote Susan's obituary, describing visits in later years to various meetings in company with Dr. Hayhurst: "I was surprised to note the number of men and women coming to her, saying: 'I do not think thee remembers me, but I went to school when thee was teaching.' Many and gratifying were the expressions of appreciation of her efforts from these, her former pupils."

When Susan was in her midthirties, she matriculated at the Woman's Medical College of Pennsylvania and in 1857 received an MD degree. She never practiced medicine, possibly because of her health, but continued teaching in Friends and other schools. In 1876, at the age of fifty-six, she was put in charge of the Pharmacy Department at Philadelphia Woman's Hospital. Later, she attended the Philadelphia College of Pharmacy and, in 1883, was, if not the first, one of the earliest women to graduate in pharmacy. She continued as chief pharmacist at the hospital for thirty years. After retiring, she continued to live at the hospital where, after a brief illness, she died on August 7, 1909, in her eighty-ninth year. She is buried in Fairhill Cemetery not far from Dr. Ann Preston (q.v.).

References: Obituary, *Philadelphia Inquirer*, August 8, 1909; Woman's Medical College of Pennsylvania, Obituary, *Transactions of the 35th Annual Meeting of the Alumnae Association . . . June 2 and 3, 1910* (Philadelphia, 1910), 27–28.

Cornelia *Brown* SILL HEURTLEY (1829–66)

Cornelia Brown, known as Cora, was born in Wyoming County in Western New York, on March 25, 1829, the daughter of the Rev. George Brown, farmer and Methodist minister, and his first wife (of three), Mary A. Thomas (d. 1845). Cora had two younger brothers, William (d. 1861) and Benjamin (d. 1869). She moved to Dansville, New York, about 1849 and, sometime thereafter married Francis Barber Sill (b. 1826), a dentist. Sill died January 30, 1857. A couple of years later, Cora went to the New York Hygeio-Therapeutic College, a chartered medical school run on hydropathic principles. She graduated on March 31, 1860, with an MD degree. While at the school she met classmate Richard Walter Heurtley, and they were married on February 20, 1866, at St. Paul's Methodist Church, in Jersey City, New Jersey. Born November 2, 1811, in Portsmouth, England, Heurtley had been married before, to Ann L'Aker. The family, including four children, had immigrated to

Boston. After the bank at which Heurtley was working failed, his wife and two of the children returned to England. A son, Percy, emigrated to Argentina and had a large family. At medical school, Heurtley was valedictorian of the class.

After graduation, the couple moved to Boston, where Richard, and medical school classmate Charles H. Estabrook established a Turkish bath business, apparently without great success. While in Boston, the Heurtleys' only child, Arthur Heurtley, was born December 30, 1860. In 1862, the family moved to 233 (later 286) Grand St., Newburgh, New York, where Richard set up practice. There is no evidence that Cora practiced. She is not listed as a physician in local directories.

Cora died of consumption on December 4, 1866. Family tradition holds that she contracted tuberculosis while nursing Civil War soldiers. Lacking any documentation for this, one also wonders whether her first husband, who died at age thirty-one, or her mother or brothers, all of whom died prematurely, might not have had tuberculosis. She is buried in the Old Town Cemetery, Newburgh. Interestingly, her tombstone says only, "Cora Brown." Her death certificate does not mention that she was a physician. Only her husband is listed in 1864 and 1865 Newburgh directories, as a homoeopathic physician. So, it seems likely that Cora did not practice medicine. Richard moved to Chicago sometime before 1874 and is listed in the 1874 Butler directory as a homoeopathic physician at 81 S. Robey Street. He married a third wife and died May 30, 1891, in River Forest, Illinois.

References: *Portrait Biographical Album of Barry and Eaton Counties, Michigan* (Chicago, 1891), 374–75; Obituary, *Western New York Advertiser* (Dansville), December 13, 1866; Personal communication from Helen Heurtley Berkeley, Rochester, NY, great-granddaughter of Cora.

Ellen J. *HIGGINS* (1828–1904)

Ellen Higgins was born in Centerville, Allegany County, New York, in 1828, the elder daughter of at least three children of Russell Higgins and his wife, Laura Trall. Russell was one of the earliest settlers in Centerville, a village located in the northwest corner of the county in the Southern Tier of Western New York. He was a farmer, and, with a partner, he erected the first local gristmill in a nearby hamlet that came to be known as Higgins' Mill. One of Laura's younger brothers, Ellen's uncle Russell T. Trall, was the well-known hydropathic physician, writer, and principal of the New York Hygeio-Therapeutic College from which Ellen would graduate in 1858 with an MD degree.

After graduating, Ellen stayed on in New York City for her entire professional career. She may have returned briefly to Centerville—the 1860 census locates her there—but the 1862, 1863, and 1864 *Progressive Annuals* list her at 15 Laight Street in New York, the address of the New York Hygeio-Therapeutic College and its associated clinic. In the 1870 census she is denoted "physician" and is living in what appears to be a boarding house. Other tenants there include a fifty-year-old professor of languages, two schoolgirls aged sixteen and eighteen, a family of four in which the woman is housekeeper, and two other people. In the 1880 census, still in New York, she is listed as a physician and is living alone. According to the history of Centerville, she "attained considerable eminence as a physician, and practiced several years in the city of New York."

Sometime between 1880 and 1892, Higgins retired and returned to Centerville. She and two of her siblings were still living in the family home in 1896. Ellen died in 1904 and is buried in the family plot in Bates Cemetery in Centerville.

References: John S. Minard, "History of Centerville, New York," in *Centennial Memorial History of Allegany County, New York* (Alfred, NY: W. A. Fergusson & Co., 1896); New York State census, 1892; US census, 1860, 1870, 1880; *Water-Cure Journal,* February 1863, 51.

Minerva *Falley* HOES (1807–85)

Minerva Falley was born February 23, 1807, in Chester, Massachusetts, the seventh of eight children (three girls, five boys) of Daniel Falley and his wife, Elizabeth Mulholland. Sometime between Minerva's birth in 1807 and that of her younger brother James, in 1813, the family moved to Oswego Falls, in Oswego County, New York. In 1825, Minerva graduated from Cazenovia Seminary, a newly established school run by the Methodists in nearby Cazenovia.

On April 19, 1833, Minerva married the Rev. Schuyler Hoes (b. 1807), who had grown up in Ghent in the Hudson Valley, attended Cazenovia Seminary, graduated in 1828, and became a Methodist minister. He was pastor of the Methodist Church in Weedsport, New York, at the time of their marriage. Hoes was also an active abolitionist. Schuyler and Minerva had four children, three daughters and a son: Margaret E. (b. ca. 1834), Mary C. (b. ca. 1835), Frances E. (b. ca. 1841), and William F. F. (Willie; b. 1847 or 1850). The 1850 census shows the family living in Fulton, Oswego County. Schuyler is listed as having personal property of $1,500, and there is a fifteen-year-old girl, Martha Gaylord, living with them, probably a domestic.

In 1853, Schuyler died. Her husband dead, and with at least two children to support, Minerva matriculated at the Female Medical College of Pennsylvania, then attended the Syracuse Medical College, an Eclectic school nearer home, and graduated on June 8, 1854, with an MD degree. Her preceptor had been W. R. Bourne, MD.

Minerva's immediate course is not known, but a year later she was in Wheaton, Illinois, just west of Chicago. "Mrs. Minerva Hoes, M.D." is one of seven faculty members listed in the 1855 and 1856 circulars of the Illinois Institute, a newly organized Methodist seminary (and precursor to Wheaton College), where she taught anatomy, physiology, and botany. She apparently soon moved on to Mt. Vernon, Linn County, Iowa, home of Cornell College. No record has been found that she served on the Cornell faculty, and she is not designated as having been a physician in Mt. Vernon.

Minerva's whereabouts between 1860 and 1875 are not known. She was in Lafayette, Indiana, at least as early as 1875, lived there for a decade, and died there March 22, 1885, at the age of seventy-eight. Whether she practiced medicine in Iowa or Indiana has not been determined. Minerva's second daughter, Mary, received her early education at Falley Seminary at Fulton, New York. She was one of the first three students to graduate in 1852. She married Nathan M. Reynolds and died in Los Angeles on May 27, 1909 (*Oswego Daily Times*).

References: *Charter and Circular of Illinois Institute* (Wheaton, IL, 1856); Cornell College (Mt. Vernon, IA), *Catalogue*, 1856–69; *Oswego Daily Times*, June 3, 1909; William Reddy, *First Fifty Years of Cazenovia Seminary, 1825–75* (Cazenovia, NY, 1877); C. W. Richmond, *A History of the County of DuPage, Illinois* (Chicago: Scripps, Bross & Spears, 1857); US census, 1850, 1860.

Mary Mitchell *HOLLOWAY* Wilhite (1831–92)

Mary Holloway Wilhite was the first woman from Indiana to graduate from medical school and the first woman doctor to practice medicine in that state. She lived in Crawfordsville, the home of Wabash College (1832). In addition to her professional duties, she was also an active reformer in matters of temperance, tobacco, care of the poor, and women's rights. Mary was born February 3, 1831, near Crawfordsville, to Judge Washington Holloway and Elizabeth King. The judge had been born in Kentucky and his wife in Virginia. They met when she was seventeen, in her hometown of Alexandria, and eloped on horseback to Kentucky, bringing with them Elizabeth's "mammy," and were thereafter estranged from her family. The Holloways later moved to Indiana, where they had several children. Mary would spend her entire adult life in Crawfordsville. As a child, Mary was a good student. At fifteen, she "united with the Christian Church" and remained an active member throughout her life. When a young woman, she taught school for several years and did sewing in the hope of becoming self-supporting.

In 1854, she entered Penn Medical University, an Eclectic school in Philadelphia; she was twenty-three and a half at the time. Some of her reasons for deciding on a medical career may be found in a letter she wrote home from school on January 11, 1856: "I am tired of being dependent on others for my bread and butter. . . . I am sure there are many rewards awaiting for me in the future. And not me alone, for ere long woman, the last and noblest work of God, will take her own position in society. Man's equal she is and ere long will prove it. In that good time that is coming we will have no men . . . practicing medicine among the female and infantile portion of the community and woman sailing from sun to sun for sixpence."

Getting to school had itself been a substantial endeavor. In an 1855 letter she describes her return to school for the fall term. She and a companion, Mrs. Purcell, took the train due south from Crawfordsville to Greencastle. As they passed through the village of Bainbridge, she saw a Mr. Shell on the station platform. "He gave me a cold bow and not even so much as the shake of the hand," presumably expressing his disapproval of her professional undertaking. Arriving in Greencastle by four o'clock, her companion went to dinner, while Mary took herself and all their baggage to the other depot where she waited until 11:30 p.m. when they boarded the train for an hour's trip to Indianapolis. There, they waited until 3 a.m., when they left on the Union & Bellefontaine line for Crestline, Ohio, northeast of Columbus. Here they connected with the Pittsburgh, Ft. Wayne & Chicago line (soon to be part of the recently organized Pennsylvania Railroad system). They arrived in Philadelphia in time for supper that evening. Mary had eaten once during the trip, early that morning.

A substantial part of the cost of Mary's medical education was borne by J. Edgar Thomson, first president of the Pennsylvania Railroad and philanthropist who was on the board of the Penn Medical University and had set up a fund for such scholarships. Mary mentions in an 1856 letter that "Mr. Thomson had been absent for some time. I have seen him but once since I came to the city. My boarding is $2.50 per week but my fire and lights are extra. A few days after he called he sent me a check for 25 dollars. I have given my last dime to my good landlady. I have no fear that my friend will see me safe through college." But, in the meantime, she needed a pair of shoes and asks her father for the price.

In that same letter she writes, "I am improving rapidly in my studies yet how much remains to be learned." The term would end in four weeks, at which time she would be "arraigned before a dreaded tribune of thirteen professors. I am struggling on and hoping for the best." On June 2, 1856, after another term, she graduated with an MD degree. On June 26, she hung out her shingle in Crawfordsville, where her practice over the next thirty-six years would concentrate on midwifery and diseases of women and children.

Obituaries and other sources attest that she cared for all who sought her help, rich or poor, black or white. At first, she met great resistance from male members of the local profession and from the public at large, but this, as it did in most communities tested, gradually abated. At her death, the local medical society resolved

> that we, as physicians, fully recognize . . . that her life has been a sacrifice for the good of others. . . . No one was too poor to obtain her services, . . . no night was too dark, no storm too hard for her not to respond to calls where humanity demanded the services of a physician or friend. . . . She began her professional life when it was thought a disgrace for a woman to aspire to anything, except domestic duties, but she lived to see woman recognized in all the avenues of social and professional pursuits where man is permitted . . . by her labors as physician and humanitarian she has built a monument more lasting than can be carved in marble slab, or written on parchment scroll, and hundreds of poor people, who have been recipients of her charity, will reverence the name of Dr. Mary H. Wilhite. (published with her obituary in an unidentified newspaper, 1892)

In addition to her professional services, Mary was very active in the community, working for temperance, against tobacco, and, on a national level, in the woman's suffrage movement. Her interest in women's rights went back to her youthful days. In 1850, she canvassed for the first woman's rights newspaper, *Woman's Advocate* (Philadelphia). In later years, as a personal friend of Elizabeth Cady Stanton, Mary A. Livermore, and Susan B. Anthony, she arranged a convention in 1869 at which they all spoke. Conscious of the plight of many children, she was a prime mover in establishing a County children's home. Over a period of at least a dozen years (1869–80), Mary wrote columns for the local newspaper, the *Saturday Evening Journal*, on medical, social, and political subjects: the use of tobacco, the curse and the cure (whiskey and tobacco), dangerous drugs, the poor and needy, dissipation and poverty, God's poor, our girls, woman's rights, woman's wrongs, the Equal Suffrage Society, woman's suffrage convention. She also wrote poems.

When she was thirty, she married Eleazer A. Wilhite, a well-known tailor of Crawfordsville. Eleven years her senior, he had been previously married and had a son. He had come to Crawfordsville from Kentucky when he was four. He took up sewing by ten. Both parents were dead by the time he was eleven. He loved music, was in a local band, and had done well in his business. By 1880, he was said to have had between $15,000 and $20,000. Eleazer and Mary had seven children, four of whom survived to adulthood. Some of the children's names are of interest: J. Edgar Thomson Wilhite, Edward Longshore Wilhite, Stanton Livermore Wilhite. Mary died February 8, 1892, of pneumonia, at her home on West Wabash Avenue, Crawfordsville.

References: H. H. Beckwith, *History of Montgomery County* (Chicago: H. H. Hill, 1881); Unidentified clippings from Crawfordsville newspaper, including an obituary and Medical Society testimonial, provided by Ann Pearce, great-great-granddaughter of Dr. Wilhite; Mary Mitchell Holloway, Typed transcriptions of two letters to her parents dated October 11, 1855, and January 11, 1856, provided by Ann Pearce; *International Genealogical Index*, 1989; Various clippings from the *Saturday Evening Journal* (Crawfordsville, IN) 1869–80; Frances E. Willard, *A Woman of the Century* (Detroit: Gale Research Co., 1967).

Mary Ann Brown *HOMER* Arnold (1824–99)

Mary Ann Homer was born February 15, 1824 (and baptized May 2, 1824), in Brimfield, Massachusetts, the fourth daughter and fourth of six children of Linus Hoar and his wife Betsey Bond. Linus had fathered three children by his first wife, who had died, the eldest of whom was ten when Linus remarried. Functionally, this was a family of nine children. The family name had been Hoar, but when part of the family moved to Homer, New York, they assumed the surname Homer. The family in Brimfield, including Mary Ann's, soon followed suit (cf. Acts of the Massachusetts Legislature, 1831, 1834, 1838). Mary's ancestors had been contributors. Six generations back, Mary's Hoar forebear, John Hoar, was a lawyer described as "distinguished for his bold, independent mind and action." His older brother, Leonard, a Harvard graduate (1650), was pastor of Old South Church, Boston, and later became president of Harvard. Mary's grandfather saw action in the Revolution.

We know nothing of Mary's education, but it was probably the standard primary schooling of the day and a seminary or academy thereafter. She attended New England Female Medical College and graduated in 1859 with an MD degree. From 1860 to 1864 she served as physician and teacher of physiology at Mt. Holyoke Seminary in South Hadley, Massachusetts. In this position she had been preceded by Sophronia Fletcher, MD (q.v.). In the Mt. Holyoke archives is a letter home from student Adelaide Winter, class of 1864: "Dr. Homer (Miss) took such care [of a student with mumps] that not one young lady caught them from her."

On July 1, 1864, Dr. Homer was married at Brimfield, to Samuel D. Arnold, an iron manufacturer then living in Minneapolis, a city to which Mary then moved. The Arnolds were well off. The 1870 census shows Samuel holding real estate worth $30,000 and with $40,000 in personal assets. The Arnold household had a domestic servant in 1870 and 1880. The 1880 census also shows the Arnolds as having two children, Jessie, aged nine, and Howard D., aged four. The fact that Mary was fifty when Howard was born and that Howard was listed as having been born in Ohio to a mother born in Rhode Island raises the possibility that the children were adopted.

According to Louis Frank's *Medical History of Milwaukee*, Dr. Arnold practiced medicine in Milwaukee from 1889 to 1908. But what of the twenty-five years before that? She is not listed in any of the standard medical directories of the period (Butler 1874, 1877; Polk 1886). That she did, indeed, practice during the later period seems supported by listings of her name as a physician in directories of the later period (Polk 1890, 1893, 1896, 1898, and 1902 Milwaukee directory). Dr. Arnold died in Milwaukee, March 1, 1899, age seventy-four.

References: Butler, 1874, 1877; Louis F. Frank, *Medical History of Milwaukee 1834–1914* (Milwaukee: Germania Publishing Co., 1915); Charles M. Hyde, *Historical Celebration of the Town of Brimfield, Hampden County, Mass.* (Springfield, MA: C. W. Bryan Co., 1879), 415–17; Massachusetts, Acts of the Legislature, 1831, 1834, 1838; Massachusetts Vital Statistics to 1850 (Brimfield), 75; Polk, 1886, 1890, 1893, 1896, 1898, 1902; Milwaukee city directories; Marriage announcement, *Milwaukee Sentinel,* July 1, 1864; Mt. Holyoke College, *Annual Catalogue,* 1860–64; US census, 1870, 1880; Adelaide White, letter dated February 25, 1862, to unknown correspondent, Mt. Holyoke College Archives, South Hadley, MA; Mount Holyoke College, *General Catalogue of the Officers and Students* (South Hadley, MA, 1911).

Eliza Clark *HUGHES* (d. 1882)

The date of Eliza Hughes's birth is not known but was probably in the later 1820s. She was born in Wheeling, then part of Virginia but, after June 20, 1863, part of the new state of West Virginia. She was a child (one of three daughters and seven sons) born to Thomas Hughes and his wife Mary. Eliza's great-grandfather, Felix Hughes, a devout Roman Catholic, emigrated from Ireland in 1732. His son, James, moved westward to Greene County, Pennsylvania (then part of Virginia), and became a large landowner. His son, Thomas, father of Eliza, moved to Wheeling, where he was a member of the City Council for thirty-two years, president of the Wheeling Savings Bank, the Wheeling Life Insurance Company, the Wheeling and Belmont Bridge Company, and a director of another local bank.

After "a thorough English and collegiate education," Eliza began to delve into the medical books of her older brother who had graduated from the Homoeopathic Medical College in Philadelphia (organized 1849, became part of Hahnemann Medical College in 1869) and started practice in Wheeling in 1853. Having decided on a career in medicine, Eliza attended lectures at Western Homoeopathic College in Cleveland and later at Penn Medical University in Philadelphia, from which she graduated in 1860. She returned to Wheeling and started practice.

Brother Alfred, apparently a Southern sympathizer in that part of Virginia soon to become West Virginia, wrote articles for the *Baltimore Exchange*, was arrested for disloyalty, and was imprisoned at Camp Chase, near Columbus, Ohio, for eight months before being exchanged for a brother of a prominent Philadelphia physician who had been captured in Virginia. A letter written by Eliza in 1862 to her brother in captivity gives some idea of her medical practice:

> Aunt Cynthia sent for me again on Saturday morning and I left home at 1 P.M., remained until [*sic*] next day at 1 P.M. got home. When I left her she could breathe with more ease and seemed better but how long it will last is impossible to tell, the family thought on Friday before I went there that she would die before morning they had all gathered around her expecting every breath to be her last. . . . I have tried a number of remedies for those smoth[er]ing and sinking spells but Nux seems to be the best in her case—if it fails what shall I resort to?
>
> Mr. Marshall's child has such an offensive diarrhoea and the remedies appear to have no effect. . . . What had I better give? Mary wants me to turn the child over to Dr. Kiger for if it dies a certificate would be required and she is afraid for me to be in the Office—as I am so closely watched since being arrested. [Whether it was Eliza's relationship to Alfred, or because she practiced homoeopathy, or something else that led to her arrest is not determined.] I don't want to bring anyone into trouble. If I could do only Office practice then I would take out [a] license as I would not have to risk expenses I could not meet, but you know persons would expect me

to come when sent for. All I want to do is to do right. If I could only see what is best for me to do.

Eliza practiced medicine in Wheeling for twenty-two years. She died unexpectedly while making a house call on the other side of the Ohio River in Portland, Ohio, on May 21, 1882. The cause of death was at first reported as apoplexy, but later it was said that she was struck by lightning. Her obituary in the *Wheeling Intelligencer* said, Miss Hughes "had attained quite an eminent position in the practice of homoeopathy, being particularly successful in treating children. Her services were in great demand for miles around Wheeling, and she had won the confidence and esteem of a wide and numerous circle of acquaintances." Eliza Hughes and Orrie Moon (q.v.) were the first women physicians who practiced medicine in Virginia as doctors of medicine.

References: Thomas L. Bradford, *Biographical Index of the Graduates of the Homoeopathic Medical College of Pennsylvania and the Hahnemann Medical College and Hospital of Philadelphia* (Philadelphia, 1918); Cleave, 439; Eliza Clark Hughes, letter dated 1862 to her brother Alfred, imprisoned at Camp Chase, Ohio, available online at "Dr. Eliza Clark Hughes," compiled by Linda Cunningham Fluherty, http://www.lindapages.com/nurses/nurses-drhughes.htm (accessed May 19, 2016); Obituary, *Wheeling Intelligencer*, May 29 and 30, 1882.

Sarah R. *Randall* HUMPHREY (b. ca. 1830–d. ca. 1865)

Sarah Randall was born in Ohio about 1830, the eldest of four children (two girls, two boys) of Richard H. Randall and his wife Sarah. The Randalls, both born in New York, had migrated to Ohio, and later to Illinois. Nothing is known of Sarah's background, childhood, or early education except that her father was a physician. In 1858, Sarah married Aaron Humphrey, MD, a resident of Tipton, Iowa. Aaron had grown up on a farm in Tipton and was a recent (1855) graduate of the New York Hygeio-Therapeutic College, where he had earned an MD degree. The couple lived in Tipton, where Aaron practiced medicine. Sarah, herself already a student at her husband's alma mater, graduated with an MD degree on April 13, 1858.

For several years thereafter the couple operated sanitaria or water-cures, first in Lancaster, Ohio, then, in 1860, in Moline, Illinois—"the cure of the great West." At Moline, one could experience water-cure, calisthenics, gymnastic exercises, and movement cure at the couple's Hygienic Retreat. By March 1863, the Humphreys were in Galesburg, Illinois, but apparently soon moved to Minneapolis to run a sanitarium there. The income tax roll for May 1865 lists Mrs. A. G. Humphrey, physician, St. Anthony, Minnesota, as paying a ten-dollar physician tax.

It is likely that Sarah died sometime between 1865 and 1868, when Aaron married Lovina Schwartzendruver. (In the *History of Knox County* [1912], it is written that Sarah had died more than fifty years earlier. This seems inaccurate in view of the tax payment.) Though lacking evidence, it seems a possibility that Sarah had tuberculosis and that the sojourn in Minnesota was to seek treatment. Sarah could have practiced but six or seven years. Aaron returned to Galesburg, where he operated the Galesburg Health Institute from 1867 until after the turn of the century. He and his wife had one son, Albert S. Humphrey.

References: *Herald of Health and Journal of Physical Culture*, October 1867, 194; Newton Bateman, *Historical Encyclopedia of Illinois and Knox County* (Chicago: Munsell, 1899), 778; US Internal Revenue Service tax rolls, Galesburg, IL, March 18, 1863, March 19, 1864, June 18, 1864, May 1865; US census, 1850, 1910; H. B. Weiss, *The Great American Water-Cure Craze* (Trenton, NJ: Past Times Press, 1967), 118.

Angenette A. *Payne* HUNT (1819–1901)

Angenette Payne was born August 10, 1819, in Madison County, New York. Nothing is known of her parents or childhood. At age twenty, on October 3, 1849, she married Dr. Nelson Hunt, of Hamilton, New York. He was born in Winhall, Vermont, and had come with his family to Madison County as a child; he was twelve years older than Angenette. Nothing is known of his education. Angenette graduated from the Female Medical College of Pennsylvania on December 30, 1851, a member of the first class.

According to Nelson Hunt's obituary, the couple at first practiced in Hamilton during the winter months and at Saratoga Springs during the summer. In 1858, they bought a failing water-cure that had been established in Verona Springs, New York, five years earlier. Together, they operated the Verona Springs Sanitarium for the next thirty-four years until Nelson's death July 2, 1892. Thereafter, Angenette ran the cure until selling it August 8, 1900, to Dr. G. N. Lehr of Utica.

On May 16, 1954, Iva L. Reveley, emerita professor of biology at Wellesley College, published in the *Utica Observer-Dispatch* a full-page article with seven illustrations about the Verona Mineral Springs, providing the most definitive information that survives. "Water-cures" located at mineral springs were popular retreats during the middle part of the nineteenth century for those seeking health or recreation.

In New York, there were well-known establishments at Elmira, Dansville, Clifton Springs, Glen Springs, Sharon Springs, and, most famous and enduring of all, Saratoga Springs. Among the less well known of these was that at Verona Springs in Oneida County, near the village of Lowell, not far from Utica. These springs, as were most of them, had been known to and used by the Native Americans. During the 1830s and 1840s, the Verona springs had been developed by a succession of proprietors.

When the Hunts bought the property, it consisted, in addition to the springs and six acres of land, of the sixty-two-room Spring House for guests (destroyed by fire in 1905), a bathhouse, a windmill to pump water for the bathhouse and the bottling room beneath it, a large barn, an ice house built into a hillside, a bowling alley, a pavilion over the spring, and a rustic summerhouse in the woods. Nelson took charge of administration, Angenette of medical care and dining room, diet being an important part of treatment.

According to Reveley, the sanitarium was "patronized most largely by persons of wealth and distinction from every part of the United States," many of whom had previously been patients of the Hunts at Saratoga. "The house was modern for its day, having running water in the kitchens, bathrooms and toilets." The major addition made by the Hunts was a farm to provide vegetables, dairy products, and poultry for the dining room. The season ran from June 1 to November 1 (and occasionally to January 1). The Hunts spent winters in New York or sometimes in Florida. The sanitarium reached its peak around 1875, declining slowly thereafter, as the Hunts grew older and water-cures lost popularity. "As far as can be ascertained," according to Miss Reveley, "neither of the proprietors carried on a general practice, but devoted themselves to working in the sanitarium, except as neighbors, in cases of accident or emergency, appealed to them for help."

Angenette Hunt moved to Rome, New York, after she sold the sanitarium. She died December 29, 1901, and is buried in Lowell, New York, Cemetery, as are her mother, daughter, and niece. In her will she left a fund of $20,000 from which the income was to provide board at the springs for "tired working girls." Though greatly diminished in principle, the fund, now administered by two Rome hospitals, was still being used in 1954 as designated by the donor.

References: Several obituary clippings for Angenette and for Nelson in the Alumnae Collection, Female Medical College of Pennsylvania Archives, Drexel University College of Medicine, Philadelphia; Article by Ida L. Reveley, *Utica Observer-Dispatch*, May 16, 1954; Obituary, *Utica Sunday Tribune*, January 5, 1902.

Harriot Kezia *HUNT* (1805–75)

Harriot Hunt, who started practicing medicine in Boston in 1835, had no collegiate medical education, although she had applied, unsuccessfully, for admission to Harvard Medical School in 1847 and again in 1850. She was given an honorary medical degree by the Female Medical College of Pennsylvania in 1853, after eighteen years of increasingly successful, if "irregular," practice. (Harvard Medical School did not accept a woman medical student until 1945.)

Harriot was born in Boston, November 9, 1805, to Joab Hunt, a ship joiner and ship merchant, and his wife, Kezia Wentworth. Both were longtime residents of Boston's North End. Joab was raised a Congregationalist, Kezia an Episcopalian. They were married in 1791 by Bishop Parker at Trinity Church. The couple were churchgoers, but Joab shortly came under the influence of John Murray and turned to the Universalist way of thinking, soon to be followed by his wife. So, the family held liberal religious views. Three years after Harriot's birth, a sister, Sarah Augusta, was born. When older, the two girls would attend Mrs. Carter's private school.

In 1827, then twenty-two, Harriot and her sister established their own private school for girls. The curriculum must have differed from the norm then prevailing. Harriot did not favor "the fashionable education father and mothers [gave] their daughters, encouraging them to acquire those peacock accomplishments" but no occupation, profession, or employment—making them dependent (*Glances*, 55). The school started with eight pupils in April and had twenty-three students by October. It continued for six years, and during that time Harriot was plagued by frequent headaches. In November 1827, her father, to whom she was very close, died of a heart attack. The family was in formal mourning for six years. The fact that Joab's estate was encumbered made the success of the school even more necessary (61–63).

"The greatest turning point of my life," she later wrote, came in 1830 when her sister became sick with what was probably tuberculosis. For the next three years, the family physician, Dr. Dixwell, "our kind allopathic physician," treated Augusta with blisters, mercurials, leeches, and four drops of prussic acid three times a day. Consultation by members of the Massachusetts Medical Society supported the regimen. After forty-one weeks of sickness and 106 professional calls, there had been no improvement.

"On the thirtieth of June, 1833, I saw a physician, Mrs. Mott, who, with her husband, had come to Boston to establish themselves in practice:—they were English people." What led to this encounter Harriot does not relate. She does tell of the criticism the family endured for employing "a quack" and expressed their own distaste for the "bombast of the advertisements the Motts printed, and the trumpeting of the certain cure that would result from their practice" (110–11). We are not told what the prescribed regimen was—presumably more physiologic and less heroic than had previously been the case—but Augusta began to improve.

"Here was my first thought of woman as a physician; and yet this was but a partial exhibition, for her husband was at her side,—giving to her position some gloss of what the world calls propriety, and you felt his power as well as hers" (111). That September, Harriot went to "write" for the Motts at their home, apparently writing letters to patients. An old friend had taken over the school. In March 1834, the three Hunts moved to the large Mott house, where they had adjoining rooms that they furnished. Harriot continued to write letters and felt a "growing consciousness that I was to be a physician" (113).

In July 1835, the Motts returned to England and the Hunts to their own home. Harriot later wrote that she and Augusta "continued [their] medical studies with unabated zeal. Our previous experiences of great use. Medical treatment rather than an investigation of hygienic laws had hitherto been our lessons. Medication we had seen rather too much" (121). Physiology became her primary interest, prevention more than cure. During all of this, the two sisters were practicing medicine in the community. That fall, they "advertised, and began, as it were, our profession" (123).

In all of its 418 pages, Hunt's autobiography reveals relatively few details of her professional practice. "I am a disciple of no medical sect," she wrote. "There is doubtless some truth to be found in every new system of medicine, however shrouded by absurdities," mentioning, specifically, Thomsonian and homoeopathic practice (171–73). She emphasized repeatedly an interest in prevention and cause, not cure but trust in Nature. "We very soon learned," she wrote, "not to trust too much to medication:—not but that we often saw it fully successful; but it did not meet our perception of the dignity of the human body" (127). Since there were, in that day, few therapeutic modalities that led to cure such a course seemed reasonable. She mentioned medicated baths and friction (30) but apparently found it difficult to engage help that could administer these properly. Daily regimen and understanding of one's physiology were the bases of her therapy.

Unlike most woman doctors of the time, Dr. Hunt apparently did not practice midwifery, on her mother's advice (135). However, the care of women was a major part of her practice. She believed that the majority of male physicians [let] their female patients remain in ignorance of the physiological laws, whose observance alone can keep them in health and enable them to transmit it to their children. . . . Diseases of women have been treated by us which few male practitioners could have treated, not only because they were beyond the reach of mere medication, and had no nomenclature in the list of maladies, but because the male practitioner could not have drawn their diagnosis, without that confession from the patient which could not be given in most cases with delicacy except to a woman. Here were women whose spiritual sufferings [had] at length poisoned their physical organizations. (153–55)

Some historians found fault that she did not embrace "scientific" medicine. But scientific medicine in that day involved anatomic dissection and the relatively new field of pulmonary acoustics—a technique then mastered by few practitioners. Science had little to offer in the realm of therapeutics and the evaluation of pharmaceuticals by blind studies. One method, promoted by James Jackson Jr. after studying abroad, had made little headway in the United States. It is not clear that the treatments offered by Dr. Hunt or Marie Zakrzewska (q.v.), professor at New England Female Medical College, varied greatly.

A Ladies' Physiological Society was formed in Charlestown (a Boston suburb) in 1843. "The formation of this society was one of the events of my life," Dr. Hunt would later write, "and gave me the first hint as to the possibility of lecturing to my own sex on physiological laws" (170). By the end of a year the group had grown from "from less than a dozen, to fifty" (177). Meetings were every fortnight. Famous speakers addressed the group. Such meetings of women became increasingly popular around the country, and Hunt spoke at many of them.

In later years, Dr. Hunt traveled frequently, not only to speak but to visit Shaker communities. Brought up a Universalist after her parents' conversion, she later became an adherent to Swedenborgian philosophy. She was also active in several social movements of the time—temperance, antislavery, women's rights. Each year, for more than twenty-five years, she accompanied her tax payment with a letter protesting taxation without representation. In her autobiography, she wrote that "Faneuil Hall was not *our* Cradle of Liberty. We had no hand in the rocking. If we *had* had, perhaps the child would have turned out better. But *men* rocked *that* cradle! There as everywhere, we have no civil rights, but those which are dependent on the will of our legislators doled out to us by ignorance, caprice, or whim" (44). And, as for the lot of the woman physician, she had this to say: "Medical 'brother' 'regularly' studied at an approved college, was accepted, recognized by the medical faculty, had an M.D. after his name—capital to start upon. Older heads to sustain him, code of laws to obey, a mistake might kill patient but not him. He studied, then practiced. *We* studied and practiced at the same time" (124).

An assessment of Dr. Hunt's career by her friend Marie Zakrzewska is of interest. Dr. Zakrzewska, a generation younger than Hunt, had her early professional training in Germany, had a medical degree from Western Reserve, and was professor at New England Female Medical College. It is not surprising that with this contrast in formal education she hardly mentions Dr. Hunt's work as a physician but emphasizes her work as a social reformer.

"There is no doubt," she wrote, "that Dr. Hunt was one of the most prominent women of the first half of this century [i.e., before 1850]. She was one of those who initiated the independent thinking and acting of women in various directions. By nature she was not aggressive, nor was she inclined to proclaim reforms, but won the appellation [*sic*] of 'reformer' later in her career." Zakrzewska emphasized Hunt's "work on the platform and in the pulpit . . . [and thought] her education was on the whole desultory, depending much upon her own inclination [and her] susceptible and versatile mind." In three and a half pages, there are only two comments on her medical practice: she "gave valuable advice on mental and physical hygiene" and offered "common sense practice." The final summary paragraph does not mention her career as a physician: she "was a woman of manifold interests, her talents were developed in many directions, she was an eloquent speaker, and was possessed of a deeply religious nature, of poetical imagination and a cheerful temperament." If Hunt advanced the science of medicine, it was by restricting the therapeutic excesses of the time. She did help many in need where science was yet to provide a solution. Harriot Hunt died January 2, 1875, at sixty-nine.

Bibliography: *Glances and Glimpses; or, Fifty Years Social, Including Twenty Years Professional Life* (Boston, 1856).

References: *Dictionary of American Biography*, 5:385–86; Harriot K. Hunt, *Glances and Glimpses* (Boston, 1856); *Dictionary of American Medical Biography* (1928), 618–19; Regina M. Morantz, "The Perils of Feminist History," *Journal of Interdisciplinary History* 4 (1974): 649–60; *Notable American Women*, 2:235–37; Marie E. Zakrzewska, "Harriot Kizia Hunt," *Woman's Medical Journal* 10 (1900): 202–5.

Emeline Morrow *HURD* Fales (b. 1825)

Emeline Hurd was born December 23, 1825, in Sparta, New Jersey, the fourth of seven children (four girls, three boys) of Charles Hurd and his wife, Mary Munson. One of her older brothers died in infancy and another at age twenty-four. Both parents were Presbyterians and Republicans. However, later family tradition is that the family was Roman Catholic. This is interesting but will require documentation. It would be rare for a Roman Catholic woman to go to medical school in mid-nineteenth century. It also was rare for Episcopalians (there were one or two). It was the liberal denominations—Quakers, Baptists, and Methodists—that made up the bulk of female medical school matriculants at that time. Perhaps her husband, Newell Fales, was Catholic, but that seems a little unlikely: he came from Revolutionary stock in central Massachusetts.

No information has been found about Emeline's childhood or early education. The *Water-Cure Journal* for July 1857 reported that Emeline, who was already denoted as "M.D.," though she had completed only one, possibly two, courses of lectures at medical school, "seems to be in general demand in Iowa. She has been practicing with good success at Iowa City, in connection with Mrs. Doctor Kimball, and has had several calls from villages in the vicinity."

The following spring, on April 13, 1858, she graduated with an MD degree from New York Hygeio-Therapeutic College. She was listed as a resident of Richmond, Iowa, at that time. One month later, on May 13, she married fellow medical student, Newell W. Fales, of Walpole, Massachusetts, a man eight years her junior. The couple joined recent classmates, the Rev. Azor Estee and his wife, Mrs. Dr. Estee, at the Petersburg (NY) Hygienic Manual Labor Water-Cure, an institution of which the Rev. Mr. Estee was proprietor.

The Faleses' only child and son, Newell Hurd Fales, known as "Nuna," was born October 29, 1859, in Iowa, so the family was by then already on its way west. Nuna, then age eight months, is listed in the 1860 census of Sacramento, California. Another source puts the family in Marysville, a community not far from Sacramento, in 1863, but they soon moved south to Cholame in the inland northeastern corner of St. Luis Obispo County, where they bought a large ranch/farm. According to family tradition both Emeline and Newell practiced medicine in the nearby village of Immusdale. This has not been confirmed. Neither Newell's nor Emeline's name is found in national directories of the period (1874, 1877, 1886), nor is either of them listed in the 1901 or 1905 *California Registry* of physicians. Whether they continued to practice in California cannot presently be determined with certainty. The village of Immusdale no longer exists, its post office was closed in 1902, and it is listed as a ghost town. The dates that Emeline and Newell died are not available. Nuna came back to Cholame (1900, 1910, 1920 census), so perhaps his parents had died by then. In 1922, after the earthquake, he sold the farm and moved to Santa Cruz.

References: Myron A. Munson, *The Munson Record: A Genealogical and Biographical Account of Captain Thomas Munson (a Pioneer of Hartford and New Haven) and His Descendants* [1637–1887] (New Haven: Munson Assn., 1895); New York Hygeio-Therapeutic College, *Biennial Catalogue*, 1855–57, 1857–59; Personal communication, February 18, 2009, from Carolle Van Someren, genealogist, Tracy, California; *Water-Cure Journal*, July 1857, 15; *Water-Cure Journal*, August 1858, 27; Harry B. Weiss, *The Great American Water-Cure Craze* (Trenton, NJ: Past Times Press, 1967), 169.

Rhoda H. *HYDE* Williams Maxcy (b. 1825)

Rhoda Hyde was born in August 1825 in New York, the second of five children (three girls, two boys) of Elijah C. Hyde and his wife, Adaline Lyman. Nothing is known about her childhood or early education. By the time Rhoda graduated with an MD degree in 1859 from New York Hygeio-Therapeutic College, the family had moved to Jersey City. Rhoda's older sister became a teacher, and two younger brothers clerks, as Rhoda had been before going to medical school (*Jersey City Directory*, 1858–59).

Once a doctor of medicine, Rhoda moved to Aurora, Illinois. Her business card appeared in the July 1860 issue of *Water-Cure World*: "Rhoda H. Hyde, M.D., Hygeio-Therapeutic Physician. Aurora, Ill." There she began the practice of "hygienic" medicine. Soon she met and, on August 11, 1861, married Solomon Williams, a farmer from the nearby village of Winfield. In 1870, the couple was living in Winfield, with a five-year-old child, May, and Rhoda's father, Elijah. The census describes Rhoda as "keeping house," a delineation common in those days even for practicing woman physicians.

The 1880 census lists Rhoda as a widow; Solomon had died the year before. May and Elijah were both gone, presumably dead, and there was a nine-year-old daughter, Fannie M., as well as Rhoda's mother, living in the household. (Rhoda must have had two other children who died: the 1900 census describes her as mother of four, one living.) Whether Rhoda continued to practice medicine after her marriage or, especially in her widowhood, is not determined. Solomon was a reasonably prosperous farmer ($15,500 in real estate, $2,000 in personal property in 1870). As is often the case with woman doctors in the early post–Civil War era, it is hard to know whether they practiced their profession or if they did, how much.

In 1880, Rhoda married Levi Augustus Maxcy. Maxcy, born in Massachusetts, had gone to California via the Horn to find gold. He found little of it but did buy a farm, married, and had two children. In 1876, his wife divorced him and took their two sons with her. In 1881, Levi leased the farm, went to Illinois to visit his sister, met Rhoda Hyde Williams, a widow with a farm and a daughter, Fannie Williams. Levi and Rhoda were married there in Illinois that same year. In 1889, Levi brought his new family to his farm in California, "a house with eight rooms and a path which led past the woodpile."

The 1900 and 1910 censuses and the 1913, 1914, and 1916 directories for Richmond, Contra Costa County, list Levi and Rhoda as residents (Fannie had married the young man from the adjacent farm). The census described each of them as having their "own income." Rhoda was ninety-one in 1916. She must have died not long after this, but a date has not been found. The only definite evidence that Rhoda practiced medicine relates to her early days in Aurora. Whether she practiced after her first (or second) marriage has not been determined.

References: Lyman Coleman, *Genealogy of the Lyman Family in Great Britain and America* (Albany, NY: J. Munsell, 1872); Vivian C. Edmonston, "The Good Old 'Daze,'" a talk given before the Contra Costa Historical Society, Danville, CA, May 14, 1870 [Edmonston was Rhoda's granddaughter]; *Jersey City Directory*, 1858–59; Richmond, CA, city directory, 1913, 1914, 1916; *Water-Cure World*, July 1860, 32; US census, 1860, 1870, 1880, 1900, 1910.

I

Anna *INMAN* (1813–87)

Anna Inman was born February 20, 1813, probably in Providence, Rhode Island, the fifth of nine children of Daniel and Abigail Mowry Inman. Daniel was a farmer. While living in Smithfield, Rhode Island, Anna attended New England Female Medical College in Boston and, in 1857, received an MD degree. Where she spent the next ten years has not been determined.

From 1867 through 1869 she held the chair of obstetrics at New York Medical College for Women, and in 1869, after Clemence Lozier (q.v.) relinquished it, the chair of diseases of women and children as well. She is not listed in the 1860 or 1868 edition of the *New England Business Directory* as a physician in Rhode Island, so she was probably living in New York City. The 1870 census denotes her as "doctress," living in Providence in a household with four other women: two twenty-three-year-old music teachers, a twenty-five-year-old dressmaker, and a fifty-year-old housekeeper. Providence directories list her as a physician from 1870 through 1881: at 11 Thomas in 1876, at 24 Benefit in 1878–80, and at 80 Prospect in 1881. She is not found in directories for 1869 or 1882. In the 1875 *New England Business Directory* she is listed under "other" physicians, at 11 Thomas, as she is also in 1878–79. Dr. Inman died, unmarried, on March 8, 1887, at the age of seventy-four.

References: Butler, 1874, 1877; Polk, 1886; *New England Business Directory*, 1860, 1868, 1875; Providence city directory, 1872, 1874, 1875, 1876, 1878, 1879, 1880, 1881; *New England Official Directory & Handbook* (Boston: C. R. Tuttle, 1878).

J

Mercy B. *Ruggles* Bisbee JACKSON (1802–77)

Mercy Ruggles was born September 17, 1802, in Hardwick, Massachusetts, the youngest of five children (two boys, three girls) of Constant Ruggles and his wife Sarah Greene Hudson. A great-uncle was a brigadier general in the Revolutionary War. At seventeen, Mercy graduated from a private school near Hardwick and began teaching in Plainfield, Massachusetts, fifty miles to the west, but soon moved back to her native area, where she continued to teach.

In 1823, she married the Rev. John Bisbee Jr. John had graduated from Brown, studied law, and was ordained a Unitarian preacher in 1821. He was a talented and eloquent speaker. A physical description of him noted hair and beard that were white on one side, with one eye blue, the other, hazel. He also had "interesting mental peculiarities" unspecified. The couple moved to Hartford, Connecticut, where John became pastor of the First Universalist Society and, shortly, to Portland, Maine, where John had a similar post. On March 8, 1829, John died of pneumonia. It had been a happy, if short, marriage. Three children had been born: the eldest, Laurelia, died in infancy of scarlet fever.

Now a twenty-seven-year-old widow with two small children (aged three and one), Mercy established a school for young ladies. It was successful, but after two or three years Mercy found its management arduous. In 1832, her younger surviving daughter, four-year-old Charlotte, died. Mercy turned to the millinery business.

In 1835, she married Captain Daniel Jackson of Plymouth, Massachusetts, and went to live in that town. The Jackson family of Plymouth were prominent shipbuilders and seamen for several generations. They were related to Charles Jackson of ether and telegraphy fame. Daniel Jackson's cousin, Lydia, who married Ralph Waldo Emerson, became a good friend of Mercy, and this introduced Mercy to the mid-nineteenth-century intellectual circle of Concord. Daniel himself was a widower with six children. Daniel and Mercy had eight more children, four of whom, twin boys and twin girls, died at birth.

In the early 1840s Mercy became interested in the practice of medicine and, in particular, in the homoeopathic method. Though she had lost six of her eleven children, most of their deaths occurred when they were infants. According to Cleave, a biographer of homoeopaths writing while Mercy was still alive, "She was constantly shocked at the violence of remedial action, and the repulsiveness of almost all medicines to the human taste and constitution; so that she conceived a fixed belief that a beneficent Creator, whose works were otherwise so perfect, had made some better way to combat the ills of the flesh; and she often expressed this belief to her family physician, Dr. Capen of Plymouth, who was of course of the allopathic school." Nevertheless, Capen provided books and encouragement and probably acted as a mentor to his patient. Gradually, Mercy developed a practice in Plymouth, providing medical services gratis to friends and neighbors. Over a period of eighteen years, her practice grew. It is said that a homoeopathic physician from Baltimore tried to establish a practice in Plymouth but that Mercy was more popular and, after the competitor left town, she began to charge for her services.

In 1852, husband Daniel died of cancer, and, by the later 1850s, her youngest child grown, Mercy, now fifty-six, enrolled at Boston's New England Female Medical College, where she was supported (1858–60) by a Massachusetts scholarship and from which she graduated with an MD degree in 1860. She moved to Boston, opened an office on May 3, and practiced medicine for the next seventeen years until her death. Her name is listed in Boston and New England business directories annually as a practicing physician. Though she declined an invitation to join the faculty of New York Medical College for Women, she did become adjunct professor of diseases of children at the new medical school at Boston University (homoeopathic), a school into which her alma mater had been absorbed.

During her years of practice in Boston, she was active in professional politics. Early, she applied for membership in the American Institute of Homoeopathy, the national professional organization of homoeopathic physicians. Membership was denied her; the bylaws did not contemplate the admission of women. She applied annually for the next ten years until 1871, when she and two other women were elected to membership. Admission to local and state societies soon (1874) followed.

Bisbee-Jackson, as she was known, was also active in other community roles—especially women's suffrage and women's rights generally, and temperance work. In 1854, by then a widow, she wrote a letter to the assessors of Plymouth Township protesting taxation without representation. She did not want women to be like men but rather "to have the same opportunities to use in a woman's way." Financially, she was well off. The 1870 census listed her as having $25,000 in real estate and $5,000 in personal property. She was living with her two children, two servants, and eight other, apparently unrelated, people.

Dr. Bisbee-Jackson died at her house at 681 Tremont Street, Boston, on December 13, 1877. The *Evening Transcript* described her as "one of the pioneers in the practice of homoeopathy in this city. . . . She enjoyed the acquaintance and correspondence of the leading homoeopathic physicians of New York and Philadelphia, and was active in advancing the healing art according to the principles of Hahnemann."

References: *Dictionary of American Biography*, 5:550–51; American Institute of Homoeopathy, *Transactions* 111 (1878): 7; Frank J. Bisbee, *Genealogy of the Bisbee Family* (n.p.: Otter Book Press, 1956); Obituary, *Evening Transcript* (Boston), December 14, 1877; Cleave, 443–44; William T. Davis, *Plymouth Memories of an Octogenarian* (Plymouth, 1906; Data on Daniel Jackson); Hardwick, MA, Vital Records; William H. King, *History of Homoeopathy and Its Institutions in America* (New York, 1905); Obituary, *Old Colony Memorial*, December 20, 1877; Jane Post, *Mercy B. Jackson (1802–1877): A Pioneering Woman*, exhibition held at Pilgrim Hall Museum, June 2004; US census, 1870; *Appleton's Cyclopaedia of American Biography*, 3:390.

Mary Reed *JENKS* (1809–88)

Mary Jenks was born April 28, 1809, daughter of William Jenks (son of Gideon) and Sophia Stackpole Austin (daughter of Charles and

Rachel Pray Stackpole). William was a contractor and builder in Portsmouth, New Hampshire; Springfield; and Boston. Sophia was the widow of Henry Austin. William and Sophia had four daughters and four sons. Mary was a dressmaker and was in chronic poor health. Not helped by either Regular or Thomsonian medicines, she turned to the water-cure. This led to improvement for her and inspired her to help others as she had been helped. She attended New England Female Medical College in Boston and graduated with an MD degree in 1854. The family was living in Springfield at that time.

Mary is listed as a practicing physician in Boston directories each year from 1856 to 1862, and in the *New England Business Directory* for 1860, which shows her at 38 Beach Street in downtown Boston. She is listed in the *Progressive Annual* for 1863 and 1864 as a physician in Boston, but information in this publication is sometimes outdated. Careful search of many subsequent editions of Boston and New England directories did not find her name. Mary is not listed in the Massachusetts Death Index 1886–90. No obituary was found in the Boston *Transcript*. Family genealogy records a death date of November 1, 1888, and also states that Mary was a doctor in Boston.

References: Boston city directory, 1850–62; *Transcript* (Boston), Obituary index, 1875–1930; Personal communication from Martha Gardner, New England College of Pharmacy, Boston; Massachusetts Death Index, 1886–90; *Progressive Annual*, 1863, 1864.

Henrietta W. JOHNSON (b. 1826)

Henrietta Johnson was born in February 1826 in New Jersey. Nothing is known of her parents, background, childhood, or early education. Sometime around 1850 she married Roland Johnson, a man ten years her senior. Johnson was a Chinese goods broker, and a prosperous one. He owned real estate worth $50,000 and had $12,000 in personal property.

Henrietta enrolled at Female Medical College of Pennsylvania and graduated in March 1853 with an MD degree. The couple later had three children: Anna H. (b. 1855) and Llewellyn H. (b. ca. 1859); the third child did not survive. Anna later became a physician and Llewellyn an artist.

In the late 1850s, the family moved from New York City to East Orange, New Jersey, and later to West Orange where, judging from census data, Henrietta practiced medicine. She is listed as being a physician in both the 1870 and 1880 census reports. Her name is also found in the *Progressive Annuals* for 1862, 1863, and 1864 as a practicing physician in Orange, New Jersey. By 1900, then seventy-three, Henrietta was a widow, retired, and living in San Bernardino, California, with her unmarried physician daughter and her son's widow and children. The son had presumably died, since daughter Anna is listed as head of household. Henrietta was still alive in 1915 and would have been eighty-nine.

References: *Progressive Annual,* 1862–64; US census, 1870, 1880, 1900.

Harriet Amelia *JUDD* Sartain (1830–1923)

Harriet Judd was born in Connecticut in 1830, moved with her family to Michigan in 1843, where she attended seminary and later went to New York Hygeio-Therapeutic College, where she received an MD degree in 1851. However, the school was not yet chartered by the legislature, hence the degree was not bona fide. She earned a second degree from the Eclectic Medical Institute in Cincinnati in 1854. At EMI she was a classmate of Alice Bunker (Stockham; q.v.). After graduating from EMI she started practice in Waterbury, Connecticut, and may have been practicing there even before she earned her MD. It is claimed that she trained at some time with both Harriet N. Austin (q.v.) and Mary Gove Nichols (q.v.).

On December 11, 1854, she married Samuel Sartain, the eldest son of a family prominent in the art world of Philadelphia and beyond. Samuel's father, born in London, was a well-known engraver. He and his wife had seven children, three of whom became either engravers or artists. There is even a Sartain Street in downtown Philadelphia. Samuel and Harriet had three children, two of whom lived to adulthood, and one of whom, Paul Judd Sartain, became a physician.

Harriet moved to Philadelphia after her wedding and set up practice as a homoeopath. She practiced from 1854 to probably around 1900. Her name appears in Philadelphia directories from 1861 to 1869 and Polk directories from 1886 to 1898. She is said to have had a large practice, the largest of any woman practitioner in Philadelphia. In developing this she was certainly helped by her introduction as a Sartain into the Philadelphia scene and also because the homoeopathic system appealed to the upper class. Among the Sartains friends were Thomas Eakins, Edgar Allan Poe, William Dean Howells, and many others in the art and literary world. Harriet supported her sister-in-law, Emily Sartain, when she went to Paris for art training. Emily later painted portraits of Constantine Hering and James Caleb Jackson.

In 1870, Harriet was elected unanimously to the local Homoeopathic County Medical Society, its first woman member, and in 1871 joined the State Homoeopathic Medical Society and the American Institute of Homoeopathy. After 1886, the year her son Paul graduated from University of Pennsylvania Medical School as a Regular, she and he shared office space at 212 Logan Square. Samuel died in 1906 and Harriet, at ninety-three, in 1923. Son Paul, in his will, established the Harriet Judd Sartain Memorial Scholarship with a $21,033 endowment, the income of which was to go a member of the graduating class who, in the judgment of the faculty, needed and was deserving of assistance for the study of medicine. The family were Spiritualists.

References: Katharine Martinez, ed., *Philadelphia's Cultural Landscape* (Philadelphia: Temple University Press, 2000); Philadelphia city directories; Polk; "Harriet Amelia Judd Sartain 1830–1923," *Sue Young Homeopathy*, http://sueyounghistories.com/archives/2008/04/16/harriet-amelia-judd-sartain-and-homeopathy (accessed June 1, 2016).

K

Sarah *KENYON* Lisk (b. ca. 1824)

Sarah Kenyon was born in New York State about 1824. Nothing has been found regarding her background, parents, childhood, or education. During 1856 or 1857 she attended New York Hygeio-Therapeutic College. No documentation has been found that she received a diploma. She is referred to as Sarah Kenyon, MD, in water-cure journals of the period and, on that evidence, is included here. At the time of her schooling, she was referred to as a resident of Schagticoke, a village northeast of Albany, New York.

A notice in the *Water-Cure Journal* reported that she "was with her cousin, Miss Cogswell, during the last days of her sickness." This, presumably, was the sister of Dr. Abigail S. Cogswell (q.v.), who would also be her cousin. After the death of Miss Cogswell, Dr. Kenyon worked for Dr. Mortimer Nevins, a water-cure physician in Peoria, Illinois. The 1860 census shows Sarah Kenyon living with the Nevins family and denotes her a water-cure physician and as having personal property valued at $200. The Nevins household included twenty-one persons and may have been a water-cure establishment. In addition to the family were, for example, a teacher, a laborer, a printer, a servant, a nurse, and a farmer.

Supporting the idea that the place was indeed a water-cure is the following notice that appeared in the February 1863 *Herald of Health*: "Married, At Peoria (Ill.) Water-Cure Nov. 17, 1862, by the Rev. D. M. Rice Mr. Alexander Lisk, of . . . Peoria Co., Ill. To Miss Sarah Kenyon, M.D., graduate of the New York Hygeio-Therapeutic College." Lisk, ten years senior to Sarah, was a moderately prosperous farmer and later a small fruit grower in nearby Richwoods, where the couple set up housekeeping and where they would live the rest of their lives. They had no children. Alexander died in 1891 and is buried in Peoria. In 1900, Sarah was living in Kenosha, Wisconsin, with a family named Bailey. No evidence has been found that Sarah practiced medicine after her marriage. She is not listed in the 1874 or 1877 Butler directory or the 1886 Polk directory. In the 1870 and 1880 census she "keeps house," although this datum is not, in itself, reliable evidence that she did not practice.

References: Butler, 1874, 1877; *Herald of Health*, February 1863, 92; New York Hygeio-Therapeutic College, *Biennial Catalogue* (New York, 1857); Polk, 1886; US census, 1860, 1870, 1880, 1900; *Water-Cure Journal* 21 (1856): 159.

Sarah C. *KLECKNER* Saltzgiver (1833–1905)

Sarah Kleckner, or Sallie, as she was known, was born in 1833, in Mifflinburg, a small rural community in central Pennsylvania and the locality in which she spent most of her life. Her parents were David Kleckner and his wife Esther Wingert. Her grandfather, John Kleckner, a native of Wurtemburg, Germany, emigrated in 1750 when he was two, grew up in Northampton County, Pennsylvania, became a blacksmith, and in 1785 settled on the six-hundred-acre farm west of Mifflinburg where he built an inn or tavern and did a bit of distilling on the side. Son David, Sallie's father, was a prosperous farmer and carried on the tavern business. Sallie was one of nine daughters in the family, all of whom received secondary education and five of whom taught school before they were married.

Sallie studied medicine with Dr. Charles Brundage of White Spring and attended the Female Medical College of Pennsylvania, from which she received an MD degree in 1861. She returned to Mifflinburg to practice. Building a practice in that village of less than a thousand people, predominantly of German background, was not easy. Sarah tried operating a drug store at the corner of Chestnut and Fourth Streets, but that failed. In 1885, she went to Ottawa, Kansas, as a medical missionary, accompanied by the local Lutheran minister, but was back in eight months.

In 1891, then fifty-eight, she married George E. Saltzgiver, a hatter in York, Pennsylvania, and the couple moved to York. "The wedding was the highlight of the social season. The marriage was held on Thursday morning at 8:00 in the Mifflinburg Lutheran Church, where 'a crowd was waiting.' Miss Emma Gutelius struck the first notes of the wedding march, and immediately" the four ushers, followed by the bride and groom, came down the aisle, proceeded to the altar rail, "the impressive marriage ceremony of the Lutheran church" followed, "and in a few minutes they were pronounced man and wife. After receiving the guests at the front of the gallery they entered the carriage in waiting and were driven to the railroad station, where, at 8:45 amid showers of rice and old slippers, they started for York, their new home. . . . Dr. Sallie, the bride, is known to fully three-fourths the readers of this paper. She has practiced medicine in our town for many years, and has made hosts of friends who are sorry to have her leave the town." After a few years, the couple moved back to Mifflinburg. Sallie restricted her practice to family and friends and became much more active in local church affairs, especially teaching Sunday school and working for foreign missions.

A letter Sallie wrote to her alma mater on the occasion of her thirtieth class reunion in 1891 gave a description rarely found of what practice was like at that time:

> I have had charge of a serious case of typhoid fever since the New Year, '91, in the person of a dear nephew, who came out of it with a skeleton of a body, but life enough to recover with careful nursing. He is now able to do a little out-door work. I was called to see him on January 2d, and found him with a pulse of 120 and a temperature of 105°. As he was likely to be ill for a long time, I did not leave him for three weeks. With the use of Antifebrin, Quinine, Veratrum Viride, Assafoetida, tepid sponging with alcohol and water, and plenty of nice fresh milk, to my great satisfaction I saw him slowly recover, and he is now likely to become right strong again. When the means used for the restoration of our patients is blessed, what a comfort it is to us. I have also had a few cases of Scarlet fever, all of which recovered. And now Obstetrical cases prevent me from being present with you this year.

Midwifery, of course, as it did with most women practicing medicine at that time, occupied the majority of her professional time.

Sallie left her library to the York County Medical Society and the York County Hospital. Probably among those volumes was her casebook, a fragment of which, covering the years 1861–63, was found years later at a mid-twentieth-century York flea market. It records that in a two-year period she delivered twelve boys and ten girls, all breech. Labor lasted from two to twenty-four hours, with an average between four and five hours.

Sarah was described as having a warm and buoyant temperament and was said to be dedicated to her work. A neighbor said she was "all doctor; strong, and good on her feet," and of "heavy frame." According to local historian Lois Kalp, "She and her husband lived in straightened [*sic*] circumstances . . . her life had been fraught with misfortune [unspecified] and influenced by the prevailing prejudice against women doctors." Sarah died June 22, 1905, and is buried in Mifflinburg Cemetery, her head facing the setting sun as she had requested. There would not be another woman doctor in Union County until the middle of the twentieth century.

References: Lois Kalp, *Silhouettes: The Historic, Memorable and Notable Women of Union County Pennsylvania 1785–1985* (Lewisburg, PA, 1985); Obituary, *Mifflinburg Telegraph*, June 30, 1905; Wedding announcement, *Mifflinburg Times*, November 30, 1891; Charles M. Snyder, *Union County Pennsylvania: A Bicentennial History* (Lewisburg, PA: Colonial Printing House, 1976), 245–46; Charles M. Snyder, *Mifflinburg: A Bicentennial History* (Mifflinburg, PA: Mifflinburg Telegraph, 1992), 38–40; Woman's Medical College of Pennsylvania, Alumnae Association, *Report of the Proceedings of the Sixteenth Annual Meeting . . . May 7 and 8, 1891* (Philadelphia, 1891), 20.

Susanna C. *KOEHLER* Worrell (b. 1832)

Susanna Koehler was born in 1832 in Pennsylvania, presumably of German ancestry. Nothing is known of her parents or childhood. In 1857, she received an MD degree from Penn Medical University, an Eclectic medical school in Philadelphia. Thereafter, she practiced medicine in Philadelphia. Her name is listed in six of the Philadelphia city directories consulted (1864–82), and she is designated in each as a physician. Each of the listings, with one exception, found her at a different address in Philadelphia. She is also listed as a physician in the 1874 and 1877 Butler medical directories.

Some time before 1874, she married James Conly Worrell, an engraver of music. They are not known to have had children, and none is listed in the 1880 census. That census also denoted Susanna not as a physician but as "keeping house." This was often the practice of census takers at that time and does not disprove Susanna's professional status. After 1882, no trace of Dr. Worrell has been found.

References: Butler, 1874, 1877; Philadelphia city directory, 1864, 1867, 1868, 1870, 1874–77, 1881, 1882, 1884, 1885; US census, 1880.

L

Amelia *Wilkes* LINES (1823–1909)

Amelia Wilkes was born on the Isle of Wight, off Portsmouth, England, November 20, 1823, the daughter of William D. Wilkes and Elizabeth Fry. According to her obituary she came to the United States when "quite young." On February 15, 1843, then nineteen and living in Painesville, Ohio, she married Oliver T. Lines, a man ten years her senior. Oliver had been born in New Milford, Connecticut, but grew up in Brooklyn and later moved to the Western Reserve, where he was in business and where the young couple would spend the first years of their marriage. The first three of their five children who survived to adulthood were born in Painesville: Frances E. (b. 1843), Richard (b. 1847), and Edward T. (b. 1853).

A biographical sketch of Amelia published in 1897 relates that about 1845, when Amelia was twenty-two and mother of one, her brother, whom she had not seen since she was two and who was a surgeon in the British navy, died. His desk "came home" to Amelia and, in one of its drawers she found a roll of diplomas signed by famous physicians, perhaps putting an idea in her head. That same year she came across an issue of a new publication, the *Water-Cure Journal*, which she studied, found interesting, and soon began practicing suggestions from it on her family, "and in a short time threw away her medicine chest." Neighbors started asking for her advice. Later, during an epidemic in Cleveland, she was said to have saved her husband's life "when the doctors had given him up." When financial reverses came Mrs. Lines often turned to the practice of hygienic treatment as a means of livelihood.

The family moved to Brooklyn, then called Williamsburg, about 1853. Mrs. Lines attended and graduated from the New York Hygeio-Therapeutic College (then known as New York Hydropathic and Physiological School) in 1854, as did Oliver in 1859. The couple lived and practiced in Brooklyn for the rest of their lives, except for a year when they lived in Plainfield, NJ (*WCJ*, June 1857).

In January 1858, the *Water-Cure Journal* reported that "Dr. Amelia W. Lines has returned to Williamsburg and taken a commodious and pleasantly situated house at no. 26 South Fourth, cor, of Second St., which is now ready for the reception of Patients and Boarders." The establishment was to be known as the Williamsburg Water-Cure. The following year, Oliver received his MD degree from the now-chartered New York Hygeio-Therapeutic College and became "the medical co-partner of his estimable wife . . . who has for several years had an

extensive practice in Williamsburg" (*WCJ*, 1859, 75). An 1863 advertisement announced that the doctors would "attend to outdoor practice too." (*WCJ*, February 1863, 51).

During these years three more children were born: Oliver (b.
1855), Mary Louise (b. 1859), and Jessie Amelia (b. 1864). There may
have been others: one source states that the couple had ten children,
so five of them, including young Oliver, must have died prematurely.
There must have been at least two more household moves; the Polk
directories list the family at 344 Washington Avenue in 1886, 1890, and
1893. When Amelia died she was living at 285 Washington Ave.

An interesting description of Amelia's views on the practice of
medicine is quoted in Mrs. Valentine's 1897 biographical sketch of her:

> It has always seemed to me that water is nature's own medicine, and
> with proper food and sunlight constitutes all that is required to adjust
> the health. Still I believe more and more in the use of medicine, as
> it is given with greater intelligence now than formerly, and there are
> certain minds which not only demand medicine, but want to realize
> they are taking something. While I believe that what I call nature's
> restorers would always be sufficient, I never persuade anyone to try
> them, as I realize any treatment must be accepted to the mind to be
> efficacious.

For the first ten years she had depended solely on water and had
used not a dose of medicine. As she grew older, her hair silvered, and
she still believed in water, but she increasingly used electricity. It was
more convenient. One was not confronted with plumbing problems.
She had the first galvanic battery in New York. She did use medicine,
but apparently sparingly. Her practice in later years was described as
homoeopathic. She also read the medical journals of all schools. Eventually, other physicians consulted with her. She saw one of her great
hopes come to pass—a city hospital controlled entirely by women—the
Memorial Hospital for Women.

In June 1900, Amelia and Oliver retired from practice and went
to live with their son in Vernon, Vermont, where Oliver died the following year with "brain trouble." Amelia moved back to Brooklyn. At
the time of her eightieth birthday, she received many accolades in the
medical press: "Dr. Amelia Wilkes Lines, who recently celebrated her
eightieth birthday, is the oldest practicing woman doctor in the world.
She is the first woman to receive a diploma in the State of New York
and has practiced in New York City since 1854." The original version
was attributed to the *New York Medical Journal* by the *Indiana Medical
Journal* from which this quote is taken. It was copied verbatim by at
least a dozen other medical journals in the months that ensued, and,

when Amelia broke her hip in 1906, even the *Journal of the American Medical Association*, in reporting the unfortunate event, accepted the claim of her priority and called her "the dean of woman physicians in the country" (April 7, 1906). It was incorrect, of course. She was not the first woman to receive a diploma in the state of New York. There were at least fourteen before her, mostly from Central and Syracuse Medical Colleges. Nor was she the dean of living woman physicians. There were at least six still living who had graduated before her: Sarah Dolley, Anna Longshore-Potts, Margaret Richardson, Sophia Harris, and Henrietta Johnson. She was, however, the first woman physician to practice in Brooklyn.

After her hip fracture she was confined to bed. Her faculties unimpaired until the very end, she died at home on September 14, 1909. Her obituary in the *Brooklyn Daily Eagle* noted her habit of reading, her large knowledge, her constant cheerfulness and her unquestioning faith. Three days later, the same paper reported her funeral: "A throng of men and women crowded the house ... [a tribute to] her absolutely unselfish character and to her always faithful counsel and skillful service." The heads of families who she had delivered, their families for whom she had cared—even great-grandchildren—came to honor her memory. Among her descendants, daughter Mary Louise became a physician and grandson, Alfred Thornton Birdsall (1871–1913), became a leading physician of Brooklyn.

References: Obituary, *Brooklyn Daily Eagle*, September 12, 1909, 34; Funeral notice, *Brooklyn Daily Eagle*, September 15, 1909, 5; Obituary of Alfred Birdsall, *Brooklyn Daily Eagle*, September 25, 1909, 1; Susan E. Cayleff, *Wash and Be Healed* (Philadelphia: Temple University Press, 1987), 72; *Herald of Health*, January 1 (1863): 3; Obituary of Oliver Lines, *New York Daily Tribune*, January 29, 1901, 4; *New York Medical Journal* 80 (1904); New York State census, 1855, 1892; *New York Sun*, March 8, 1906, 7 [broken hip]; Polk, 1886, 1890, 1893; US census, 1890; Mrs. M. T. Valentine, *Ephraim McDowell, M.D. the Father of Ovariotomy* (New York: McDowell Publishing Co., 1897), 217–19 [biographical sketch of Dr. Lines]; *Water-Cure Journal*, June 1857, January 1858, 1859, 75; *Water-Cure Journal*, February 1863, 51.

Adeline *Sadler* LITTLEJOHN (1813–1903)

Adeline Sadler was born March 13 (or 18), 1813, in Massachusetts. Nothing is known of her parents, background, or childhood. As a young woman she taught in New York State, including, it is said, at Ingham University, in Leroy, New York. (Ingham, the first chartered woman's university in the United States, opened as Leroy Female Seminary in 1837, was chartered as Ingham Collegiate Institute in 1852, and as Ingham University in 1857.)

On May 1, 1837, in Cattaraugus County, New York, Adeline was married to Philo B. Littlejohn, by the Rev. A. S. Allen. Adeline was then living in Cuba, New York, a village in Allegany County, adjacent to Cattaraugus County on the east. The couple must have soon moved west, because in 1839, they left Quincy, Illinois, with several other couples, headed to Oregon as Presbyterian missionaries to the Indians there. The group had no institutional church sponsorship, and the project was not a successful one. For a while, the Littlejohns lived with the Marcus Whitman family, apparently because Adeline and Narcissa Whitman had been friends back East. (It was said that Adeline and Narcissa were the only two people in the missionary group who were on a first-name basis, the others still practicing the formality they had known back East.)

While the Littlejohns were living in Oregon, their young son was drowned in a millrace. They later had three more children, Almira C. (b. 1844), Julia L. (b. 1845), and Leverett Julius (b. 1846), all born in Oregon Territory. In 1846, the family returned to the States. The 1850 census found them in New Hudson, Allegany County, New York, close by Cuba, New York, and denoted Philo as "Oregon missionary."

Sometime prior to 1859, the Littlejohns had moved west to Delhi, Iowa, where Philo was a farmer. Adeline, then in her midforties, enrolled at New York Hygeio-Therapeutic College (her youngest, son Leverett, was by then thirteen), and graduated with an MD degree in 1859. Curiously, though Leverett's name appears on the 1856 Iowa State census, he is not listed as part of the family in the 1850 or 1860 federal census.

With the coming of the war, Philo enlisted as a private in Company K, Thirty-Seventh Regiment, Iowa Infantry. Adeline worked in Memphis as a nurse. Son Leverett, age nineteen, enlisted February 26, 1864, in Company B, Fourth Cavalry Regiment, was taken prisoner June 11, 1864, and died February 10, 1865, as a prisoner at Andersonville, Georgia.

After the war, the family remained at Delhi at least as late as 1886. Philo died there on February 25, 1886. Though federal and state census reports for 1860, 1870, 1880, and 1885 consistently record Adeline as "keeping house," it seems likely that she practiced medicine during those years. The documented support for this assumption is the fact that the Internal Revenue Service rolls for 1862 and May 1865 each record her as a physician who paid, each time, a tax of ten dollars. After Philo's death, Adeline moved to Humboldt, Iowa, where she lived with daughter Almira and her husband, Calvin Clark, a feed barnkeeper. Adeline died there on July 6, 1903, just short of ninety years old.

References: Hubert H. Bancroft, *The Works of Hubert H. Bancroft* (San Francisco: Bancroft, 1886), 1:1834–48, 2:1848–88; Charles H. Carey, *History of Oregon* (Chicago: Pioneer Historical Publishing Co., 1922), 350; Cattaraugus County (NY) Marriages, 1837–65, transcribed by Lynn Tooley, http://www.newhorizonsgenealogicalservices.com/ny-marriage-cattaraugus-early.htm (accessed May 19, 2016); Obituary, *Humboldt County Republican,* July 10, 1903; Iowa State census, 1856, 1895; John F. Merry, *History of Delaware County, Iowa, and Its People* (Chicago: S. J. Clarke Publishing Co., 1914); US census, 1850, 1860, 1870, 1880, 1900; US Internal Revenue Service tax rolls, Iowa, 1862, 1865.

Hannah Elizabeth *Myers* LONGSHORE (1819–1901)

It is remarkable that Hannah Myers and two of her four sisters all became doctors of medicine. In addition to Hannah, there was Mary Frame Myers (Thomas) (1816–88, q.v.) and Jane Viola Myers (1831–1918, q.v.). Not only that, Hannah's husband Thomas Longshore's younger sister, Anna M. Longshore (later Potts, q.v.) became a physician, as did the wife of his older brother Joseph, Rebecca H. Reynolds Longshore (q.v.). Joseph himself was to play a large role in the early development of medical education for women, having been a prime mover in the founding of both the Female Medical College of Pennsylvania and Penn Medical University.

Both the Myers and the Longshore families were Quakers, and the Myerses were early settlers. Hannah was the first of the five girls and two boys born to her parents. At the time of Hannah's birth, May 30, 1819, in Montgomery County, Maryland, and until she was fourteen, her father Samuel taught school in Washington. He was paid $21 a month and managed to save $200 in five years. The family were followers of Sylvester Graham's teaching, emphasizing Graham bread and vegetables in their diet. Hannah went to Quaker schools. In 1833, the family moved to a farm in New Lisbon, Columbiana County, Ohio, to escape the distasteful proslavery atmosphere they found in Washington. Hannah continued her education, with hopes of going to Oberlin, but this did not come to pass. When she was twenty-two, she married Thomas E. Longshore, a teacher, and moved to the Philadelphia area where he lived.

During the first eight years of their marriage, Hannah and Thomas had two children, a son who became a physician and a daughter who would be active in the Pennsylvania Society for Woman's Suffrage. The interest that Hannah had shown in biology and dissection of small animals from quite early in her life flowered again under the tutelage of her brother-in-law, Dr. Joseph S. Longshore. She was given access to his medical library. In 1850, she matriculated in the first class at Female Medical College of Pennsylvania, one of eight students, and in 1851 graduated with an MD degree. Years later the graduation scene was described in a newspaper: "A corps of armed policemen was one of the details of that commencement; and a mob of many hundred young men students from rival institutions was another. But the latter dispersed like a shadow on the horizon when the actual crisis came, and all was order when Dr. Joseph Longshore stepped to the stage for a memorable oration."

Starting practice was no easier. In order to establish a practice in Philadelphia, Hannah gave popular lectures, first on medical education of women before a Quaker group over which Lucretia Mott presided, followed by a series of lectures to women on physiology and hygiene. Even better, she gained a reputation by curing a patient with dropsy who had been given up on by several other physicians. Thus established, she would conduct a busy practice over the next forty years. She liked doing minor surgery and reducing dislocations, especially. The maximum charge for this procedure was $3. Even so, she did well financially. When she died, daughter Lucretia inherited $100,000.

There was opposition, of course. Most physicians would not consult with her, and some druggists would not fill her prescriptions. She dealt with the latter problem by carrying her own pharmacy in a little black bag. It is said that she was absent because of sickness but twice during her professional life. She drove her own horse, and she liked to drive it fast! Her daughter, Lucretia Longshore Blankenburg, later described some of the indignities endured by members of a woman doctor's family, among them having Hannah labeled "indecent and immodest" because she gave lectures on the female genital system. Even her colleague Ann Preston (q.v.) criticized her for driving her own horse when making house calls. It wasn't "ladylike."

During her career she was also active as a teacher. In 1851 and 1852, she was demonstrator of anatomy at the newly organized New England Female Medical College in Boston. (The claim is made that she became thereby the first female faculty member at a medical school, a position she shared with Lydia Folger Fowler [q.v.].) In 1853, she was demonstrator of anatomy at the Female Medical College of Pennsylvania, and from 1853 to 1857 she taught at Penn Medical University, another Philadelphia medical school established by Joseph Longshore and colleagues who had broken away from the faculty at Female Medical College of Pennsylvania. PMU was Eclectic and coeducational. She also continued to give popular lectures on physiology and hygiene.

Hannah continued to practice until 1892, when she was seventy-three, retiring then on what was said to be a good competency. When she was eighty, she, her daughter, and her sister, Dr. Jane Myers, who lived with her, went to Europe, where they spent more than two months. In the archives of the Medical College of Pennsylvania is a record of an interview with Hannah's daughter from which the following details are excerpted: Hannah weighed two hundred pounds, loved ice cream, and smoked a pipe. Her daily routine was office hours 8–10 a.m. After lunch she would rest a bit and then go out after 3 p.m. She never went to table if there were patients in the office. Her husband kept the books and compounded the medicines. When she started reading homoeopathy several years after graduation, her alma mater was not pleased. She and Dr. Ann Preston, the dean, did not get along too well. Dr. Longshore had advanced views on many matters that got her into trouble.

Early biographer H. B. Elliott describes her as "constitutionally extremely diffident. For many years she was so easily embarrassed that she dreaded and shunned society, beyond the limited circle of a few friends. To appear in public as a lecturer, and to visit strangers professionally, always required a struggle against this timidity and the habit of reserve." She did not adopt the Quaker costume or language, but was "plain in her mode of speech and dress." She was "direct, unhesitating, and informal in her approach to a case; unpretending, and yet evidently assured in the exercise of her judgment; with a peculiar mingling of personal modesty and professional positiveness, she inspires patients with immediate trust."

Hannah died in Philadelphia October 18, 1901. Her Quaker background, her liberal and sympathetic husband, and her own interests and determination were surely essential to her success. (If it were possible, it would be interesting to compare Hannah's practice with that of the other "leading" Philadelphia female physician of the time, Harriet Judd Sartain [q.v.].)

References: Undated interview with her daughter Lucretia Blankenburg in the archives of the Female Medical College of Pennsylvania, Drexel University College of Medicine, Philadelphia; *Dictionary of American Medical Biography*, 1:459–60; "H. B. Elliott," *Eminent Women of the Age* (Hartford, CT: S. M. Betts & Co., 1868), 542–44; *National Cyclopaedia* (New York, 1894), vol. 5 [this article is essentially the same as that in Willard and Livermore]; *Philadelphia Evening Bulletin,* June 23, 1899; *Notable American Women 1607–1950*, 2:426–28; Frances E. Willard, *A Woman of the Century* (Buffalo: C. W. Moulton, 1893), 471–72.

Note: There is said to be an autobiography of Hannah Longshore among the papers of the Longshore family 1819–1902. Not seen.

Rebecca H. *Reynolds* LONGSHORE (1836–1918)

Rebecca Reynolds was born December 22, 1836, in Pennsylvania, the fifth of nine children (six girls, three boys) of Israel A. Reynolds, a farmer, and his wife, whose name is not known. The mother must have died between 1846, when her last child was born, and the 1850 census enumeration in which her name does not appear. Rebecca was thirteen in 1850. Nothing is known of her childhood or early education.

Rebecca had already married Samuel C. Longshore, a farmer, before she graduated from Penn Medical University in 1861 with an MD degree. The marriage probably took place in 1860 or 1861: Samuel appears to be single and living in a boarding house in the 1860 census. Samuel's older brother, Thomas Elwood Longshore, had married Hannah E. Myers (q.v.), who became a physician. Hannah's two sisters, Mary Frame Thomas (q.v.) and Jane Viola Myers (q.v.), both became physicians. Samuel's younger sister, Anna Longshore Potts (q.v.), was a doctor. So, the profession of medicine seems to have played a large role in the family.

Whether Rebecca and Samuel had children is uncertain. No listing for the couple was found in the 1870 census; in the 1880 census no children are listed, though by then the children might have left home. It is also possible that Samuel, who was thirty-nine when he married Rebecca, had been married before, to a woman named Sarah Ann Case.

No information has been found about the years 1860–80. In the 1880 census Rebecca is listed as being a physician, so she was probably practicing medicine. Samuel and Rebecca were then residents of Columbus, Platte County, Nebraska, where Samuel was a miller. Martha Reynolds, one of Rebecca's younger sisters, was living with them. By 1900, Samuel must have died; Rebecca was back in Unionville, Pennsylvania, living with the family of a different sister, and is denoted "physician" in the census for that year. In the 1910, she is living in San Diego, California, owns her home, and appears to be caring for a woman ten years her senior. The census calls her a "nurse." She must have been in California at an earlier period because she registered as a homoeopathic physician living in National City, California, on December 6, 1888. Her sister-in-law, Anna Longshore-Potts, had moved to National City earlier in the 1880s. Rebecca died at her home in National City, April 17, 1918, at the age of eighty-one.

References: *Census of Women Physicians November 11, 1918* (Rochester, NY, 1918); Medical Society of the State of California, *Official Register and Directory of Physicians and Surgeons in the State of California,* 17th ed. (n.p., 1905); National City, CA, city directory, 1917; *San Diego Sun,* April 18, 1918, 11; US census, 1850, 1880, 1900, 1910.

Anna Mary *LONGSHORE*-Potts (1829–1912)

Anna Mary Longshore was the youngest of ten children and fourth daughter of Abraham Longshore and Rhoda Skelton. Her older brothers, Joseph and Thomas, were both married to physician wives, and Joseph was a prime mover in organizing the Female Medical College of Pennsylvania and, later, Penn Medical University, an Eclectic and coeducational institution.

Anna was born in Bucks County, Pennsylvania, April 16, 1829. She was twenty years younger than her brother Joseph. She graduated in the first class from Female Medical College of Pennsylvania, December 30, 1851, started practice in her hometown, Langhorne, but later moved to Philadelphia, where she remained until the early 1860s. She is listed in *McElroy's Philadelphia City Directory* as a physician as late as 1861. In 1857, she married Lambert Potts, and they had at least one son, Emerson J. Potts, who, in turn, had two sons, William L. and Charles J. Potts, both of whom lived in San Francisco.

Rather peripatetic after leaving Philadelphia, she moved to Toledo, Ohio, for a year in the early 1860s, then opened a sanitarium in Geneva, Illinois, remaining there until 1867, when she moved on to Adrian, Michigan, where she practiced general medicine for about nine years. While there, she began giving private lectures to her patients, turning her emphasis to prevention rather than treatment of bad health. In 1876, she gave a course of public lectures that was so well received that she appears to have given up practice and turned full-time to the lecture circuit.

At first, the lectures were given in small towns, but gradually it was in larger communities that she spoke. In 1881, she gave a lecture in San Francisco and subsequently in other large cities along the Pacific coast, from Seattle to San Diego, enlightening the people on "love, courtship and marriage." In 1883, supported by a staff of seven, she sailed for New Zealand, where she spoke to packed houses in major cities. By November of that year, she was in Sydney, speaking to an audience of 4,500 in the exhibition building, after an introduction by the US consul. Then, on to the other cities of Australia. Reports in the press described her efforts as "a brilliant success" and said that she was "enthusiastically received."

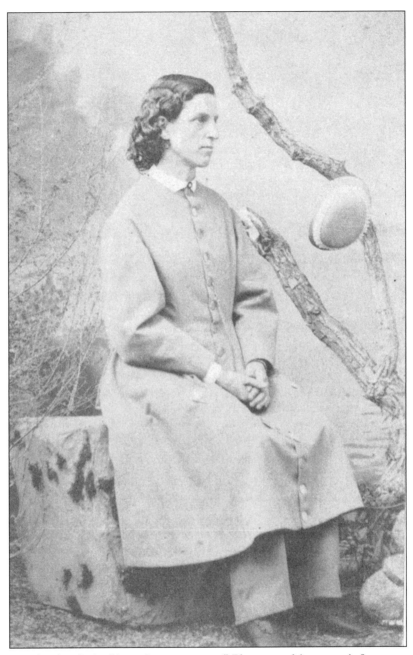

Harriet Austin in "American costume." Photographic portrait from the Albert Leffingwell papers, Atwater Collection of American Popular Medicine, Edward G. Miner Library, Rochester, NY.

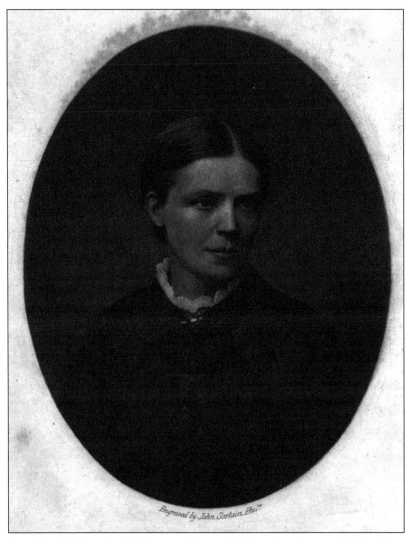

Engraved by John Sartain. Phil.ᵃ

Emeline H. Cleveland. Engraved portrait from the Atwater Collection, Edward G. Miner Library, Rochester, NY.

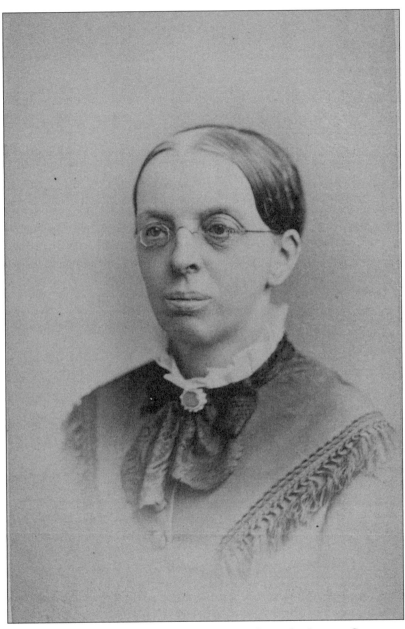

Mary Scarlett Dixon. Photographic portrait from the Legacy Center Archives, Drexel University College of Medicine, Philadelphia.

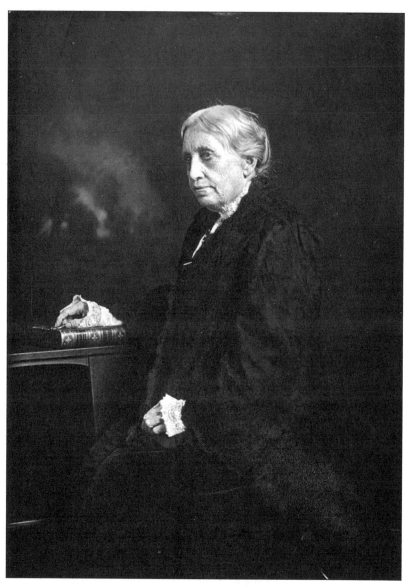

Sarah Read Adamson Dolley. Photographic portrait from the archives of the Edward G. Miner Library, Rochester, NY.

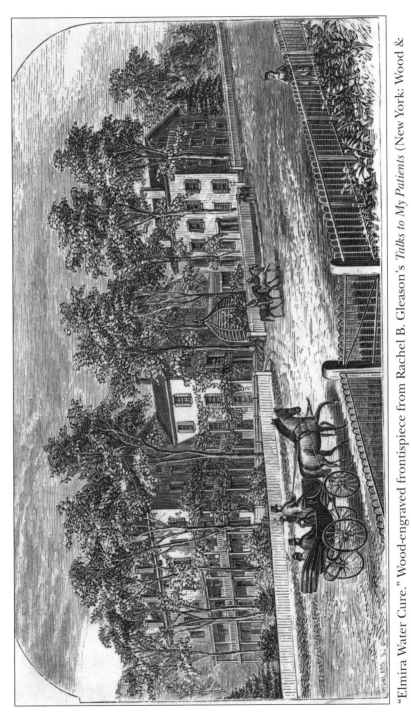

"Elmira Water Cure." Wood-engraved frontispiece from Rachel B. Gleason's *Talks to My Patients* (New York: Wood & Holbrook, 1870).

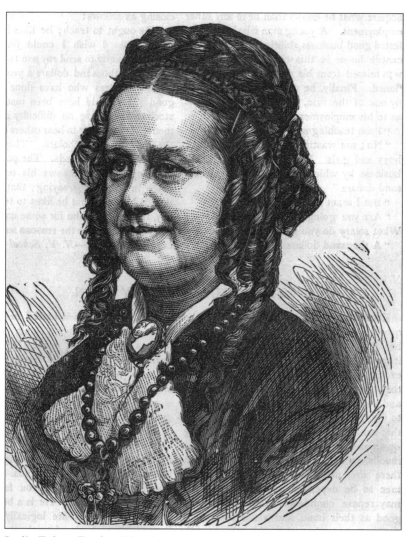

Lydia Folger Fowler. Wood-engraved portrait from *The Illustrated Annuals of Phrenology and Health Almanacs* (New York: Fowler & Wells, 1884, [1880 almanac]), 23.

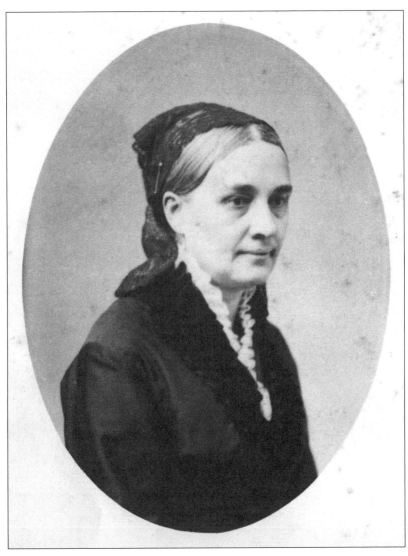

Rachel Brooks Gleason. Photographic portrait from her *Talks to My Patients*, 5th ed. (New York: Wood & Holbrook, 1874).

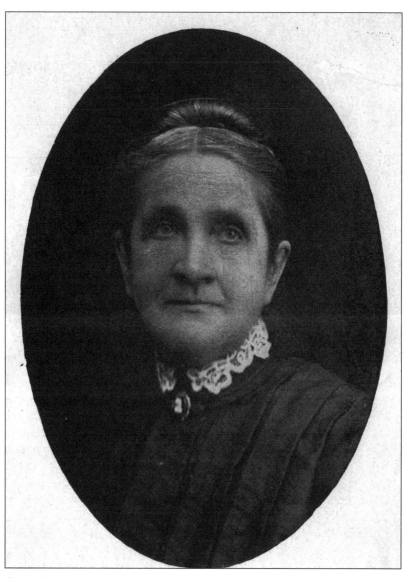

Cordelia A. Greene. Photographic portrait from her *Art of Keeping Well* (New York: Dodd, Mead & Co., 1914).

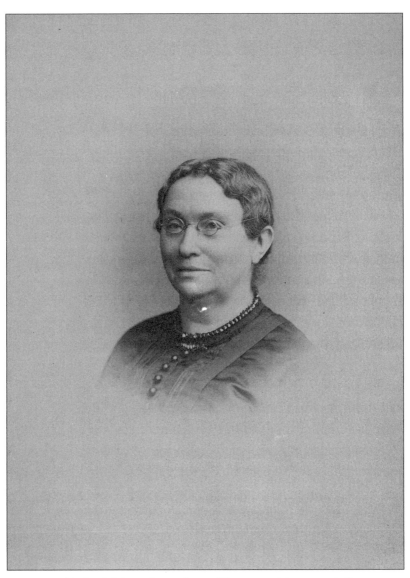

Hannah Elizabeth Myers Longshore. Photographic portrait from
the Legacy Center Archives, Drexel University College of Medicine,
Philadelphia.

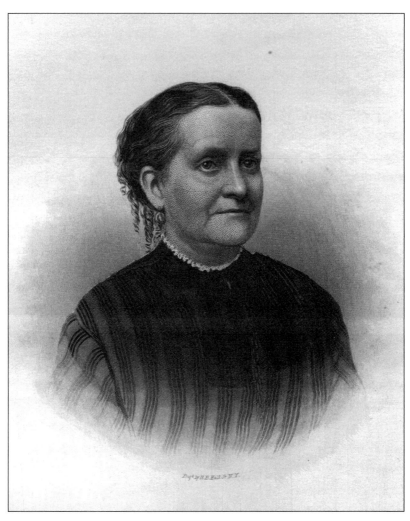

Clemence S. Lozier. Steelengraved portrait in *Eminent Women of the Age*
(Hartford, CT: S. M. Betts & Co., 1868).

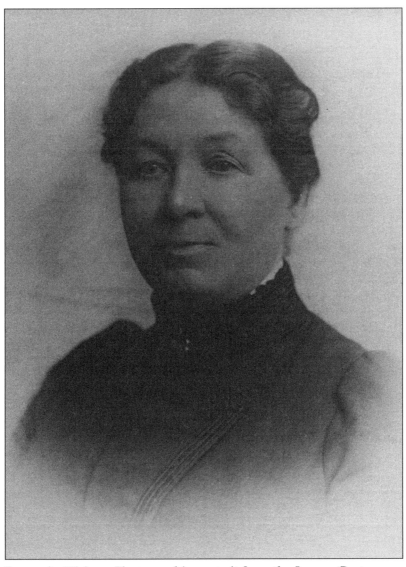

Samantha Nivison. Photographic portrait from the Legacy Center Archives, Drexel University College of Medicine, Philadelphia.

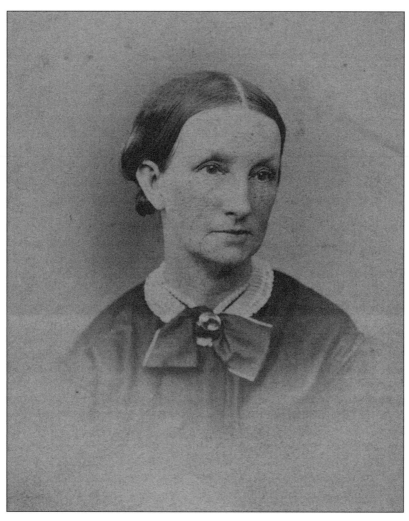

Ann Preston. Photographic portrait from the Legacy Center Archives, Drexel University College of Medicine, Philadelphia.

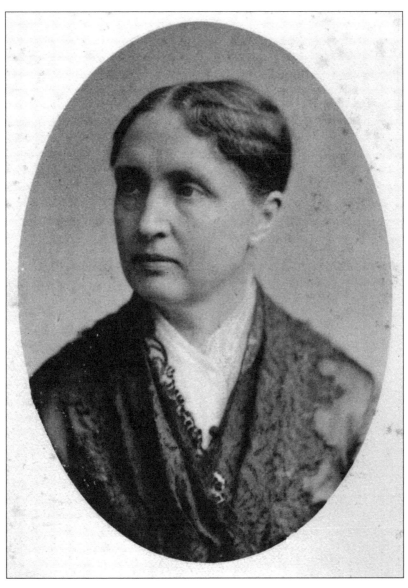

Alice B. Stockham. Photographic portrait from her *Tokology, a Book for Every Woman* (Chicago: Sanitary Publishing Co., 1883).

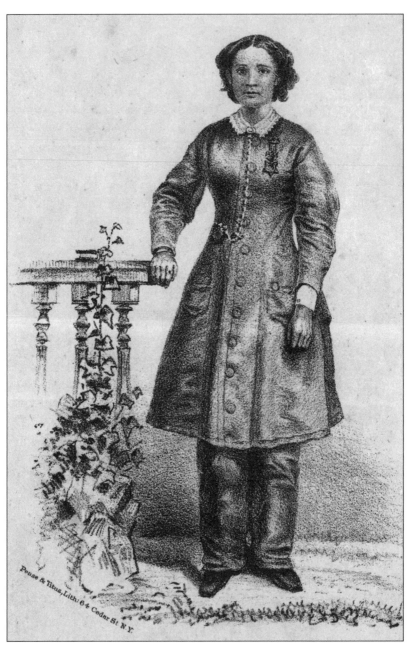

Mary E. Walker. Lithographed portrait from her *HIT: Essays on Women's Rights* (New York: American News Co., 1871).

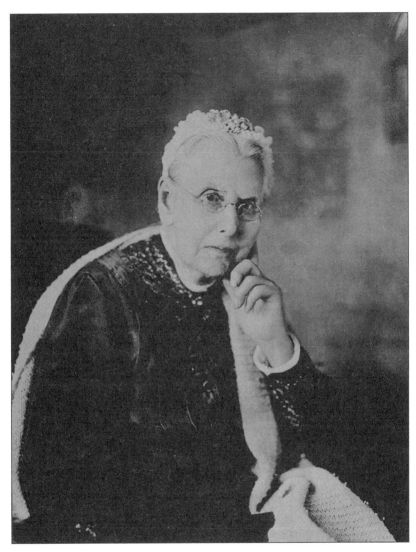

Marie Zakrzewska. Photographic portrait from the Legacy Center
Archives, Drexel University College of Medicine, Philadelphia.

The following year she was off to England. On the night of February 17, 1885, she spoke to 3,500 people in St. James Hall. The London lectures continued for five months, after which she spoke in provincial cities, returning periodically to London to repeat the lectures there. In London she stayed at the home of Lady Claude Hamilton, where many receptions were held. After almost three years, she returned to the United States, appeared at Tremont Temple in Boston, Chickering Hall in New York City, and finally returned home to California. Still later, she would make a round-the-world lecture tour that included India.

Dr. Potts must have moved to California about 1880; at least that is when she registered there as a physician. Her home base became National City, near San Diego, and it was in this area that, during her absences, she had built a sanitarium on Mt. Paradise. Newspapers reported the progress of the venture in some detail. In July 1883, she sent word from Australia that work was to commence and the site was graded and trees planted forthwith. In August the word was that the building was to be started and finished before she returned. The cornerstone was laid August 24. The sanitarium, however, which was to cost $20,000–$25,000, did not open until 1889, after Anna returned.

Dr. Longshore-Potts is last listed as a physician in the Polk medical directory for 1893 and presumably retired from professional life about this time. Her lectures had made her a wealthy woman. She died in San Diego on October 24, 1912, with senile debility.

Bibliography: *Marriage: Based on Conjugal Love* (Adrian, MI, 1872); *Love, Courtship and Marriage* (London: Author, 1887); *Discourses to Women on Medical Subjects* (London: Author, 1887; *The Logic of a Lifetime* (Alameda, CA: Author, 1911).

References: *Census of Women Physicians November 11, 1918*; Clippings etc. in the archives of the Female Medical College of Pennsylvania, Drexel University College of Medicine, Philadelphia; *McElroy's Philadelphia City Directory for 1861* (Philadelphia: E. C. & J. Biddle & Co., 1861); San Diego Public Library, newspaper clippings, 1881–89; Obituary, *San Diego Union*, October 25, 1912, 16; Frances E. Willard, *A Woman of the Century* (Buffalo: C. W. Moulton, 1893).

Laura A. LORD (b. ca. 1825)

Laura and her husband, Varnum Augustus Lord, practiced medicine and dentistry in Gowanda, New York, from 1852 until at least 1864. The village of Gowanda, located in the southwest corner of New York State, incorporated in 1848, straddles Cattaraugus Creek, so that part of it is in Cattaraugus County and part in Erie County. After 1864, the Lords disappear; no trace of them has been found.

From the 1855 New York State census we know that Varnum was born in Connecticut about 1822, his wife in Monroe County, New York, about 1825, and their son Albert in Michigan about 1841. So, the family had spent some time in Michigan before returning to Western New York. Nothing else has been found about their family backgrounds, their parents, childhood, or early education. Son Albert did become a dentist.

The Lords were living in Gowanda when both Varnum and Laura attended lectures at the recently organized Eclectic Syracuse Medical College. Varnum claimed to have graduated with an MD degree in 1852 and Laura in 1853. In the absence of adequate records, it has not been possible to substantiate this.

Some idea of their practices may come from advertisements and a long letter from Laura in contemporary Gowanda newspapers. There is a notice in which Varnum claimed twelve years' experience in dentistry, that he had lately "visited all the principal cities and associated with many of the best dentists in the United States," and is now prepared to offer the best in scientific dentistry—"setts [*sic*]" of teeth made from pure gold or plated silver, to replace "old carious teeth, filled with animal and vegetable matter in a state of putrefaction, producing foeted [*sic*] breath, deranging the stomach, giving place to dyspepsia . . . sending thousands to a premature grave." Beneath this is a somewhat smaller advertisement for the services of the couple as physicians & surgeons. Curiously, this advertisement has the following header:

> sevastopol taken by the allies! *V.A. Lord Associated with Laura A. Lord*
> physicians and surgeons. Announce to the citizens of this village that they will attend to all calls in their profession. Mrs. Lord, from long experience and extra instructions received while at medical college, on diseases incident to females, is happy to say to her female friends that the long looked for day has at length dawned when her sex can have an educated female physician to treat them in a scientific manner. From 6 to 10 female patients can be accommodated with board and treatment at her residence, on reasonable terms.
> (*Gowanda Chronicle*)

A little over two years later, Laura and Varnum are still in the same location, but Varnum was also advertising, both as dentist and as physician in separate ads, with his brother (not named) as a partner. Laura's notice reads, "Mrs. Laura A. Lord, Physician, is permanently located in Gowanda, N.Y. *All reports to the contrary notwithstanding.* Office in Plumb's Block" (*New Yorker*).

In the same issue of that newspaper was a three-thousand-plus-word "Card to the Public," from Laura A. Lord, MD. In this rambling essay Dr. Mrs. Lord denies rumors that she is leaving (or has left) town. She refutes "the variety of illegitimate stories which have received publicity. . . . Our professional reputation speaks for itself. . . . It will bear scrutiny and investigation. We have a good practice and among the first families in the village and country." Further on, she defends women's right to transact their own business and says they are entitled to participate in "trades and professions. . . . Nor have we ever intended to practice for a pittance because we were a woman." The major portion of the letter deals with the role of women as accoucheurs: "Nowhere between the two lids of the Bible does it intimate the name of a male accoucher [*sic*]." The entire piece gives the impression that Dr. Lord was doing a thriving baby delivery business to the displeasure of her male peers, and that business, of course, was the bread and butter of the medical profession in those days.

The Lords, including brother, Orlando, and son, Albert, continued to advertise in the local newspapers during the rest of the 1850s. The last ad found was for Laura in August 1864 (*Gowanda Reporter*). Their names do not appear in the 1870 or 1880 US census, in the Butler medical directories for 1874 or 1877, or in the 1886 and 1890 Polk medical directories. Nor is there any mention of them in Leonard's detailed history of Gowanda.

References: I. R. Leonard, *Historical Sketch of the Village of Gowanda, N.Y.* (Buffalo, 1898); *Gowanda Chronicle,* June 30, 1855; *Gowanda Reporter,* September 10, 1858, and August 31, 1864; *New Yorker* (Gowanda), October 27, 1857; US census, 1850, 1860.

M

Janet C. *MACLEAN* Fowle (b. ca. 1835)

Janet Maclean was born about 1835, in Sparta, Georgia. Nothing has been found about her parents, background, childhood, or early education. In 1859, Janet graduated with an MD degree from Cleveland's Western Homoeopathic College. The following February 21, she married classmate and fellow graduate, Orrin C. Fowle of Hillsdale, Michigan. The 1860 census, enumerated later in June of that year, records Janet and Orrin living in Hillsdale with a family named Riddell. Orrin is listed as a physician, but Janet, as was often the case in census reports, had no occupational designation. She was pregnant at the time and on December 11, 1860, was delivered of the couple's only child, Carolyn N. Fowle.

The marriage was short lived. Orrin and Janet were divorced even before Carolyn was born, and the couple returned to their respective parental homes. Orrin spent the rest of his life in Moscow, Hillsdale County, Michigan, a community of four hundred souls, where he practiced medicine and lived with his mother and two younger sisters. He is listed in both the Butler and Polk directories. The 1880 census, however, lists him only as a farmer. He died in 1915 and is buried in Old Soldiers Cemetery in Moscow. He never remarried.

Janet returned to Georgia, where Carolyn was born. No evidence has been found to support the idea that she practiced medicine. She often went by her maiden name, but she did stay in contact with the Fowle family. Carolyn, who was born in Covington, Georgia, married Henry Talbot Walker Jr., in Boston, December 31, 1880, had four children, and lived until 1933. Attempts to locate her living grandchildren in 2012 were not successful.

References: Butler; Polk; Marriage announcement, *Federal Union* (Hancock County, GA), February 7, 1860; US census, 1850, 1860, 1880, 1900.

Elzina C. MAYO

No information has been found regarding Elzina's parents, background, or early education. When Elzina Mayo and her husband, Joseph, graduated from Eclectic College of Medicine in Cincinnati in 1857, they were residents of New York State. Soon after receiving their medical degrees they moved westward. The 1865 IRS tax roll located them in Morrison, Illinois, where they each paid a ten-dollar physician tax, one of the taxes imposed during the Civil War. Joseph paid several additional taxes: ten dollars as a retail dealer (he later ran a drug store, so he may have already been in this business), twenty-five dollars as a liquor dealer, five dollars for having a gold watch, another five dollars because of his carriage, and, in addition, another tax because of his income. So, the Mayos seem to have been well off.

Sometime before 1879, the couple moved farther west, settling in Sedgwick, Kansas, a farming and trade center of five hundred inhabitants (1882) that had been laid out in 1870. Here, the couple continued to practice medicine and run a drug store. The following entry (and illustration), taken from the *Harvey County Atlas* (1882), describes a small, two-story, gabled frame building, with a square façade and lean-to porch, typical of early western commercial structures. "This is the oldest building in Sedgwick, moved here from the former Park City site, 8 miles southwest of Sedgwick. It is one of only two known remaining buildings from the original site of the 1870s. It was originally a dram shop saloon." After being moved to Sedgwick in 1880, it "was used as a drug store and doctor office. Some of the doctors using the building were Drs. Mayo and wife." The building now houses the Sedgwick Historical Museum.

The 1885 city directory of Sedgwick lists Dr. Joseph Mayo as a druggist at 519 Commercial and his son George H. as a clerk in the shop. No mention is made of Elzina. Joseph died January 30, 1886, at the age of ninety. The date of Elzina's death has not been determined. The couple had at least one child, George H. Mayo, born April 11, 1844, married Katie E. Montague, and died July 20, 1910.

References: W. E. Dockson, comp., *Directory of the Cities of Newton, Halstead and Sedgwick, Harvey County, Kansas* (Newton, 1885); John Edwards, *Historical Atlas of Harvey County Kansas* (Philadelphia: J. P. Edwards, 1882); Internal Revenue Service tax roll, Morrison, IL, 1865.

Helen *Walker* McANDREW (1826–1906)

Helen Walker was born February 6, 1826, in Kirkintilloch, Scotland, the daughter of Thomas Walker and his wife, Margaret Boyd. As a young adult she moved from Paisley to Glasgow where she learned the bookbinding trade. At church, she met William McAndrew, who had come from Perth to engage in his work as a cabinetmaker. The two were married in 1849 by Fergus Ferguson and immediately set out for America and an eleven-week honeymoon in steerage from Clyde to Sandy Hook. With them they brought volumes of Burns, Bunyan, Shakespeare, and the Bible that Helen had bound, as well as William's tool chest.

Upon arrival at the Battery in Manhattan, the young couple debarked. They were met by a friendly stranger with a Scottish brogue who offered to help them find lodging, shouldered William's tool chest, and disappeared forever into the crowd. Another Scot persuaded them that New York was a "squeezed orange," an island already overcrowded, and urged them to move to the city of the future—Perth Amboy, New Jersey. There they found grass growing in the streets and decided that the future was too far distant. Next they tried Baltimore, but there they got themselves into trouble "for teaching negroes to read. The neighbors don't like it. It is not respectable." Friends deserted them and they headed west.

After saving enough money for their passage, they boarded a long white packet boat that was towed up Chesapeake Bay to Havre de Grace. Here their tugboat was replaced by a trio of mules in tandem, directed by a mule boy. They entered a lock at the mouth of the Susquehanna Canal, which ran parallel to the barely passable river to its east. Thence north to the Juniata River just above Harrisburg, where they headed westward. "Our watery road winds among the mountainous hills along the blue Juniata. Day after day we sit upon the yellow deck and watch the landscape unfold." Finally, the navigable portion of the river ended and they had to portage over the Allegheny Mountains. "A huge cradle rides down the mountain on an iron track. . . . It slides under the canal-boat." After the boat was tethered, "A man waves his arms toward an engine-house up the mountain. . . . The packet ascends the mountain . . . and then, head foremost, down the western slope" back into the water, downstream to Pittsburgh, and then down the Ohio River to another canal and from there to Cleveland. The rail portage between Holidaysburg and Johnstown was considered one of the wonders of the world and was the crucial link in Pennsylvania's attempt to compete with the Erie Canal. From Cleveland, passengers changed to a side-wheeler that took them to Detroit.

Ultimately, the couple settled in Ypsilanti, a village west of Detroit near Ann Arbor. Mrs. McAndrews took up nursing as a source of income and found that she was so good at it that she decided to attend medical school. By this time she had had Thomas, the first of her two sons, born in 1852. She engaged a "colored mammy" to look after her family, took the steamer to Buffalo, the Erie Canal to Albany, and a Hudson River steamer to New York, where she enrolled in the New York Hygeio-Therapeutic College (1855). To pay for her passage, she helped the cooks aboard the steamers and the canal boat. While in New York she worked at a book bindery to support herself. McAndrew graduated on October 25, 1855.

Starting her practice back in Ypsilanti was not easy. According to her son, writing years later, the local view was that being a woman physician "isn't nice; it isn't respectable. The men physicians turn up their noses. The town doesn't think it likes this sort of thing. Only negroes and poor whites came into her office." The situation changed, however, after Dr. McAndrew "cured" the chronically ill wife of Samuel Post, a prominent local citizen. Post was a dry goods merchant who had become prominent in local Republican political circles. The Regular doctors, including consultants from Ann Arbor, had failed. McAndrew's cure involved opening the bedroom windows, putting medications down the drain, serving "plain and tasty dishes," moving the bed so the patient could see the lawn and trees, and being told each day that she looked better. Regimen and psychology played a larger role in her practice than did materia medica.

Having graduated from a hydropathic medical school, McAndrew opened in 1870 a water-cure on Huron Street with an adjacent swimming pool in the river itself. The institution included vapor baths, shower baths, mineral baths, and sitz baths. This was probably next to the octagonal house that William had built earlier for the family and as an office for his wife. A few years later, the local Ypsilanti Paper Company dug an eight-hundred-foot well to supply water for its paper-making operation. The water had a peculiar taste and was soon reputed to have remarkable therapeutic qualities—including the cure of patients with cancer and rheumatism. One had but to drink three or four glasses a day, "no matter how nauseating," take sponge baths twice a day with tepid water, and apply moist packs to affected parts. A second well was dug about six months after the first by a private company, and from this new well Dr. McAndrew was able to have water piped to her Rest for the Weary establishment at eight dollars a barrel.

Dr. McAndrew was listed as practicing in Ypsilanti in both editions of Butler (1874 and 1877) and in the Polk directories for 1886, 1890, 1893, 1896, 1898, and 1900. She is found on federal census rolls for 1850, 1870, and 1900, and paid tax as a physician to the Internal Revenue Service each year between 1862 and 1866 inclusive, an unusually consistent record not found for any other woman physician of the period.

Her husband William died in 1895. Originally a cabinetmaker, he is labeled a furniture dealer in the 1870 census, with $8,000 in real estate and $8,500 in personal property, so he seems to have prospered. Helen, usually listed as a homoeopathic physician, reported $12,500 in real estate and $1,200 in personal property. In addition to her son Thomas, who married and went into the furniture business, the couple had a second son, William (b. ca. 1864). William provided much of the information here recorded.

The McAndrews were much involved in social movements of their day: abolition, temperance, woman's suffrage, and coeducation at the University of Michigan. Mr. McAndrew helped hide runaway slaves in barns and drove them by night under hay to the river, where they were rowed to Canada. Together, the couple organized a juvenile temperance society. They invited Susan B. Anthony, Frances Willard, and Mary Livermore to lecture in Ypsilanti and hosted them in their home. The McAndrews were quiet and modest. William is said to have used a lowercase *i* when writing of himself. "Both had singular courage. None of their acquaintances [could] recall ever seeing either of them exhibit any trace of fear or nervousness on any occasion" (Mann, 54). Dr. McAndrew died October 26, 1906.

References: Internet article on Helen Walker McAndrew; John T. Mann, Ypsilanti, *A History in Pictures* (Chicago: Arcadia Publishing, 2002); Bertha Selman, "Pioneer Women in Medicine," *Medical Woman's Journal* 54 (1947): 51–54, 64; Parts of this entry for Dr. McAndrew is based on a biographical memoir written by her younger son, William, and published originally by the Ypsilanti Business and Professional Women's Club; Charles R. Pattison, "Ypsilanti: Its Past, Present and Future (Part III)," *Ypsilanti Commercial,* May 24, 1871, *Ypsilanti Gleanings,* October 1981, http://ypsigleanings.aadl. org/ypsigleanings/13884 (accessed May 19, 2016); Polk medical directories for 1886–1900; US census 1850, 1870, 1900; US Internal Revenue Service tax rolls 1862, 1863, 1864, 1865, 1866; *Water-Cure Journal* 27 (1859): 38.

Olive *Frisbie* McCUNE (1828–1907)

Olive Frisbie was born August 17, 1828, in Delhi, Delaware County, New York, the second of twelve children of Erastus Frisbie and his wife Elizabeth Lee. Nothing is known of her childhood or early education. On April 19, 1853, at twenty-four, she married William Story McCune, of nearby Andes, New York. Six years later, on March 3, 1859, she and her husband graduated from the New York Hygeio-Therapeutic College with MD degrees. Olive was already mother of one child, a daughter, Maude, born June 17, 1854.

Returning to Delhi, the couple leased a property at Fish Lake, about seven miles to the east of Delhi, in the township of Bovina. Fish Lake was a 164-acre lake whose water came entirely from underground springs; there was no inlet, but the outlet had flow sufficient to operate a grist mill that had once been there. In a building at lakeside, the two doctors established the Fish Lake Water-Cure, where they offered "air, light, temperature, exercise, sleep, and cheerful mental impressions." Each guest was asked to bring six large towels, two woolen blankets, and a comforter. Room, board, and treatment was five or six dollars a week. Treatment was offered for spinal and liver disorders, rheumatism, neuralgia, and "female complaints."

The following advertisement appeared in an 1859 issue of the *Water-Cure Journal*: "Drs. W. S. and Olive F. McCune have an establishment already prepared for the reception of invalids, in Delhi, N.Y., called Fish Lake Water-Cure, a beautiful, retired, and salubrious locality." Three years later, the journal was pleased to publish reports of cases from Fish Lake (May 1862, 103).

Olive's father, Erastus, died at the cure in 1861. A few weeks earlier, Olive had had her second child, a son named William Erastus, who would himself later become a physician. The water-cure probably continued to operate until 1865, when Olive's husband died of small-pox in April of that year.

In 1868, now forty and a widow with two young children (ages fourteen and six), Olive moved to Brooklyn and established a practice there: "Mrs. O. F. McCune, M.D. has taken rooms at No. 49 Hicks Street, Brooklyn, where she will attend calls. Patients visited at their houses. All forms of diseases treated. Special applications of Electricity and Swedish Movements." (*HOH* [successor to *WCJ*], May 1868).

Earlier that same year, Dr. McCune, in a letter to the *Herald of Health* (January 1868) expressed herself forcefully on a practice she thought discriminated against women:

> Why must we have that odious epithet, *female*, so constantly sounded in our ears? One cannot read anything about women but the word is used every third line. Why not say *men* and *women*, instead of men and *females*? Some of our most learned men talk and write this manner. It is female duties, female teachers, female editors, female speakers, female doctors, etc., till, for one, I wish the word was banished from our language. Cultured as well as uncultured people talk in this manner. Pray don't use the term any oftener than you do its opposite, *male*. In speaking of the sex, do use that best of all general terms, *women* and you will by so much elevate the sex.

Seven years later, in each issue of the *Herald of Health*, from January through March 1875, Dr. McCune announced her removal to a new location: "Mrs. O. F. McCune, M.D., has opened an office at 387 Pacific St., corner of Bond, Brooklyn, N.Y. Her large experience in all forms of women's and children's diseases enables her to promise relief after many others have failed. She makes a special use of electricity."

By December of that year, she had moved to 79 Henry Street, near Orange Street. Olive practiced medicine in Brooklyn for thirty-seven years. Her name is found in directories regularly, listed as a practicing physician: *New York Business Directory* for 1882, Polk Medical directories for 1886–1902, and the AMA medical directory for 1906. She is listed as a homoeopath. Her son, William Erastus, who graduated in 1885 from New York Homoeopathic Medical College, is said to have practiced with his mother. However, he is listed at a different address in the 1886 Polk directory. He died in 1889. His sister, Maude, died in 1890.

Olive continued to practice until 1906, when she was struck down by a horse, receiving injuries from which she never fully recovered. In September that year, she went to visit a niece in Binghamton, was taken ill while there, gradually failed, and died on January 3, 1907. She had outlived all but two of her eleven siblings. She was "well and favorably known. She was a prominent member of Plymouth Church. . . . She was a woman of strong character and intellect, retaining her faculties until near the end of her long and useful life."

References: *American Medical Directory*, 1906; Obituary, *Delaware Republican*, January 12, 1907; Nora G. Frisbie, *Edward Frisbie of Branford and His Descendants* (Baltimore: Gateway Press, 1984), 1:639, 2:68–69, 574–75; *Herald of Health*, January 1868, 32; *Herald of Health*, May 1868, 37; *Herald of Health*, January, February, and March 1875; New York Hygeio-Therapeutic College, *Biennial Catalogue*, May 1, 1857–May 11, 1859; *New York State Business Directory*, 1882; Polk, 1886–1902; John Raitt, *Ruts in the Road* (n.p.: Author, 1985), vol. 3; *Water-Cure Journal* 27 (1859): 75, May 1862, 103.

Eliza Jane *Hall* McQUIGG (1816–87)

Eliza Jane Hall was born November 16, 1816, on a farm near Westtown in rural Orange County, New York, the fourth of ten children of Lewis Hall and Mary Cory (seven girls, three boys). Both parents had Revolutionary ancestors. Eliza's older brother, Jonathan, and younger sister, Susan Emily (q.v.) became doctors of medicine, as did two of her nephews. On March 16, 1839, then still living in Orange County, she married Edmund Hobart McQuigg. The couple settled in Barton, Tioga County, on the shores of the Susquehanna between Elmira and Binghamton. Two children were born there: Frances (b. June 25, 1841) and Mary Elizabeth (b. December 25, 1842). In August 1846 Eliza and Edmund separated. As would come out in later court proceedings, Edmund "did not treat his wife kindly. . . . He cursed at her, he damned her," he made her cry. Eliza, on the other hand, never treated her husband "any other way than kindly." This was the testimony of Edmund's sister, who had lived with the couple for several weeks. Eliza, for her part, said that she was compelled to leave Edmund "because of his guilt of open an[d] notorious adultery, and because of his cruel, and inhuman treatment of he[r]." Edmund had persuaded Eliza to sign over all her property to him and during the six years between separation and divorce so arranged things so as to protect that property from any claim Eliza might have upon it. Claiming desertion, Edmund divorced Eliza in Indiana in 1854, where it was "easier and cheaper" to do it. Edmund kept the children, who lived with his relatives or at school. Eliza's later unsuccessful attempt to have the divorce decree voided led to a substantial trial record from which much of this biographical information is drawn.

Eliza, in the meantime, moved from one place to another. She went to Cuba with one of her sisters and tutored in a Spanish family. She went to Green Bay, Wisconsin, where her older brother, Dr. Jonathan, lived. She visited Chicago. She traveled down the Mississippi River with two of her sisters to New Orleans, where the three taught painting. She visited Natchez, St. Louis, and the state of Texas. In the early 1850s, she attended Syracuse Medical College, a short-lived Eclectic school, from which, she said, she received a "Diploma as a Physician." (It has not been possible to document this because the records are incomplete.) From there, in November 1852, she went to New York City, sailed to and crossed Panama, and sailed again to San Francisco, arriving there January 5, 1853, still with the surname McQuigg, which she soon dropped. The following May 1, 1854, her third child, Charles Victor Hall, was born.

In San Francisco she was soon employed as a physician at a local water-cure establishment operated by Dr. S. M. Bourne. In the February 25, 1853, issue of the *Daily Alta California* was the following advertisement: "Home for the Sick at 118 Dupont St. southeast corner of Pine," in which the virtues of the home and the use of water as therapy are extolled, the various "pathies" rejected, and the doctors "simply proceed at once to assist nature in effecting her own cure." No drugs are required. Dr. Bourne is assisted by Mrs. E. J. Hall, MD. Eliza Jane's name appears the following year in the San Francisco directory as a practicing physician at Portsmouth House and in several, but not all, years subsequently. Eliza Jane ran an advertisement of her own in the *Daily Alta California* at least fourteen times between July 13 and August 3, 1853: "Mrs. E. J. Hall, M.D., Physician, Surgeon and Accouchess. Success warranted in the cure of diseases peculiar to woman. Mrs. H. has had much experience in the treatment of diseases incident to children. Residence, Montgomery st. west side, between Pacific st. and Broadway."

Sometime during these years she became associated with Eliza W. Farnham (q.v.). In Dr. Farnham's deposition in the divorce retrial, she said, "During the time she [Eliza Jane] was with me at this and other places she was my companion and assistant, I was lecturing." The two visited eight or ten places during a six- or seven-week period. Farnham said further, "She practiced chiefly in San Francisco where she was settled but also did business in the places we visited."

In 1856 or 1857, Eliza Jane attended the New York Hygeio-Therapeutic College. In the biennial catalog of that school, she is listed as already an "M.D.," which would seem to support her contention of having a Syracuse degree. On returning to San Francisco, she became matron at the British Hospital, an institution supported by the British government from 1852 until 1859. In 1859 and 1861 directories there are listings for Eliza Hall, widow, furnished rooms, and Mrs. Eliza Hall, laundress, at 204 Sutter. Whether these refer to Dr. Eliza is unclear. But in a later advertisement, Dr. Eliza offered five furnished rooms, with gas and free baths at fifteen dollars a month in association with an advertisement that ran in June and July of 1862 in the *Daily Alta California*:

> Mrs. E. J. Hall, M.D. is prepared to treat all forms of Diseases, in all stages, upon natural principles, with confidence of success, especially in all such cases as have been given up by the regular Faculty. The sick, of all ages and conditions, will be expected to place themselves wholly under her care, without restriction or interference from any other parties. The poor will be treated without charge. Compensation asked will be moderate in all cases. Her treatment is peculiar and simple, and aims to cure in the shortest possible time. Baths administered to patients without extra charge. 625 Market street.

An adjacent advertisement read, "free baths! free baths! by mrs. e. j. hall, m.d., 625 Market street, Opposite Montgomery. To all the sick in all the Charity Hospitals, and to all Children in the different Orphan Asylums and Charitable Institutions, every Wednesday and Saturday, from 10 A.M. to 5 P.M. Free Bathers furnish their own towels and soap. reserved baths for persons in health." The 1862 San Francisco directory lists "Mrs. E. J. Hall M.D., physician and electrochemical baths, 625 Market and 127 Stevenson."

Eliza may have given up medical practice after this. Her listing in the 1863 directory is the last in which she is denoted "M.D." However, she is not described there as a physician but rather as a widow and proprietress of the patent Volcanic Smelting Furnace, which she had apparently invented or at least modified so that she had three patents on various components. A local newspaper reported in December 1862 that the furnace was "a complete success. The furnace was yesterday filled with copper ore and in twenty minutes after the fans commenced playing the metal was separated from the rock and commenced flowing off. This appears incredible, but it is nevertheless true; and it is easy to see that the importance of the discovery cannot be exaggerated. It will completely revolutionize mining enterprise not only on this coast but wherever minerals are found. In charging this furnace only about two bushels of charcoal, to one bushel of ore are used, while in other furnaces about ten bushels of fuel would be required." A year or so later, the furnace won a premium at the exhibition of the Mechanics

Institute of the City of San Francisco and the report of this was accompanied by a detailed description by Dr. Eliza of how the furnace was designed and operated.

Not much is heard about the furnace over the next few years, and it is not clear whether Eliza was still living in San Francisco or had moved to Los Angeles. In April and May 1869 a new advertisement appeared in the *Daily Alta* offering advice on its use and the sale of rights to use it. One was to apply to "eliza j. hall, m.d., at the Water-Cure, 637 California street, opposite St. Mary's Cathedral." Dr. Hall is listed as the proprietress. This certainly suggests that she was still living in San Francisco and was operating a water-cure establishment.

Sometime after this Eliza and her son, Charles Victor, moved to Los Angeles. Eliza's younger daughter, Mary Elizabeth, also joined them. The 1870 US census shows Eliza Jane, Mary Elizabeth (known as Libbie), and Charles Victor all located in Los Angeles. Libbie, who legally changed her maiden surname to Hall in 1861, married Capt. William Moore of Los Angeles sometime in the 1870s. Charles Victor attended the University of California at Berkeley (1867–70). He must have been a bright lad; he was only thirteen at matriculation. He was in real estate and later the oil business. No information has been found about Eliza's professional or business activities after she moved to Los Angeles. Perhaps she had prospered with her volcanic furnace. In any case, in 1881 she deeded 157 acres of land near the present-day USC campus to son Charles Victor and, according to family lore, was the owner of mineral mines in California. Eliza Jane died in Los Angeles on March 22, 1887, at the age of seventy and is buried at Angelus Rosedale Cemetery in Los Angeles.

References: Advertisement for Volcanic Smelting Furnace, *California Medical Gazette Advertiser*, May 1869; Advertisement for Dr. Bourne's water-cure, *Daily Alta California*, February 25, 1853; Advertisement for Mrs. E. J. Hall, MD, *Daily Alta California*, July 19–August 3, 1853; Advertisement, *Daily Alta California*, June 26, 28, and July 12, 18, 1862; *Daily Alta California*, March 31, 1869; Editorial puff for Volcanic Smelting Furnace, *Daily Alta California*, April 14, 1869, et seq.; Clifford Hall, "Descendancy Narrative of Lewis (Robert) Hall," 2014, typescript [Mr. Hall is a great-great-grandson of Eliza Hall]; Indiana State Archives, *Eliza Jane McQuigg vs. Edmund McQuigg*, Marion County Circuit Court, 1858, box 473, folder 069, location 42-S-7, accession number 2007236; *LeCount & Strong's San Francisco Directory for the Year 1854*; *Marysville Daily Appeal*, December 31, 1862; Mechanics Institute of the City of San Francisco, *Report of the Fourth Industrial Exhibition* (San Francisco, 1864); New York Hygeio-Therapeutic College, *Biennial Catalogue*,

1856–57 and 1858–59 (New York, 1857, 1859); *San Francisco Directory,* 1854, 1858, 1862, 1863; *Water-Cure Journal,* June 1853, 137; Letter from Dr. G. M. Bourne.

Ellen J. *MELLON* (b. ca. 1832)

Ellen Mellon was born somewhere in Pennsylvania about 1832, exact location not known. Her parents were both born in Ireland. She graduated with an MD degree from Penn Medical University in 1856 and was a resident of Philadelphia at that time. Her name is found in eleven Philadelphia city directories between 1867 and 1887, listed each time as a physician. Her name is not listed in Butler's medical directories (1874, 1877) or in Polk's medical directories (1886, 1890). She probably practiced medicine in Philadelphia from 1856 until at least 1887. No death date or obituary for her has been found. Remarkable is the fact that she remained at the same address (2425 Callowhill) from 1867 to 1887, possibly longer. This was quite unusual for the time. She did not marry.

References: Philadelphia city directories, 1867, 1868, 1878, 1879, 1880, 1881, 1882, 1883, 1885, 1886, 1887; US census, 1870, 1880.

Myra *King* MERRICK (1825–99)

Myra King was the first woman doctor to practice in Ohio. She founded both a medical school and a dispensary in Cleveland. Born August 15, 1825, in Hinkley, Leicestershire, England, she came to the United States with her parents when she was one year old. The family settled in Boston. At the age of eight, she began working in the local cotton mills, and she was later to boast that she was self-supporting since that time.

In 1841, the family moved to Ohio and settled near Elyria, where, on February 19, 1848, at the age of twenty-three, she married Charles Henry Merrick. The couple soon moved back to the East, to near New Haven, Connecticut. According to Ingham's history, Myra studied in New York City at Hyatt's Academy Rooms, then took a course at Nichols's Hydropathic Institute, and soon started the study of medicine with Dr. Levi Ives of New Haven as her preceptor. Soon, she matriculated at Central Medical College, an Eclectic school in Rochester, New York, and, in June 1852 received an MD degree. Her graduation essay, entitled "Chemistry in Its Relation to Medical Science," won a prize from the state Eclectic Medical Society. While still in medical school, Myra and another student, with their professor, Dr. L. C. Dolley, were a committee on the practicality and manner of awarding prizes (*Buffalo Medical & Surgical Journal*, 1899). After graduation, she went to Cleveland and opened an office on Miami Street, then a fashionable residential street. For a brief period she moved back to Elyria but soon returned to Cleveland, where she stayed the rest of her life.

The Merricks had two children, Richard Lester (b. 1854), who lived in Cleveland, and Arthur B. (1861–64). In 1859, Charles became postmaster of North Eaton, the village in which the couple had been married. In 1861, he went off to war and was a hospital steward for three years. In his absence Myra managed his lumber business. Sometime between then and September 17, 1882, when Charles married Helen May Finley and moved to Washington state, where he was again a postmaster, he and Myra must have been divorced. (According to LDS records, a Charles Henry Merrick had two children in Chicopee, Massachusetts, in 1865 and 1874 with Ellen Augusta Bullens. Whether this was a different Merrick or whether Myra's husband had still another mate is unknown.)

During the Civil War Myra went to Lorain, Ohio, but returned to Cleveland after the war was over and built a large practice among wealthy and influential citizens, including many of the prominent officials of the Standard Oil Company. She was the family physician of John D. Rockefeller. She "bore an enviable reputation in the art of healing" (*News Herald*). "She was an earnest student and kept in close touch with the best medical thought in all corners of the globe. . . . Her skill and womanly tenderness endeared her to all patients" (*Plain Dealer*). She is said to have introduced in Cleveland the use of the Walcher position, a maneuver occasionally used to engage the head of the fetus with the pelvic brim. "Her serene confidence in herself that was far removed from all vanity" led to her overcoming male professional opposition. "In due time . . . she stood shoulder to shoulder with the best physicians in the city [and] she overstepped most of them in a pecuniary way and her practice, largely, was among a wealthy and exclusive class that gave her an income far up in the thousands" (*Plain Dealer*).

Dr. Merrick was active in the community. During the war she organized a relief society for the care of the sick and wounded. In 1867, after the Western Homoeopathic College stopped accepting women and with support from her prosperous patients, she established the short-lived Homoeopathic College for Women and was its president for a time. The school merged with WHC in 1870 to become the Homoeopathic Hospital College of Cleveland, a school that did accept women. In 1879, she founded the Free Medical and Surgical Dispensary for Women and Children at the corner of Woodland Avenue and Erie

Street; she was the dispensary's first president, and this was perhaps her favorite accomplishment. The institution cared for 57,270 patients in fourteen years, and of that number 1,322 were surgical patients. She was a member of the American Institute of Homoeopathy and of the Unity Church.

In 1890, she retired from practice, handing over responsibility for her patients to her daughter-in-law, Dr. Eliza J. Merrick. Six weeks before her death at seventy-four, she developed serious heart trouble. She died November 10, 1899, at the home of her son, who, with her daughter-in-law, survived her. She was also survived by a foster daughter, Mrs. Frank Friend.

References: *Buffalo Medical & Surgical Journal* 39 (1899): 385; Obituary, *News Herald* (Cleveland), November 11, 1899; Obituary, *Plain Dealer* (Cleveland), November 11, 1899, 3; Mrs. W. A. Ingham, *Women of Cleveland and Their Work, Philanthropic, Educational, Literary, Medical and Artistic* (Cleveland: W. A. Ingham, 1893), 315–30; *Dictionary of American Medical Biography*, 2:516–17; *Ohio State Archeological & Historical Quarterly* (Columbus) 49 (1940): 315–97.

Maria *MINNIS* Homet (1820–92)

Maria Minnis was born June 20, 1820, near Phelps, Ontario County, New York, the youngest child of Samuel Minnis and his wife Sarah Horton. She began teaching school when she was sixteen years old and did this for several years. During this time she read medical books and studied with Dr. Caleb Bannister. At age thirty, she went to Terrytown, Pennsylvania, a village along the east branch of the Susquehanna River in the Wyalusing Valley, where she continued her studies with her mother's cousin, Dr. George Firman Horton (Rensselaer Polytechnic Institute, 1827; hon. MD, Rutgers, 1829). Then, on to Female Medical College of Pennsylvania in Philadelphia, where she received an MD degree, graduating in the school's second class in 1853.

Returning to Terrytown, she set up in practice in a rural area, partly to disprove the commonly held opinion that women could not endure the hardships of a country practice. "This determined me to take a practice in the country, for, I thought, *alma mater* would be glad to have this obstacle removed." She "settled in a small village in Pennsylvania, with the Susquehanna river on one side and the mountains on the other."

We know a bit about her practice because, in 1964, her grandniece, Elizabeth Homet, gave to Maria's alma mater (later known as Medical College of Pennsylvania) her diploma and a ledger Maria had started in the 1850s, in which she recorded the name of each patient, the nature of the patient's problem, the medicine given, and the charge for the service, as well as other expenses she incurred. She bought a horse for $25, paid $1.25 to have the horse shod, $1 for the horse's blanket and a sidesaddle. She had $94.20 worth of medicine shipped for $3.10 from New York. She bought a gallon of alcohol for 85 cents and some quinine for a quarter. She charged $3 for an obstetrical visit, presumably a delivery, 50 cents for other visits, 12 1/2 cents for pulling a child's tooth, and $1.25 for setting a broken collarbone. Payment was often in butter or grain. Her practice covered both sides of the river, and she made many trips by ferry, crossing both from Terrytown to Wyalusing and, later, upstream from Homet's Ferry to French Town. The cost was 12 1/2 cents one way.

> I often rode ten miles in the night as well as in the day. I made friends, and my practice increased rapidly. The second year I bought a carriage with side lamps, which was much more comfortable than riding on horseback. . . . Everyone had a friendly greeting for me. The poor and the rich alike opened their doors to me. If I had a hard day's ride, I was sure to have invitations to stop to dinner, and have my horse fed, and often my horse would be left in the stable, and a fresh one brought out for my use the rest of the day. Of course, these many acts of kindness could not banish the care and anxiety, and, above all, the great responsibility with which I ever felt burdened; but they did seem to give to the snow some warmth, they seemed to make the swollen creeks less violent, the mountain precipices less danger-ous. . . . I practiced in the village three years, and averaged three dol-lars per day. Then I married, and removed about two miles on the other side of the river on my husband's farm. Here it was much eas-ier; my husband never allowed me to harness my horse, and if I had a call in the night he always drove for me.

Maria married Edward Homet on November 13, 1856. He was the son of a locally prominent farming family and did surveying as well as running his farm. Earlier Homets (pronounced O-me) had come to the area in the 1790s as émigrés from France after the Revolution and settled in Azilum, a planned expatriate community farther upstream at another bend in the Susquehanna River, near Towanda. Many émigrés later moved south or, after Napoleon granted them amnesty, back to France. The Homets stayed.

Edward had designed and built the house in which he and Maria lived, overlooking a bend in the river. There is a touching letter from Maria to Edward, written three weeks before their wedding, at a time when Edward was putting the finishing touches on the new Italianate style house: "Dear Edward, I want to come and see you on Saturday evening next. Can I come? I thought I would ask you to come down but when crossing the river yesterday I saw you on top of the house or on nothing, for I could not see what supported you, and I thought how tired you would be so I said to myself—I will not ask him to come down. Then I thought I would like to know, at the close of the week, whether you had escaped all danger." She goes on to describe the seamstress making her wedding dress, working at the other end of the table on which she was writing. She expresses the hope that nobody will get sick for a week or two, but then goes back to her concern for Edward: "If you only keep well and no accident happens to you. . . . But don't your head get dizzy, when up so high? [he was working on the cupola] Then it might make you lame too. I think I will bring a little of the medicine you spoke of [whiskey?] but you must take it at night or you might not be able to climb so well. I am glad you are not afraid [of climbing]. . . . But I must confess it made me tremble a little to see you up so high. But you are doing your duty and I trust no harm will come to you."

Edward and Maria lived the rest of their lives in the house that Edward built. They had one child, a daughter named Lucy, born eighteen months after they were married. Maria continued to practice for a few more years. "After practicing thirteen years, my family thought they needed me at home, and that I needed rest. I therefore gave up practice. I now go out occasionally, but my visits are gratuitous." Looking back, she was glad that she was a doctor. "She never lost that keen sense of the ridiculous which she said was part of her Irish wit, and which she always declared helped her to bear with some of the trials of her early practice."

Maria died February 4, 1892, at seventy-one. In her obituary in the *Wyalusing Rocket* was written, "For many years she was a practicing physician and was known so well throughout this part of the country that it is only necessary to say that her extended practice and success as a physician speak well for her. She was a quiet and good neighbor, highly esteemed by those who knew her." She was a staunch Methodist. She is buried in the Homet family cemetery in Homet's Ferry. Her daughter, unmarried, lived with her father in the big house until her own death in 1907. Edward died the following year.

References: Woman's Medical College of Pennsylvania, *Report of the Proceedings of the Seventeenth Annual Meeting of the Alumnae Association* (Philadelphia, 1892), 25–26; *Towanda Daily Review*, February 11, 1964; Maria Minis, letter dated October 23, 1856, to Edward Homet, Homet's Ferry, PA, Archives of the Female Medical College of Pennsylvania, at the Drexel University College of Medicine archives, Philadelphia;

Maria Minnis, medical ledger, Archives of the Female Medical College of Pennsylvania, at the Drexel University College of Medicine archives.

Frances G. MITCHELL

Frances Mitchell was born in England. Nothing is known of her parents, background, or early education. She was a resident of Philadelphia when she enrolled in the Female Medical College of Pennsylvania, from which she graduated with an MD degree on December 31, 1851, one of eight members of the school's first class. According to Alsop, she returned to England after graduation. The annual announcement of the Woman's Medical College of Pennsylvania for 1890 records her death as being between 1885 and 1890.

References: Gugliema F. Alsop, *History of the Woman's Medical College, Philadelphia, Pennsylvania, 1850–1950* (Philadelphia: J. B. Lippincott, 1950), 35; Woman's Medical College of Pennsylvania, *Annual Announcement for 1890* (Philadelphia, 1890).

Augusta R. *MONTGOMERY* Nelson (1828–98)

Augusta was born in New York State April 17, 1828, the fifth of seven children of Martin and Eliza Montgomery. The 1850 census finds her in Darien, Genesee County, New York, where she is living with her mother and younger brother George. Eliza had $3,500 in property, a reasonable sum for that day.

Augusta attended the Female Medical College of Pennsylvania and graduated with an MD degree on January 27, 1853, with the second class to come from that school. On May 21, 1856, she married Robert W. Nelson, MD, an Englishman, born in 1816, licensed by the Royal College of Physicians in 1838, who came to the United States in June 1852 and settled in Buffalo, not far from Darien. In 1854, he received a diploma from the Medical Society of the State of New York.

After their marriage, the couple moved to St. Louis, where they stayed for five years before moving in 1861 to Bloomington, Illinois. They were probably both practicing at this time. In 1862, Robert became an assistant surgeon in the army and was assigned to the military hospital at Mound City in southern Illinois, on the banks of the Ohio River, just north of Cairo and the confluence of the Ohio and Mississippi Rivers. There, a large brick building had been taken over by the government and turned into one of the largest and best military hospitals in the west. It could accommodate from 1,000 to 1,500 patients. Wounded from the Battles of Belmont (November

1861), Fort Donelson (February 1862), and Shiloh (April 1862) were brought there.

Probably in 1862, Robert was transferred to a still newer military hospital at Island #10, about forty miles downstream, opened in 1862 after the island was captured by Union troops. Named for being the tenth island in the river south of the confluence of the Ohio and the Mississippi, it was a large sand bar about two miles long and a half mile wide, heavily forested, located at the base of a giant loop in the river, about where Kentucky, Tennessee, and Missouri meet. The sharp loop made it necessary for boat traffic to slow considerably and be therefore more vulnerable to gunfire. Heavily fortified, the island was important in controlling river traffic. After a two-month siege, it fell to Union forces on April 7, 1862. A military hospital was established on the island, and the Nelsons were in charge of it. (The sources are conflicting on this point. One says they were both there, another implies that mother and son were at home in Bloomington and that they "removed from Bloomington to Lansing, Mich., in 1863, on account of the health of [the] son, a lad of five years, who, during a visit with his mother to the army while at Island No. 10, had contracted severe illness.")

In June 1864, Robert resigned his commission, "completely worn down by arduous duty," and went to Lansing. The record shows that Robert became a homoeopath in 1862 and Augusta in 1868 (Pettet). They do not appear to have been "establishment" homoeopaths: they were not members of the American Institute of Homoeopathy and are not mentioned in Cleave or King. However, Robert does have two bibliographic entries in Bradford's *A Clinical Assistant; Being Reliable Gleanings from Practice* and what is probably a second edition of the same work, *A Clinical Assistant: Being an Index of Diseases, Their Symptoms and Homoeopathic Treatment.*

While in Lansing the homoeopathic members of the local profession established the Michigan Homoeopathic College (1871), and Robert was chosen professor of obstetrics. He lectured for two seasons. The school closed in 1873, partly at least because the state legislature was not willing to give it financial support.

The 1874 Butler directory places Robert in Dewitt, Michigan; and the 1877 Butler, the 1877–78 Pettet, and the 1878 Lansing directories all show both Nelsons to be in Lansing, with a home and office at 28 Washington Avenue, practicing as homoeopathic physicians, electricians, and proprietors of electro-therapeutic baths. Sometime after this they moved to Utah, but, twenty years later, when Augusta died in Oregon, the Lansing newspaper took note of the fact that she "had resided in this city, where she was well-known among the older residents."

The first Polk directory in 1886 lists the Nelsons as being in Ogden, Utah, and Robert is listed as there in 1890. By 1893, Robert had apparently died, and Augusta had moved to Denver. Perhaps the Charles D. Nelson (MD, Harvard, 1891) living there was her son. Augusta is still listed in Polk as a practicing physician. In 1894 she moved to Portland, Oregon, where she lived with her eldest son until her death. She is listed as a practicing physician there in the 1896 and 1898 Polk directories. She died, apparently of a heart attack, March 27, 1898.

References: Thomas L. Bradford, *Homoeopathic Bibliography of the United States from the Year 1825 to the Year 1891, Inclusive* (Philadelphia: Boericke & Tafel, 1892); Thomas L. Bradford, *A Clinical Assistant; Being Reliable Gleanings from Practice* (Chicago, 1879); Thomas L. Bradford, *A Clinical Assistant: Being an Index of Diseases, Their Symptoms and Homoeopathic Treatment* (Chicago, 1882); Butler, 1874, 1877; Samuel W. Durant, *History of Ingham and Eaton Counties, Michigan, with Illustrations and Biographical Sketches* (Philadelphia: Ensign, 1880); Lansing city directory, 1878; Obituary, *Morning Oregonian*, March 28, 1898; *Lansing Journal*, April 1898; Death certificate, Oregon State Archives, 79A-37, Ctn. 4; J. Pettet, *The North American Homoeopathic Directory for 1877–78* (Cleveland: Robison, Savage & Co., 1878); Polk, 1886, 1890, 1893, 1896, 1898; US census for 1850.

Orianna Russell *MOON* Andrews (1834–83)

Orie Moon, as she was known, was born August 11, 1834, in Scottsville, Virginia, a village about fifteen miles south of Charlottesville, to a prominent local family. Her father, Edward H. Moon, was a merchant. Her mother was Anna Maria Barclay. She was the second of eleven children, seven of whom lived to adulthood. Her older brother, Thomas, studied medicine at the University of Pennsylvania but apparently did not earn a degree, perhaps because he died of cholera in 1855; he is not listed in the University catalog. Her next-younger sibling, Charlotte, was a Baptist missionary in China for forty years.

Wishing to follow in her brother's footsteps, she went to Troy (New York) Female Seminary and thence to the Woman's Medical College of Pennsylvania, from which she received an MD degree in 1857. After graduating, she went to Paris for hospital training and then to Jerusalem, where her mother's brother was a missionary. There she practiced medicine for a year and a half, treating children with ophthalmia especially. One of her adult patients, an Arab chieftain who recovered, is said to have given her an Arab blessing to the effect that she have many children, and only sons. On returning to America she probably set up practice in Scottsville.

With the outbreak of the Civil War, Orie was commissioned a captain (surgeon) in the Confederate army, said to be the only female officer. After the Battle of Bull Run, she became a nurse in the Confederate hospital in Charlottesville. Here she met, and married on November 24, 1861, John Summerfield Andrews of Memphis, an 1859 or 1860 graduate of Shelby Medical College and assistant surgeon at the hospital. They had twelve children (all sons!), six of whom lived to adulthood.

After the war, husband and wife practiced together, first in Tennessee, then in Alabama, and finally back in Scottsville where, in 1879, they opened a hospital in Viewmont, Orie's childhood home. Orie died in Scottsville, December 26, 1883. Her husband died sometime after 1886, the last year in which he was listed in the Polk medical directory. It is claimed, apparently correctly, that Orie was the first woman MD south of the Mason-Dixon Line. In his autobiography, *A Doctor's Experience in Three Continents*, Edward Warren, who was surgeon general of the Confederacy and who knew Orie, wrote of her the following:

> I met also for the first time that *rara-avis* in the field of Southern medicine, a female physician, in the person of Miss Moon, a native of Albemarle County, Virginia, and a graduate of the Woman's Medical College of Philadelphia. She was a lady of high character and of fine intelligence, and, though she failed to distinguish herself as a physician, she made an excellent nurse, and did good service in the wards of the hospital. Unfortunately for her professional prospects she fell in love with one of our assistant surgeons, and compromised matters by marrying him and devoting herself to the care of her own babies— like a sensible woman. Imagine, if you can, the position of this young lady, with much of native modesty and refinement in her composition, in a hospital of wounded soldiers, and with only medical officers as her companions, and you will have eliminated a most potent argument against the inappropriateness of a woman becoming a doctor. In my humble judgment, no one possessing a womb or endowed with the attributes of femininity ought to dream of entering the ranks of the medical profession, and Dr. Moon's experience at Charlottesville teaches a lesson in this regard which her aspiring sisters would do well to heed and appreciate.

The possibility of matrimony and the probability of maternity— the ends for which women were created—raise a barrier in the path of those who would thus enter upon the domain of medicine, which they should regard as nature's protest against their intrusion. In a word, women were made not to administer drugs nor to amputate limbs nor to engage in the arduous and exciting incidents of a doctor's career, but to fill the sacred *role* of sister, wife and mother—to render homes happy, and to sustain, cheer and comfort men in the struggle of life.

References: Philip Alexander Bruce, *History of Virginia* (Chicago: American Historical Society, 1924), 6:418–19; Anna Mary Moon, *Sketches of the Moon and Barclay Families* (Chattanooga, 1939); Edward Warren, *A Doctor's Experiences in Three Continents* (Baltimore: Cushings & Bailey, 1885), 279–80.

Note: Dr. Moon is not listed in *Virginia Surgeons in the Civil War*, appendix 2, 393–420. John S. Andrews is listed as assistant surgeon, July 19, 1861, in hospital at Charlottesville, resigned February 4, 1862.

Martha Harris *MOWRY* (1818–99)

Martha Mowry was born June 7, 1818, in Smithfield, Rhode Island, the second child of Thomas Mowry, a Providence merchant, and Martha Harris. She had a brother, six years her senior. Her father was said "to do his own thinking," and her paternal grandfather had been prominent in local affairs. Her mother died when Martha was eight weeks old. Young Martha was brought up by her father's sister, "a cultured woman, of literary tastes."

By the time Martha was grown, she had attended six or seven different private schools in Providence: those of Miss Sterry and Miss Chace, Miss Walker's academy, Friends' Yearly Meeting Boarding School (1827–31), Miss Latham's Select Boarding School, and Miss Winsor's Young Ladies Boarding School. At this last school, where she spent four years, she developed some kind of heart trouble (said to have been aggravated by overexertion in running 1 1/4 miles to escape a strange man who was pursuing her and two classmates). She left school but continued to study: mathematics, Greek, Latin, Hebrew, and ancient philosophers. Then back she went to Green Street Select School in Providence, after which she continued study on her own, emphasizing languages and oriental literature.

In 1844, at the age of twenty-six, she decided to study medicine, which she did with a series of doctors in Providence and nearby communities (Drs. Briggs, Fowler, Fabyan, Mauran, and DeBonnerville). In the winter of 1849–50, now thirty-one, she was asked to take charge of a medical school in Boston, a position for which she had further training from Dr. Cornell and Mr. Gregory. (This school, not yet chartered, was to be the nucleus of what would later be New England Female Medical College.) Martha had also become a well-known lecturer on physiological subjects and, in 1851, was awarded a silver cup by the

Providence Physiological Society. In the early 1850s she advertised regularly in the *Water-Cure Journal.*

In 1853, obviously well known and recognized for her training and experience, she was called upon by representatives of the Female Medical College of Pennsylvania, who, it is said, examined her medical knowledge. It must have been satisfactory: a week later she was awarded an MD degree from the school and, that fall, was appointed professor of obstetrics and the diseases of women and children. She spent but one year in this position, whether by her choice or the school's is not known, and returned to Providence, where she practiced medicine for the next forty years. Her practice emphasized, no doubt, midwifery and pediatrics, as was usually the case for women in that day. The following advertisement appeared in the *Providence Daily Journal* on October 9, 1855: "Martha H. Mowry, M.D. Office 22 1/2 South Main St. Miss Mowry's duties as professor at the Female Medical College of Philadelphia [*sic*] . . . having closed for the season, has resumed her practice in Providence, and can be found at her office, 22 1/2 South Main St. Office hours from 8 to 10 a.m., from 12 to 3, and from 6 to 7 p.m. Visits made to patients in the city or country." Similar notices appeared in the 1855 and 1856 *Rhode Island Almanac.* By 1880, she started to reduce her workload and, after 1882, no longer took night calls.

Martha was active in other spheres, especially the women's rights movement. She was present at the Woman's Rights Convention, held October 23 and 24, 1850, in Worcester, where she gave "a neat finished address near the close of the Convention, evincing a fearless and truthful spirit." She was also on the Central Committee, along with Wendell Phillips, William L. Garrison, and William H. Channing, of Boston, and Gerrit Smith, of Peterboro, New York. She took part in several Congresses of the Association for the Advancement of Women in the 1880s and 1890s, was on the Reforms and Statistics Committee, and was later a vice president. She was a trustee of Woman's Educational and Industrial Union of Providence and a member of the Rhode Island Woman's Club. Martha died, unmarried, at the age of eighty-one, in Providence, in August 1899. She is buried in Smithfield Cemetery.

Note: Martha Mowry was not a student at Female Medical College of Pennsylvania. She received an MD degree after being examined by a committee and prior to becoming a professor at the school. There is a photograph of her in Willard and Livermore's *American Women.* There is a photograph of her tombstone on the Internet at findagrave.com.

References: Richard M. Bayles, *History of Providence County, Rhode Island* (New York: W. W. Preston & Co., 1891), vol. 1, ch. 4, "The

Profession of Medicine"; Seebert J. Goldowsky, "Rhode Island's First Woman Physician," *Rhode Island Medical Journal*, November 1971, 546–49; *Providence Daily Journal*, October 9, 1855; *Rhode Island Almanac*, 1855, 1856; Harriet H. Robinson, *Massachusetts in the Woman Suffrage Movement*, 2nd ed. (Boston: Roberts Bros., 1883); Frances E. Willard, *American Women*, newly rev. (New York: Mast, Crowell & Kirkpatrick, 1897).

Jane Viola *MYERS* (1831–1918)

Jane Viola Myers was the youngest and least well known of the Myers girls, all three of whom became physicians. Her oldest sister (actually a half sister), Mary Frame Myers Thomas (q.v.), born 1816, practiced in Richmond, Indiana; her older sister, Hannah Myers Longshore (q.v.), born 1819, was a prominent practitioner in Philadelphia. Jane Viola, twelve years younger than Hannah, was born January 29, 1831, in Sandy Spring, Maryland, where her Quaker father taught school. In 1833, the family moved to New Lisbon, Ohio, a Quaker community in which they hoped to escape the distasteful proslavery atmosphere of the Washington area.

In 1854, still a resident of New Lisbon, Jane Viola graduated from Penn Medical University in Philadelphia with a doctor of medicine degree, as her eldest sister Mary Frame would do two years later. Sister Hannah had graduated from the Female Medical College of Pennsylvania in 1852. Upon finishing medical school, Jane Viola remained in Philadelphia, opened an office next door to Hannah's, and practiced medicine for thirty-five years until her retirement. She is listed as a physician in Philadelphia directories from 1861 through 1894, briefly at 1116 Callowhill and thereafter at 1326, later (1879) at 1328 Arch Street. She also succeeded her sister Hannah as instructor in anatomy at Penn Medical University. She never married. In her later years she involved herself in public welfare activities.

Jane Viola was described as "smaller in stature [than Hannah], demure, and with a sympathetic attitude to her patients." In 1870 she was living with Hannah and Hannah's husband and daughter, as she was in the 1890s when she, Hannah, and Hannah's daughter Lucretia Blankenberg took a two-month trip to Europe. Jane Viola died at eighty-seven on August 27, 1918, in Philadelphia.

References: Obituary, *JAMA* 70 (1918): 1393; Elizabeth Bass, "It Runs in the Family," *Journal of the American Medical Women's Association*, February 1954, 45; Lucretia Blankenberg, undated interview in the archives of the Medical College of Pennsylvania, at Drexel University College of

Medicine, Philadelphia; *Census of Women Physicians, 1918*; Philadelphia city directories, 1861–94; US 1870, 1880, 1900.

N

Samantha S. *NIVISON* (1833–1906)

Samantha Nivison, one of twelve children of Nathan Nivison, a prosperous farmer, and his wife, Catherine White, was born May 30, 1833, in Jacksonville, Tompkins County, New York. Nathan bought and sold several farms, always at a profit. He sent four of his five daughters to Lima Academy, in nearby Lima, New York.

Samantha grew up on a farm—Peach Orchard Point—on the east side of Seneca Lake, near Watkins (known today as Watkins Glen). Later, the family moved to nearby Mecklenburg; it was this place that Samantha really considered home. After leaving Lima Academy, Samantha went to Female Medical College of Pennsylvania. She graduated March 10, 1855.

The years immediately following medical school were spent giving lectures on health and physiology. She spent three years as a physician at the newly opened Clifton Springs Water Cure, then set up practice in Mecklenburg. In 1862, she opened the first of three water-cures with which she would be associated. This one was at Dryden Springs, near Ithaca, at the southern end of Cayuga Lake. In the early years, it prospered, as did several other water-cures in Central New York State: Elmira, Dansville, Clifton Springs, Verona, and Chittenango. The springs at Dryden had been known for many years. The coming of the Southern Central Railroad, from Owego to Auburn, combined with the springs, made the otherwise isolated village of Dryden a commercially viable location for a health resort. The price of room and board and treatment was from ten to twenty dollars a week, depending on the location of one's room. For some years the place prospered. By 1872, the rates were twelve to twenty-five dollars a week.

In April 1863, Dr. Nivison was one of twenty-nine woman incorporators of the New York Medical College for Women, organized by Clemence Lozier (q.v.). During 1868–69, Dr. Nivison was busy planning a much grander establishment for patients: Cascadilla Place, to be located on the shores of Cayuga Lake, at the northerly edge of what is now Cornell, a university then still in the planning stages. Several letters between Dr. Nivison and Ezra Cornell concerning Cascadilla Place have survived, and the project apparently had Cornell's support. It was to be much more than a water-cure, encompassing a nurse training school and a medical school, as well. For whatever reason, the plan was never realized, probably for lack of funding and the fact that it got lost in the momentum of getting Cornell up and running. Today, Cascadilla Hall at Cornell is the only reminder of Dr. Nivison's dream.

While visiting the 1876 Exposition at Philadelphia, Dr. Nivison met persons who directed her interest to Hammonton, New Jersey, which was to become the site of her next venture—another sanitarium—which opened about 1878. Five years later, she built a separate two-story building nearby which was to be a home for foundlings, an undertaking supported by Andrew D. White, president of Cornell, and by the Episcopal bishops of New Jersey, Pennsylvania, Ohio, and central New York. Dr. Nivison had long had an interest in abandoned and orphaned children. She had raised three girls and four boys as her wards. One of the boys was mentioned as her adopted son in her will, although the formalities of adoption had not been completed.

In the Children's Home, as it was called, disaster struck the following spring. Between March 1 and May 15, twenty-one of the children died, of measles it was reported. The dead infants were buried on the grounds, but the deaths were not reported to the authorities. The news hit the *New York Times*, which sensationalized the tragedy. It was the low point in Samantha's life.

Dr. Nivison was described as a "large, plumpish, tall, slightly mannish" person who was inclined to walk fast and purposefully. She was apparently slow to make friends and had a somewhat aristocratic air about her. She had great dreams and expectations. But, in the words of her biographer, Samuel A. Cloyes, "As a physician, Dr. Nivison was a good one. As a business woman, however she was not so successful." Her high purposes and idealism were not matched by practicality. All of her enterprises were underfunded and overburdened with debt. The "cure" at Dryden Springs was perhaps her most successful venture. In 1889, she had established a bottling plant there from which to market the spring waters. At the turn of the century, she sold the Dryden Springs complex to New York City interests, but the deal fell through. The sanitarium closed in 1903. Twelve years later it burned to the ground. Dr. Nivison returned to Hammonton, where she continued to receive patients. She died there on December 19, 1906, during an asthma attack. She is buried in Mecklenberg, New York. Her biographer called her "a rather curious, yet withal a glorious, person" and wrote that "those who knew her most intimately often referred to her, behind her back of course, as that 'grand old gal.'"

References: Samuel A. Cloyes, *The Healer: The Story of Dr. Samantha S. Nivison and Dryden Springs, 1820–1915* (Ithaca, NY: DeWitt Historical Society, 1969); Samuel A. Cloyes, "Chronology of the Life of Samantha S. Nivison, M.D.," ca. 1978, typescript; Full-page advertisement for Dryden Springs Place, *Ithaca Directory and Tompkins County Business Directory for 1873–4*; *New York Times*, March 19, 1880, p. 8, col. 4; *New York Times*, January 4, 1884; *New York Times*, June 5, 1884.

O

Helen *Bartlett* O'LEARY (1830–1916)

Helen Bartlett was born May 30, 1830, in Maine, daughter of Frederick Bartlett and his wife Lydia Dunham. Years later, applying for membership in the Daughters of the American Revolution, she traced her lineage to Sgt. Joseph Bartlett, who had joined the Revolutionary army as a private in 1775 and served many enlistments during the war.

Sometime in the early 1860s Helen married Canadian-born Arthur O'Leary. O'Leary, according to the 1860 census, was a lecturer in phrenology, with $5,400 in real estate and $5,585 in personal property. The O'Learys had one child, Helen B., born in 1856. In 1861, Helen graduated from Penn Medical University in Philadelphia, with an MD degree. She was then a resident of Massachusetts and appears to have returned there. The 1863 and 1864 *Progressive Annuals* record her as a practicing physician in Massachusetts, city unspecified. Later directory entries (Polk 1890 and 1893) claimed that she was professor of anatomy in 1865–66 at the Woman's College of Physicians and Surgeons of New York. The only medical school for women in New York at that time, however, was the homoeopathic New York Medical College and Hospital for Women.

The 1870 census locates the family in Iowa City, Iowa, where Arthur is listed as a doctor of hydropathia and holding $37,600 in real estate and $30,000 in personal property. The family has a domestic servant and a twenty-five-year-old boarder, George W. Allen, a hydropathic doctor with $6,000 in personal property. Curiously, Helen is listed not as a doctor but as "keeping house." However, she was probably practicing medicine. Not a few women in this period known to be practicing were thus denoted, reflecting either the prejudices of the census taker or the discretion of the woman doctor.

Helen and Arthur returned to Boston sometime between 1875 and 1879. By the time of the 1879 *Boston Almanac*, they are both listed as physicians living at 75 Chester Square. Helen is listed in the 1880 census and is described as "physician." In 1888, Helen was president of the Ladies' Physiological Society of Boston. In the 1893 *Boston Almanac* listing, she is living at 56 Berkeley, as a physician; Arthur is not and has presumably died. The 1895 official roll of practitioners of medicine in Massachusetts lists Helen as having registered before January 1, 1895. By 1900, now seventy and probably retired, Helen was living with her daughter and son-in-law in Brookline. She had practiced medicine for more than thirty years. She died March 4, 1916, in Wollaston, Massachusetts, and is buried in Mount Auburn Cemetery in Cambridge. A physical description of her appeared on her 1889 passport application: high forehead, blue eyes, aquiline nose, dark hair, and long face.

References: Official list of practitioners of medicine as of December 31, 1904, in Massachusetts, *Public Documents of Massachusetts: Being the Annual Reports of Various Public Officers and Institutions for the Year 1904* (Boston, 1905), doc. no. 56; National Society of the Daughters of the American Revolution, vol. 6, Washington, DC, 1898, 254, #5734; US census, 1860, 1870, 1880, 1900; US passport application, Helen Bartlett O'Leary, July 31, 1889.

P

Elizabeth Ann *PACKARD* Johnson (1828–1905)

Elizabeth Packard was born in Brockton, Massachusetts, on May 15, 1828. She was the second of eight children and eldest of three daughters of Josiah and Betsey Denny Bolton Packard. Her father was a shoemaker. Between the years 1854 and 1857, then a resident of North Bridgewater, a village near Brockton, and supported by a state scholarship, she attended the New England Female Medical College in Boston. She graduated in 1857 with an MD degree. Four years later, in 1861, she married Nahum Johnson, a thirty-seven-year-old West Bridgewater shoe manufacturer. The couple had at least two sons.

Though she is listed as a doctor of medicine in the *Massachusetts Register* for 1858, at 34 Bowdoin Street, Boston, and as a physician in the *Progressive Annuals* for 1863 and 1864, her name is not listed as a physician in either the Brockton or the Bridgewaters in the *New England Business Directories* for 1860, 1868, or 1875; the Butler medical directories for 1874 and 1877; or the 1886 Polk medical directory. Nor does Kingman's *History of North Bridgewater* describe her as a physician. However, she is listed as a physician in the 1869–70 and 1872–73 North Bridgewater city directories, so it seems likely that she practiced medicine. Nahum died sometime before 1878; that year Elizabeth is listed in the Bridgewater directory as Nahum's widow. Elizabeth died, March 2, 1905, at home in Brockton, at seventy-six years of age with congestive heart failure, a broken hip, and their sequels. Her death certificate listed her occupation as "at home," not as "physician."

References: Bureau of Vital Statistics, Boston; Butler, 1874, 1877; Church of Latter-Day Saints, *International Genealogical Index*, 1988 ed.; Bradford Kingman, *History of North Bridgewater* (Boston: Author, 1866), 609; *Massachusetts Register for 1858*; Polk, 1886; *New England Business Directory*, 1860, 1868, 1875; *Directory of North Bridgewater*, 1869–70, 1872–73; *Progressive Annual*, 1863, 1964.

Huldah *Allen* PAGE (1816–66)

Huldah Allen was born April 16, 1816, probably in Vassalborough, Maine, the fourth of eight children of Cornelius Allen and his wife, Margaret Knight. Vassalborough, a community ten miles north of Augusta, was one of three major Quaker settlements in Maine and was designated a quarterly meeting. After the death of Huldah's mother in 1833, the family moved to Augusta. On September 24, 1848, then thirty-two, Huldah married William P. Page. Two years later, according to the 1850 census, she was living with the family of a younger sister in Hallowell, suggesting that her marriage was already in trouble. In 1862, she divorced Mr. Page and resumed her maiden name. The couple may have had a child, Linney Page, who died in infancy.

In April 1858, then forty-two and a resident of Augusta, Huldah graduated from New York Hygeio-Therapeutic College, where she had been a student for at least two sessions and where she had apparently distinguished herself. According to the December 1857 issue of the *Water-Cure Journal*, she was the class leader in chemistry and physiology and had delivered the introductory lecture at the opening of the fall session that year.

In October 1859, Dr. Page became professor of physiology and hygiene at her alma mater. She also was lecturing on health and hygiene back in Maine. It was reported in the *Water-Cure Journal* for October that year that "Dr. Page [was] in the field . . . lecturing to the people of Maine with good acceptance. She is an excellent speaker." Noting that people were dying as a result of the medicines they were taking, Dr. Page said she would "explain the subject in a series of lectures, in Columbian Hall, in the afternoons next week, as advertised in your paper" (*Bath [ME] Times*). Her topics were to include curing and killing, summer diseases, fevers, and consumption, among others.

In 1863, she is listed on the IRS tax roll as a resident of 52 Morton Street in New York City. At that she paid a ten-dollar tax as a physician. It was also the year that she was appointed professor of physiology and hygiene at New York Medical College and Hospital for Women, newly organized by Clemence Lozier, MD (q.v.). Her practice must have been reasonably successful: in 1864 she subscribed fifty dollars to the college fund at the medical school. Though a resident of New York, this was probably during the school term, because she was also listed as a resident of Augusta at this time. *Progressive Annuals* for 1862, 1863, and 1864 list her as a practicing physician in Augusta.

How much of her time she spent in New York and how much in Maine is not known. According to reports in the *Herald of Health,* successor to the *Water-Cure Journal,* she was still giving public lectures in March of 1863 and, during that spring, contributed several items to the journal: "Advice to Ladies," "What the Maine Ladies Say," and "The Craft in Danger." There is mention of her in the *Herald of Health* in 1865, and, in 1866, she published a report on the treatment of smallpox.

Huldah died that same year, January 1866. The vital records of Augusta report a death date of January 5 and give her age as forty-seven years, nine months, which would make her birth date March 1819 rather than April 15, 1816. Maine State Archives records her death date as January 15, 1866, and her age at death as forty-nine, giving a birth year of 1817. No obituary, cause of death, or burial site has been found. Her estate, according to the probate record dated February 1866, listed her older brother Johnson and sister Sarah as next of kin. Her estate was valued at $350.

References: Ethel C. Conant, *Vital Records of Augusta Maine to the Year 1892* (Portland, ME, 1934); Samuel T. Dale, *Windham in the Past* (Auburn, ME, 1916), 292; *Herald of Health,* March 1863, 130–31; *Herald of Health,* April 1863, 174; *Herald of Health,* June 1863, 227, 254; *Herald of Health,* May 1864, 189; *Herald of Health,* January 1865, 124, 148; *Herald of Health,* January 1866, 23; Rufus M. Jones, *The Society of Friends in Kennebec, Maine* (New York, 1892); Marquis F. King, *Changes in Name by Special Acts of the Legislature of Maine 1820–1895* (Portland, ME?: M. F. King, 1901), 46; *Progressive Annual,* 1862, 1863, 1864; US census, 1830, 1840, 1850; US Internal Revenue Service tax rolls, New York City, February 1863; *Water-Cure Journal,* December 1857, October 1859, 57–58.

Esther (Hettie) *Kersey* PAINTER (1821–89)

Hettie Kersey was born in 1821 in Chester County, Pennsylvania, the daughter of Joseph Kersey and his wife, Charity Cope, and granddaughter of Jesse Kercy (*sic*), a prominent Quaker preacher. Hettie had at least one brother, James. Her parents died when Hettie was young, and she was adopted by an aunt and uncle, Mordecai and Esther Hayes, of Chester, both of whom were active in humanitarian work. Nothing is known of Hettie's childhood and early education.

She married Joseph H. Painter, a man fourteen years her senior, and they had two sons, J. K. and L. M. Painter. The couple moved to Ohio, where they were involved in temperance work, the suffrage movement, and smuggling fugitive slaves. In 1852, they returned to Philadelphia, later moving across the Delaware River to Camden, New Jersey. Toward the end of the 1850s, Hettie enrolled at Penn Medical University, from which she graduated in 1860 with an MD degree.

With the coming of the Civil War, Hettie became involved with the Union army as a nurse and manager. She established the first military hospital south of Washington and across the Potomac. This was probably in the vicinity of Manassas, in a theological seminary; there she had a staff of forty men assigned to her by General Philip Kearney. After the First Battle of Bull Run, attending the New Jersey Volunteers, she followed the army, working in hospitals and on the field, commissioned by the governors of both New Jersey and Pennsylvania, aided by a special railroad pass and an order that the army was to assist her. She managed hospitals, nursed soldiers, wrote letters for them, and saw to the distribution of medical and commissary supplies. After the war she continued to work in hospitals, often accompanying sick and wounded soldiers to their homes, until temporary hospitals were emptied.

For a time she practiced medicine in Washington but in 1868 went west to visit her two sons, J. K. in Cheyenne, Wyoming Territory, and L. M. in Corinne, Utah Territory, both of whom were involved in the Union Pacific Railroad. (J. K. had been a telegrapher during the war, and, on one occasion when Hettie visited him, she was quite impressed with the new technology when seeing him relay a message from General Sherman to President Lincoln.) While in the West, her health declined, and she spent some time there recovering, mostly in Salt Lake City, and, on recovery, built up quite a practice among prominent Mormons and even some members of the California governor's family. But, sick again, she moved eastward to Lincoln, Nebraska, where her husband was editing a semimonthly agricultural periodical called the *Nebraska Patron.*

In a year or so her health improved, and she proceeded to establish an infirmary for the chronically sick, said to be the first such institution in the West and one to which patients came from many distant parts of the country. An advertisement in the *Lincoln City Directory* for 1881–82 described the establishment: "This is an Institution opened under the management of Mrs. Dr. H. K. Painter, and fills a want long felt in this new country. The location is on high, rolling ground, commanding a view of the East, North and West, while to the South, the beautiful city of Lincoln is spread out like a map. The infirmary is large and roomy, and constructed wholly on principles conducive to Health. Here the weary invalid can find rest."

Dr. Painter died on August 9, 1889, in Lincoln, after a short bout with cardiac symptoms, probably a coronary occlusion. She is buried in Wyuka Cemetery. Said her obituary, "In the death of Mrs. Dr. Painter the old soldiers have lost a true friend, one ever ready to do good for the veterans in times of peace as she did a quarter of a century ago amid the clash of arms." The Daughters of Union Veterans in Nebraska named two of their tents in her honor, in 1890, H. K. Painter Tent #1, and in 1936, Tent #37. A year before her death she was granted a federal pension. Personally, Hettie was described as a petite woman with a kind smile and the confident, inspiring manner of a true physician.

References: Obituary, *Daily Nebraska State Journal*, August 9, 1889; *History of the State of Nebraska* (Chicago: Western Historical Co., 1882); *Lincoln City Directory*, 1880–81, 1881–82; *Sunday Journal and Star* (Lincoln, NE), March 25, 1975, photograph; Nebraska Daughters of Union Veterans, Nurses, photograph; US census, 1880; United States Statutes at large, vol. 25, July 9, 1888, An Act Granting a Pension.

Note: In *Nebraska History*, 1942 (23:72), is a photograph labeled "Dr. Hettie K. Painter niece of John Brown (with her daughter)." The accompanying text states that (1) she saw her husband dragged from his bed and murdered before her eyes, (2) that the daughter was adopted, (3) that Dr. Painter was a spy for the Union, and (4) that she was a niece of John Brown. None of these claims is supported by any other source consulted. Mr. Painter was known to be living in Lincoln, Nebraska, in the 1880s.

Louisa Fearing *Coffin* PARKER (1813–1906)

Louisa Coffin was born in January 1813, in Wareham, Massachusetts, the daughter of Valentine C. Coffin and his wife Sarah F. Nye. Like Lydia Folger Fowler (q.v.), who was born in Nantucket, and Alice Bunker Stockham (q.v.), Louisa traced her ancestry to Tristram Coffin, one of the founders of Nantucket. No information regarding Louisa's childhood or early education has been found.

On June 6, 1830, at the First Congregational Church in Nantucket, Louisa married Isaac Holmes Parker, a machinist. The 1900 census reports that the couple had ten children, four of whom were alive in 1900. The only two identified were Josephine (b. 1846), who married Charles Thurston, and Isaac Clinton Parker (b. 1850), who was a decorator and did not marry. The premature deaths of so many children may have been a motivating factor in Louisa's desire to become a physician.

She attended two or three lecture courses at New England Female Medical College in Boston between 1856 and 1861, graduating in 1861 with an MD degree. She proceeded to establish her practice in Boston. The *Progressive Annuals* for 1862, 1863, and 1864 locate her as a physician on Walnut Place; Boston business directories for 1872 and 1875 at 173 West Seventh Street; and the 1877 Boston city directory at 160 West Seventh. By 1880, Isaac had retired. How much longer Louisa practiced is uncertain.

In the 1890s, by then a widow and in her late seventies, Louisa had moved to New Bedford, where she did not apparently practice medicine, and by 1900 to Weymouth, where she died of "old age" at ninety-three on May 8, 1906. Her death certificate called her a "physician." She is buried in Rochester, Massachusetts, a village close by her birthplace, Wareham.

References: Obituary, *JAMA* 46 (1906): 1548; *Boston City Directory*, 1877; *Boston Directory*, 1872, 1875; *Massachusetts Register & Business Directory*, 1867; Nantucket, MA, *Vital Records to the Year 1850* (Boston, 1925); *New Bedford and Fairhaven Directory*, 1893–97; *New England Business Directory*, 1868; *Progressive Annual*, 1862, 1863, 1864; US census, 1880, 1900.

Susan *PARRY* (1826–90)

Susan Parry was born December 10, 1826, in Buckingham, Bucks County, Pennsylvania, in a rural ancestral homestead of the Parry family. Her parents, Charles Parry and Phoebe Fell, were descended from Welsh and English forebears, respectively, who had come to America two centuries earlier. They had all been members of the Society of Friends. Whether Phoebe had siblings is unknown. She lived her entire life in Bucks County. She was a good student, liked books, and later taught school. After her father's premature death, she moved to Philadelphia, continued to teach school, and, having decided on a medical career, attended lectures on scientific subjects in preparation for that.

In 1858, when she was thirty-two, she graduated from the Female Medical College of Pennsylvania with an MD degree and started practicing medicine in Bucks County. The 1864 *Progressive Annual* places her in Lahaska, a small community near Doylestown. Her obituary, however, reports that she practiced in Newtown from 1861 to 1869. In either case, she moved to Doylestown in 1869, where she practiced for twenty years. She is not listed in the Butler directories (1874 and 1877), but she is in the first Polk medical directory of 1886. In 1883, she became a member of the Bucks County Medical Society, the second woman to be elected to that body.

Affected with chronic pulmonary disease for several years, she retired from practice. She died, unmarried, in Doylestown, on February 12, 1890, at the age of sixty-four, and is buried in the Friends' Burying Ground in Buckingham.

References: Woman's Medical College of Pennsylvania, Alumnae Association, *Report of the Proceedings of the Sixteenth Annual Meeting, May 7 and 8, 1891* (Philadelphia, 1891), 29–30; J. H. Battle, *History of Bucks County, Pennsylvania, 1887* (Spartanburg, S.C.: Reprint Co., 1985), 865; Obituary, *Bucks County Intelligencer* (Doylestown), February 14, 1890; Polk, 1886.

Sarah E. *PAUL* Sandt (1837–98)

Sarah Paul was born July 4, 1837, in Mt. Holly, New Jersey, the daughter of Mifflin Paul, of Seabright, New Jersey. Nothing is known of her mother, her background, childhood, or early education. In 1861, she graduated from the Female Medical College of Pennsylvania, said to be the top student and youngest student in her class (not verified). On October 25, 1867, then thirty, she married George B. Sandt. Sandt's first wife, Caroline V., had died in June 1866, leaving two children. The 1870 census places the family in Trenton, New Jersey, Ward 1, where George was a hay dealer and Sarah was listed as a physician, holding $10,000 in real estate and $500 in personal property. The 1880 census shows them living in Ocean, Monmouth County, New Jersey, with four children: Walter, twenty-three; Carrie W., eighteen; George M., twelve; and Paul R., nine. Son George M. later became a physician and practiced in Trenton for many years. Father George is listed as a hotel proprietor, and the family apparently lived in the hotel because the census names sixty-three men and twenty-two women living in the same household. In the 1880 census, Sarah is no longer denoted a physician, and her name was not listed in the 1874 or 1877 Butler medical directories. Sarah died in Wernersville, Pennsylvania, on February 2, 1898, at the age of sixty.

References: Butler, 1874, 1877; US census, 1870, 1880.

Jane *PAYNE* (1825–82)

Jane Payne was born September 1, 1825, in Bristol, England, the eldest daughter of the Rev. Henry Payne and his wife Ann. In 1832, the family came to the United States, lived in New York City for four years, and then moved to Springfield, Ohio. Miss Payne attended a young ladies' seminary at Hamilton, Ohio. After graduating she became a teacher at a seminary in Cincinnati, moving later to Piqua and then Troy. In 1852, the family moved to Mt. Vernon, Ohio, when Jane's father became rector of St. Paul's Episcopal Church. Jane, now twenty-seven, came with them.

Two major health problems had befallen Jane during her childhood. When three years old she contracted measles, which led to the loss of sight in one eye completely and partially in the other. She was unable to read in an ordinarily lighted room and often required others to read to her when studying. Later, while still young, she dislocated a hip. Whether this was improperly reduced or because of other complication, she remained lame the rest of her life and was able to walk only short distances at a time, and that unsteadily.

Sometime in the 1850s, she went to Dr. Trall's water-cure in New York City for treatment. While she was there she became interested in reading many of the medical books that were available in the institution's library. Apparently, she had earlier entertained the idea of becoming a physician, and, according to her obituary, "she was often heard to say, if she were a man, she would be a physician." The experience at Dr. Trall's strengthened her desire to do this. On returning to Mt. Vernon, she became a student in the office of her personal physician, Dr. John R. Russell.

Amelia Bloomer, of dress reform fame, and her husband, Dexter, had moved to Mt. Vernon from Seneca Falls, New York, in 1854, and there they continued publishing periodicals, including a woman's rights newspaper, the *Lily*. This made Mt. Vernon, at least for the year they were there, a national center for reform and surely must have had some influence on Jane Payne. Also, both her father and her medical preceptor were supportive of the movement, unusual, at least for an Episcopal priest of that day.

For formal lectures and a degree, Jane went to the Female Medical College of Pennsylvania in Philadelphia, graduating in 1861, first in her class. Among her classmates was Sarah Kleckner (q.v.). Now Dr. Payne, she returned to Mt. Vernon and established a practice that would continue for almost twenty years. Initially, there was opposition. In a later resolution, written at the time of Dr. Payne's death, the Knox County Medical Society wrote that "she commenced her duties as a physician in Mt. Vernon under very embarrassing circumstances. She had to contend with the prejudices of the community against a female physician, and with the experience and reputation of old and acknowledged teachers in the profession; but, with that earnestness and perseverance that characterized her as a student, she obtained a lucrative business, despite all adverse circumstances."

The use of the word "lucrative" is interesting: Was it intended as a sly criticism, or did it show what doctors thought important in that day? Whatever the case, Dr. Payne's office was never in the fashionable part of town but, rather, "squarely in the midst of the factory district, the Irish immigrant boarding houses, and the tiny Black community clustered around the town's gas works. In her first year of her ministrations she advertised free medicine three days a week, and promised to promptly answer country calls" (Hesler).

Perhaps one of the happier things to befall Dr. Payne was the responsibility she took in raising the orphaned children of both a brother and a sister. Added to her lameness, blindness, and professional opposition now came a new problem: in 1868 she developed some kind of cancer, later removed by surgery at Cincinnati in 1871. In 1880, the tumor had recurred and she went to London for treatment. She returned, continued to practice, but the problem recurred and grew "with alarming rapidity," soon leading to her death at home on March 11, 1882. She had cared for her patients until four months prior to this.

Dr. Payne's funeral was held at St. Paul's Episcopal Church, and, remarkably, members of the Knox County Medical Society attended in a body. In spite of inclement weather, the service was "largely attended." Said her obituary, "Dr. Payne was a woman whose benevolence was of an exalted type. She was ever thinking of and doing for others. . . . She brought more than medicine and medical skill to the homes of the poor. Wherever she found destitution and want, she labored to relieve it as she did the bodily pain." She is buried in Mt. Vernon's Mound View Cemetery.

References: Obituary, *Democratic Banner* (Mt. Vernon), March 17, 1882; Lorle Hesler, "A Lesson in Courage," *Columbus Dispatch Magazine,* March 2, 1975; Knox County Medical Society, "Resolution Regarding the Death of Dr. Payne, Adopted March 13, 1882," in *Constitution and Report of the Proceedings of the Seventh Annual Meeting, March 17, 1882,* by Woman's Medical College of Pennsylvania, Alumnae Association (Providence, RI, 1882), 18–19; Obituary, *Mt. Vernon Republican,* March 16, 1882.

Sarah Brooks *Felt* PETTINGILL (1810–77)

Sarah Felt was born May 16, 1810, in Charlestown, Massachusetts, the eldest of eight children (five girls and three boys) of Jacob Felt and his wife Betsy Neagles (or Nagles). The family was well off. Mr. Felt was a merchant who, on a trip to Tennessee in 1808, was struck by the yellow color of some soil he encountered, took a sample of it to New York City for analysis, and found that it was yellow ochre. He leased the land on which it was located, and made a fortune. This was the first discovery of ochre in the United States. Later, he made another soil discovery, this time a special clay, and became a dealer in clay for pipes. Still later, he was in the iron forging business.

Ultimately, Felt became a physician and moved to Portsmouth, New Hampshire, where he practiced for a number of years. On her mother's side, Sarah was related to Dr. John Brooks (1752–1825), physician, Revolutionary army officer, governor of Massachusetts, and president of the Massachusetts Medical Society.

Sarah's education was at home by a governess; later she completed the literary course at Charlestown Seminary. When she was seventeen she was married (August 16, 1827) to John Pettingill Jr., a Charlestown merchant. The couple had nine children, seven of whom lived to adulthood. The first three were born in Charlestown. In the early 1830s, Mr. Pettingill became sheriff of Merrimack County, New Hampshire, and the family moved to Concord, where they lived for about eighteen years and where Mr. Pettingill had mercantile interests in addition to his official position.

Sarah's last child was born in 1848. For two years after this, according to Cleave, she was away from home in spring and fall for reasons not specified. For her health, the family moved to Philadelphia, which became their permanent home. Husband John went into the real estate business.

In 1856, now forty-six years old, and her youngest child eight, Sarah decided to go to medical school and matriculated at Penn Medical University, graduating with an MD degree in 1860. From that time until her death seventeen years later, she practiced medicine in Philadelphia, emphasizing the care of women. Her name is listed as a practitioner in standard medical directories each year. At some point she was converted to homoeopathic practice and tried to enroll at Hahnemann Medical College, but she was allowed only to audit lectures on practice and materia medica, sitting behind a screen that hid her from sight of the male students. She was said to be the first woman homoeopathist in Philadelphia. In 1871, the first year women were accepted, she was elected a member of the American Institute of Homoeopathy, as were Mercy B. Jackson (q.v.) and Harriet J. Sartain (q.v.).

One son, John Brooks Pettingill (MD, University of Pennsylvania, 1870), became a surgeon in Chicago. A daughter, Eliza Felt Pettingill (MD, Female Medical College of Pennsylvania, 1865), also became a physician and practiced with her mother. Another son became a dentist. A grandson, George Andrews Barrows (MD, Hahnemann, 1892) practiced medicine in Philadelphia. Sarah died March 29, 1877, suddenly and unexpectedly, while riding a Philadelphia trolley. Husband John, who was blinded by cataracts for the last twenty-five years of his life, died in Asbury Park, NJ, in 1894, where he was probably living with his oldest daughter or his dentist son.

References: Obituary, *Transactions of the American Institute of Homoeopathy*, 1893, 152–53; Butler, ?; Polk, ?; Charlestown, Massachusetts Vital Records; Cleave, 107; John E. Morris, *A Felt Genealogy* (Hartford, CT: Case, Lockwood, Brainard & Co., 1893); Obituary, *Philadelphia Inquirer*, March 30, 1877; Funeral notice, *Philadelphia Inquirer*, April 4, 1877; Charles H. Pope, *A Pettingill Genealogy*, ed. Charles I. Pettingill (Boston, 1896).

Dolly Ann *PORTER*

Miss Porter was listed as a resident of Fabius, Onondaga County, New York (near Syracuse), when she graduated from Syracuse Medical College on February 16, 1854. A month earlier, her residence given as New York City, she was listed as a delegate to the fifth annual meeting of the New York State Eclectic Medical Society, held January 10, at the Medical College.

After graduation Dolly Ann stayed on as a student for the spring-summer session of the school but was also establishing a local medical practice. In the *Syracuse Standard* for May 19, 1854, the following item appeared: "A lady physician named D. Ann Porter advertises in the *Chronicle*, offering her services as Physician and Surgeon to the citizens of Syracuse. She will pay particular attention to diseases of her own sex and those of children. Residence No. 60 South Warren St."

In October 1854 Dr. Porter's business card appeared in local newspapers. In January 1855, she was again listed as a delegate to the now sixth annual meeting of the New York Eclectic Medical Society. No further trace of her has been found. Her name does not appear in Syracuse city directories from 1851 to 1860 or in the Syracuse newspaper database after 1855.

References: *Syracuse Medical & Surgical Journal,* 1854, 5–6; *Syracuse Medical & Surgical Journal,* 1855. 12; *Syracuse Standard,* May 19, 1854.

Maria W. PORTER (1823–88)

Maria Porter (maiden surname unknown) was one of the first woman doctors to practice medicine in Iowa. She was born in Nottingham, England, April 16, 1823. Her mother died when she was still an infant. Her father brought her to the United States when she was nine years old. Her early schooling was at New Brighton (PA) Seminary. From youth, she was an ardent church worker. In 1845, when she was twenty-two, she married Nathaniel Porter of Allegheny City, a man fifteen years her senior, himself an immigrant from England. By the time of the 1850 census, the couple had two children and were living in Derry, a village in southwest Pennsylvania. During the 1850s, the family grew to five children. During the late 1850s Maria, in addition to caring for five small children, studied medicine with Dr. J. P. Dake in Pittsburgh and a Dr. Lane of Blairsville and attended two lecture courses at the Female Medical College of Pennsylvania in Philadelphia, graduating in 1859 with an MD degree.

In 1860, Maria moved with her family to Davenport, Iowa, where she lived and practiced medicine the rest of her life. She inaugurated her practice with a series of public medical lectures to the community, a method of advertising commonly used at the time. Such lectures were given from time to time thereafter. Husband Nathaniel is last listed in the Davenport city directory in 1861 and had presumably died. Whether Maria was motivated to become a physician in anticipation of his death is not known. In any case, Maria was left with five children, aged five to fifteen, to support. They all grew to adulthood. The two boys became printers, and one of the girls married a printer. Another girl became matron of the Davenport Orphans Home, and another spent her life in China as a missionary.

In 1870, Maria embraced the homoeopathic method of practice. She became a member of the Hahnemann Medical Association of Iowa. Though there is little information about the nature of her practice, as is usually the case, there is ample evidence that she did practice medicine. Davenport city directories list her as a physician from 1861 through 1885, as do Iowa medical directories for 1878 and 1880, Butler medical directories for 1874 and 1877, and the Polk medical directory for 1886. As a physician, she also paid the federal income tax of $6.67 in 1863, and $10 annually for the next three years. (In two of those years she was also taxed $1 for having a carriage, $1 for having a watch, and $2 for having a piano.)

During the Civil War, Maria was an active worker on the home front, especially with the Soldiers' Aid Society. The following description appears in her obituary:

> With her horse and buggy she visited constantly the various camps in and about Davenport, carrying to the soldiers various useful articles from the Aid society, and visiting the sick in the hospital. She was well known among the soldiers and a hearty welcome always met her when she drove into camp. Even her horse and buggy were enthusiastically regarded by the soldiers. At one time some new recruits of the rougher sort, attracted by the then not so common sight of a lady driving alone, intercepted her. Immediately some soldiers sprang forward with the exclamation: "Get away from there—we can't get along without that horse and buggy." During the entire time that the soldiers were encamped about Davenport her house was filled with the wives and children of the departing soldiers.

Dr. Porter was active in establishing the Soldiers' Orphans Home near Davenport, as well as in temperance work and missionary work of the Methodist church. She was secretary for the Women's Foreign Missionary Society of the Methodist Episcopal Church for the Upper Iowa Conference and at the time of her death was president of the Des Moines branch of the Women's Foreign Missionary Society that included both Iowa and Missouri. "Her ability as a public speaker and presiding officer often brought her before the public." She "peacefully fell asleep" September 8, 1888, at the age of sixty-five, surrounded by her family. She had practiced in Davenport for twenty-eight years, raised five children, and was a community leader.

References: Butler, 1874, 1877; Obituary, *Davenport Democrat*, September 10, 1888; Davenport city directories, 1861–85; Obituary, *Medical Advance* 21 (1888): 567–68; William H. King, *History of Homoeopathy and Its Institutions in America* (New York: Lewis Publishing Co., 1905), 1:387; Charles H. Lothrop, *The Medical and Surgical Directory of the State of Iowa for 1878 and 1879* (Clinton, Iowa, 1878); *Medical and Surgical Directory of the State of Iowa, for 1880 and 1881* (Clinton, Iowa, 1880); Polk, 1886; US census, 1850, 1860, 1870, 1880; US Internal Revenue Service tax rolls, 1863–66.

Ann *PRESTON* (1813–72)

Ann Preston was born December 1, 1813, in West Grove, a Quaker community in Pennsylvania, not far from Philadelphia. Her father, Amos, was a Quaker minister. Amos and his wife Margaret had nine children.

Ann was the second and eldest of their three daughters; both sisters died before reaching adulthood. Life in West Grove was intellectual, religious, and active in support of temperance, abolition, and woman's rights. Ann went to a local Quaker school and later briefly to a Friend's boarding school in Chester, Pennsylvania. She soon returned home to care for her six younger brothers and to run the household because of her mother's chronic and increasingly poor health. Throughout the 1830s, Ann was largely housebound, though she did teach school for a while, wrote reports and addresses for the local antislavery society, was active in the local temperance movement, published a book for children, *Cousin Ann's Stories* (1849), and attended lectures sponsored by the local literary group.

In the 1840s, Ann turned to teaching physiology and hygiene, lecturing to groups of local women and, in 1847, became apprenticed to a local physician. In 1850, at age thirty-seven, her brothers grown, she matriculated at the newly opened Female Medical College of Pennsylvania, having been rebuffed by other medical schools, received a medical degree the following year, returned for a third (postgraduate) course, and in 1853 was appointed professor of physiology and hygiene at the school. She spent the remaining nineteen years of her life at the college. Her career was primarily as teacher and administrator, secondarily as physician. She apparently saw patients, but only in her office, partly because of her own poor health. She had suffered probably from what today is called rheumatoid arthritis.

Ann's tenure on the faculty was not without challenges. In 1858, the Philadelphia County Medical Society formally ostracized the school, which meant that its students could not go to any of the public teaching clinics in Philadelphia hospitals. In response, Dr. Preston formed a committee and herself raised a large portion of the funding to establish a woman's hospital in association with the college, at which clinical training could be provided for women students. In 1861, with the onset of the Civil War, the school shut for a year, but the hospital opened with a staff of five male physicians and Emeline H. Cleveland, fresh from surgical training in Paris, as chief resident. In 1863, Preston inaugurated a nurse training school.

In 1866, Dr. Preston was appointed dean, the first woman to be a medical school dean, and two years later, finally, was able to gain the right for her students to attend the general clinics at Philadelphia General Hospital (Blockley) and a year later at Pennsylvania Hospital as well. But medical students and many physicians in the community were not happy with this arrangement, claiming that medical coeducation was immodest and immoral. They were loud in the expression of their disapproval. Dr. Preston responded firmly in a written statement that said that where it was moral for women to be as patients, it was moral for them to be as doctors. Was she suggesting a boycott? In any case, things calmed down. In the meantime, several patrons had paid off the debts of the medical school. Its future looked more promising.

Ann Preston was described as of slight frame, womanly, serene, and unwavering. She never married. In 1871, her rheumatoid arthritis became again more active. She died at home on April 18, 1872, at the age of fifty-eight. She was succeeded as dean by Emeline Horton Cleveland.

Bibliography: *Introductory Lecture to the Course of Instruction in the Female Medical College of Pennsylvania, for the Session 1855–56* (Philadelphia, 1855); *Valedictory Address to the Graduating Class of the Female Medical College of Pennsylvania, for the Session of 1857–8* (Philadelphia, 1858); *Introductory Lecture to the Class of the Female Medical College of Pennsylvania, October 18, 1859* (Philadelphia, 1859); *Nursing the Sick and the Training of Nurses: An Address Delivered at the Request of the Board of Managers of the Woman's Hospital, at Philadelphia, May 21st, 1863* (Philadelphia, 1863); *Valedictory Address to the Graduating Class of the Female Medical College of Pennsylvania, at the Twelfth Annual Commencement, March 16, 1864* (Philadelphia, 1864); *Women as Physicians* (Philadelphia, 1867); *Valedictory Address to the Graduating Class of the Woman's Medical College of Pennsylvania, at the Eighteenth Annual Commencement, March 12th, 1870* (Philadelphia, 1870).

References: *Notable American Women, 1607–1950*, 3:96–97; H. B. Elliot, in *Eminent Women of the Age*, by James Parton (Hartford, CT: S. M. Betts & Co., 1868); Pauline Foster, "A Biography: The Struggle to Obtain Training Acceptance for Women Physicians in Mid-nineteenth Century America" (thesis, University of Pennsylvania, 1984; not consulted); *Dictionary of American Medical Biography* (Westport, CT: Greenwood Press, 1984), 608; *A Cyclopedia of American Medical Biography* (Philadelphia, 1912), 2:291–92; Frances E. Willard, *A Woman of the Century* (Buffalo, 1893).

R

Janet *Bailey* RABON (1824–1915)

Janet Bailey was already married to Joseph Rabon when the two arrived from England aboard the ship *American Empress* on August 12, 1852. They were steerage passengers. He was twenty-seven, she was

242 ᷿ Biographical Dictionary of 222 Graduates

twenty-eight. Joseph was a gardener. The couple went to Cleveland, where they settled. They had no children, and, by 1868 at least, Janet was a widow. It seems likely that Joseph's death occurred in the late 1850s, thus motivating Janet to attend medical school, which she did. In 1860, she graduated from the Western Homoeopathic College in Cleveland. It is not clear whether her degree was doctor of medicine with emphasis in midwifery or was limited to midwifery. In 1896, she registered as a doctor of medicine in conformance with Ohio's registration law.

Between 1868 and 1904 she was listed in twenty different directories as a physician and as a midwife, living at six or seven different locations during that period. In the directories she is described variously as Dr. Janet Rabon, Mrs. Dr. Janet Rabon, or Mrs. Joseph Rabon, physician. Curiously, the 1894 directory says she "removed to Bangor," in southwestern Michigan, but she was back at her prior (1893) address in 1896. She is also listed in the Butler medical directory for 1877 and the Polk medical directory for 1886.

Over the years, her household arrangements varied. Listed in the 1870 census are two young couples living in her house, one with a small child, as well as a twenty-two-year-old housekeeper, her mother, and her nine-year-old son. In the 1880 census Dr. Rabon is referred to as Janette Rabon, a homoeopathic physician, and has her teenage niece and nephew living with her. She is listed in the first (1896) report of registered physicians in Ohio. By 1900, now at Trinity Church Home, she is still listed as a physician and is said to not be unemployed, so she may have been practicing even then, though this seems unlikely; she was seventy-six. (Found on the Internet, quite by accident, was the following: "Ruby V. Lannert was born on 25 Mar. 1890 in Cleveland, Cuyahoga Co, OH, US. Born at home at 79 Beech St. Midwife was Janet Rabon, M.D.") In 1905 or 1906, Dr. Rabon retired. She lived at Trinity Church Home until her death October 9, 1915, at ninety-one. Her funeral was held in the Church Home chapel. She is buried in Lake View Cemetery.

References: American Medical Association, *Directory of Deceased American Physicians 1804–1929* (Chicago: AMA, 1993), 2:1269; Butler, 1877; Cleveland city directories, 1868, 1871, 1872–76, 1878, 1882, 1885, 1887, 1893, 1894, 1896, 1900, 1903, 1904, 1906, 1907, 1910, 1914; New York passenger lists 1820–1957; Ohio, State Board of Medical Registration and Examination of Ohio, *First Annual Report* (Columbus, 1897), 57; Polk, 1886; US census, 1870, 1880, 1900, 1910; Lannert Family Society, Four-page history including John Adam Lannert and Mary Arting, their children, and grandchildren. Ruby V. Lannert was the second of

three children of John and Mary Lannert. http://freepages.genealogy.
rootsweb.ancestry.com/~heritagecrossroads/lan (accessed September
6, 2012; no longer available)

Marenda *Briggs* RANDALL (1815–76)

Marenda Briggs Randall, of Woodstock, Vermont, was thirty-eight years
old when she matriculated at Penn Medical University. Born in 1815,
the only child of Luther Briggs and Hope Simmons, she lost her mother
when she was twelve years old. At nineteen she married Nathaniel
Randall III, then a Woodstock jeweler. They had five children, but the
first two died in infancy. It was an unhappy marriage almost from the
start, apparently because Nathaniel was both controlling and insistent
on a stay-at-home wife. Marenda had hoped to escape a controlling
father by marrying, but she found her husband equally dominating.
Throughout her life, Marenda sought independence, first from her
father, then from her husband. Apparently her husband's intellectual
superior, she tried to interest him in various activities, among which
were utopian communities and, later, Spiritualism.

She wrote two letters in 1843–44 to Cassius Clay, lawyer, Kentucky
legislator, and US ambassador to Russia during the Civil War. The first
was in response to an antislavery article he had written for the *Herald of
Freedom* (though his family were slaveholders), and three months later,
she wrote expressing her own spiritual and philosophical values, giving
one the idea that she was not an average housewife.

About this time, in her late twenties, she became interested in
social experiments. Marenda and the children went to live at a newly
formed utopian community in Western New York—the Skaneateles
Experimental Community—one of about forty such communities
that sprang up in the United States in the 1840s. If the project was a
success, Nathaniel, who stayed in Woodstock to run the jewelry business, would join them later. The community was in Mottville, just
north of Skaneateles, and under the leadership of John Anderson
Collins (1810–1900), a noted abolitionist. Collins had put up $5,000
and had a $10,000 mortgage on the place. Members shared living
quarters and worked on the farm, in the sawmill, or the print shop.
Marenda was in charge of education. Collins did not believe in religion, civil government, or in marriage. Though not all cohabiting
members were married, it was not a free-love community. Nevertheless, the neighbors considered the place a Babel. Though economically viable, factional disputes led to dissolution of the community in
May 1846. Quincy Johnson, a "long-headed tonguey lawyer" from Syracuse, along with Collins, made off with half the property. Marenda

had left before this end. Her husband had come to visit and, sensing that it was Marenda's money the community coveted, or perhaps because of the free-love reputation of the place, persuaded Marenda to return to Woodstock, where the couple had two more children, Eliza M. (Lizzie) and Eloise Olive.

About 1850, Nathaniel, then forty-one, decided to become a physician. He attended the medical school in Woodstock and received an MD degree in 1851. He became interested in Thomsonian botanic medicine but ultimately practiced homoeopathy. In the meantime, Marenda embraced Spiritualism, to which she remained devoted the rest of her life, becoming a practitioner and a lecturer. In September 1853, after nineteen unhappy years of marriage, Marenda matriculated at Penn Medical University in Philadelphia, with a goal of becoming self-supporting and of helping to "liberate" her fellow wives. She probably chose Penn because it was coed and, being Eclectic, was more liberal than most other schools. It also was popular with Spiritualists (at least seven are known to have graduated from the school). Nathaniel took her to school; the children (ages twelve, seven, and two) were to live with him. Marenda and her husband were apparently separating. They did not live together thereafter. Once Marenda earned her medical degree and became self-supporting, the children were to live with her.

In her journal, on September 5, 1853, Marenda wrote:

> So here I am, far far away from that home where everything I could reasonably wish save a kind husband; from that home where I have left three precious children to be cared for externally by those I cannot approve, until I can qualify myself to support them, and yet I feel happy and free. . . . I am now to take care of myself, and why should I not? Why should I be bound and led? . . . Why should I not have the liberty to improve [my] ability by use? I will at least try, and if I fall, my sisters shall have the benefit of my experience. (Richberg)

Over the ensuing days there are many more entries on "woman the slave." It is clear, too, that Marenda's concern was not voting rights but rather equality in marriage.

Little is known of her studies and daily life at medical school. She probably wrote about these things in her journal, but it has not been possible to locate that document. In October 1853, Marenda wrote, "Life flows smoothly on . . . all are kind, and I am happy . . . my duties are various, complicated, numerous, and I may say arduous: yet they are all pleasant and attractive and easy of accomplishment. My studies are all easy and everything is yet joyous."

During the year, Marenda spoke to various groups on the subject of woman's rights and about Spiritualism. She once addressed the state legislature in Harrisburg, urging an appropriation that would make it possible for a woman from each senatorial district in Pennsylvania to attend medical school. In spite of all these distractions she graduated, in 1854, with highest honors, receiving a note from the dean to that effect.

Marenda returned to Woodstock and started medical practice. She was probably the first woman doctor of medicine to practice in Vermont. In 1857 she and Nathaniel were divorced. The children apparently went to live with her. The 1860 census lists only Eliza at home. George, by then nineteen, was probably on his own. Also listed is four-year-old Olive Howard (Steward?). This child, born in Pennsylvania, was said to be Marenda's natural child.

Vermont directories confirm that Marenda was a practicing physician in Woodstock from 1859 to 1865. According to grandson Donald Richberg, as a physician, she put her husband "in the shade." An article by Mary Grace Canfield in the *Vermont Standard* (Woodstock) provides an unusual amount of detail about the extent of Marenda's practice. Canfield was able to interview descendants in at least eight families who had used Marenda's professional services for problems such as diphtheria, lung fever, asthma, and, of course, midwifery.

In 1864, Marenda's twenty-four-year-old son, George, was killed at the Battle of the Wilderness. Late the following year Marenda, Eloise, and Olive moved to Hammonton, New Jersey, where they planned to raise cranberries. Eliza had married. Marenda continued to be active in Spiritualism circles and as a practitioner of Spiritualism and medicine. She also founded a society of women called Scientific Conversazione. The cranberry venture was not a success, and, in 1875, the family of three moved to Chicago. There, Eloise married an attorney. Olive became a painter. Marenda died the following year, August 31, 1876. Though Marenda practiced medicine in Woodstock for eleven years and probably for ten more in Hammonton, was well-known in Spiritualism circles, and was involved in woman's liberation and abolition activities, there is no mention of her in any of the Woodstock histories consulted for this sketch.

References: Ann Braude, *Radical Spirits: Spiritualism and Women's Rights in Nineteenth-Century America*, 2nd ed. (Bloomington: Indiana University Press, 2001), 149–50; Mary Grace Canfield, *Vermont Standard* (Woodstock), August 15, 1935 [article providing interviews with the descendant members of families that had been patients of Marenda Randall]; *Progressive Annual*, 1863, 1864; Marenda Briggs Randall, autobiographical journal (location of original unknown), quoted extensively in Eloise Richberg, "Marenda Randall," a typewritten essay written for an English composition class in 1946, at the Woodstock Historical Society [Mrs. Richberg was Marenda's great-granddaughter]; Marenda B. Randall, two manuscript letters dated Woodstock, VT, December 26, 1843, and Skaneateles, NY, March 11, 1846, to Cassius Marcellus Clay, Lexington, KY, Cassius Clay Papers, Carnegie-Vincent Library, Lincoln Memorial University, Harrogate, TN; Donald R. Richberg, *My Hero: The Indiscreet Memoirs of an Eventful but Unheroic Life* (New York: Putnam, 1954) [Richberg was Marenda's grandson]; US census, 1850, 1860; US Internal Revenue Service tax assessment lists, September 1865; *Walton's Vermont Registers*; *The Skaneateles Communal Experiment 1843–1846: A Paper Read before the Onondaga Historical Association, Feb. 13, 1953* (Syracuse, 1953); Windsor Vermont city directories, 1863, 1864, 1865, 1866; *Vermont Directory and Commercial Almanac*, Rutland, 1860, 1861.

Mary J. *Smith* REYNOLDS (1824–1915)

Mary Smith was born May 22, 1824, in Wooster, Ohio, daughter of Dr. John Smith of New Jersey and his wife, Sarah Buttles from Connecticut. Nothing has been found about her childhood or early education. On March 30, 1848, Mary married Benoi O. Reynolds (b. 1824) at Marsailon, Ohio; Benoi was a native of Sempronius, Cayuga County, New York. The couple had two children: James C. (b. 1849) and Willis S. (b. 1851). Benoi would soon graduate from Rush Medical College (1851). The family had moved first to Ives Grove, Racine County, Wisconsin, then to Delavan, then Elkhorn, and finally, in 1865, to Lake Geneva, where they spent the rest of their lives. While they were in Elkhorn, Mary enrolled at the Female Medical College of Pennsylvania. She graduated with an MD degree in 1861.

Her sons then twelve and ten, respectively, she returned to Elkhorn and started to practice medicine, probably taking care of her husband's patients during the Civil War. He was surgeon to the Third Wisconsin Cavalry Volunteers. After the war, the family moved to Lake Geneva, where Mary and her husband practiced for many years. They are both listed as being active practitioners in the 1874 and 1877 Butler medical directories and in the Polk medical directories from 1886 through 1902. Meantime, their son John C. (MD, Rush, 1870) had started practice in Lake Geneva. Though Mary's name continued to be listed in Polk, she wrote that she retired in 1892. In a letter to classmate Sally Saltzgiver (q.v.) in 1895 she reported giving up practice three years earlier, handing over responsibility for her patients to her husband and son. "She felt that three doctors in one house were too many."

Benoi, who was a member of the Wisconsin State Medical Society, the Wisconsin State Board of Health, the American Public Health Association, and at one time vice president and attending physician at Lake Geneva's Oakwood Springs Sanitarium, died January 19, 1911. Dr. Mary died at home on October 22, 1915. Her funeral was at the Congregational Church, of which she had long been a member. Her obituary described her as "a woman of noble impulses and fine character, a considerate Christian woman."

References: Butler, 1874, 1877; Obituary from an unidentified Lake Geneva newspaper numbered 44, no. 31, 1915; Polk, 1886–1902; *Progressive Annual*, 1864; Woman's Medical College of Pennsylvania, *Report of the Proceedings of the Thirteenth Annual Meeting of the Alumnae Association of the Woman's Medical College of Pennsylvania, May 9th and 10th, 1895* (Philadelphia, 1895), 151; Woman's Medical College of Pennsylvania, *Transactions of the 41st Annual Meeting of the Alumnae Association of the Woman's Medical College of Pennsylvania* (Philadelphia, 1916), 35.

Sarah Ann *RICE* (1823–87)

Sarah Rice, like both her parents, was born in Marlborough, Massachusetts, on July 17, 1823, the sixth of eight children, fourth daughter, of Jonathan and Betsy Brigham Rice. On her mother's side she was a third cousin, once removed, of Peter Bent Brigham. In 1859, then thirty-six, she received an MD degree from Penn Medical University, an Eclectic School in Philadelphia. She returned to Marlborough, where she practiced medicine the rest of her life. She is listed in various directories as a physician in Marlborough 1867–85. She died, unmarried, in Marlborough on January 7, 1887, of "capillary bronchitis."

References: Marlborough, Massachusetts, Vital Records; *Massachusetts Register for 1867*; Middlesex County (MA) directories for 1873, 1875, 1878, 1882–83, 1884–85; *New England Business Directory*, 1868; *Progressive Annual*, 1863, 1864.

Margaret *Phillips* RICHARDSON (1816–1909)

Margaret Phillips was born October 27, 1816, in Radnor Township, Delaware County, Pennsylvania, the daughter of John Phillips and his wife Barbara Colflesh. Her parents were of Welsh descent, members of the Baptist Church, and her father was a farmer, first in Radnor and later in Juniata. The couple had seven children, a son and then six daughters, of whom Margaret was the eldest. "Her youth was devoted to acquiring an education such as the paid schools of the day afforded" (*Norristown Daily Herald*).

On September 12, 1839, Margaret married Abraham Richardson, a fellow townsman. They had one child, a son, John Phillips Richardson, who later graduated from the University of Pennsylvania Medical School, began practice in Norristown, served in the Civil War, and later practiced in Philadelphia and New York City. Abraham died in 1841, two years after the couple were married, leaving Margaret with an infant son to raise.

Ten years later, Margaret entered the recently organized Female Medical College of Pennsylvania, graduating in 1853 with an MD degree. Thereafter, she practiced for four years in Juniata County before moving to Norristown in the summer of 1857. She registered in 1881 as a physician, as the law then required. She practiced in Norristown until three years before her death, when she fell and broke her hip. She died on May 15, 1909, of pneumonia, at the age of ninety-two years, six months, nineteen days.

Throughout her professional career she kept casebooks, of which there were ultimately four volumes. When she died, she left these and her diploma to her alma mater. Though these cannot presently be located, a summary of her obstetrical cases was found. Between 1853 and 1896 she delivered 447 babies, 38 of whom were twins. Her peak years were 1859–71. During these years she delivered 17, 19, 18, 41, 37, 52, 45, 45, 38, 28, 22, 18, and 15 babies, respectively. After 1878, there were one to three babies a year, except in three years when there were four babies delivered and one year with five. No mention is made in this summary of infant or maternal mortality.

References: Obituary, *Norristown Daily Herald* (PA), May 15, 1909; Obituary in Woman's Medical College of Pennsylvania, *Transactions of the Thirty-Fourth Annual Meeting of the Alumnae Association of the Woman's Medical College of Pennsylvania, May 27 and 28, 1909* (Philadelphia, 1909), 25–26; Papers of Margaret Phillips Richardson, Medical College of Pennsylvania archives at Drexel University College of Medicine archives, Philadelphia, acc. 293, obstetrical casebook, 1853–96.

Emily *RIDGEWAY* Robbins (1832–1903)

Emily Ridgeway was born in Philadelphia in 1832. No information has been found regarding her background, parents, or early education. She graduated from Penn Medical University in 1859. Evidence of what she did in the three years immediately following her graduation is contradictory. One source says that she practiced medicine at 1324 Brown Street in Philadelphia. Another places her as a practitioner at Ft. Madison, a village in southeastern Iowa.

In 1862, Emily married medical school classmate, Charles W. Robbins, MD. The couple set up practice in northeast Philadelphia. For the next thirty-plus years they were at one of three locations on Richmond Avenue, an economically modest neighborhood. In later years, at least, they are listed in directories as homoeopathic practitioners. They are both listed as practicing physicians regularly in Philadelphia and Polk medical directories from 1865 until the end of the century. Around the turn of the century, they retired to May's Landing, New Jersey, a village between Vineland and Atlantic City. Emily died at the age of seventy-one, on August 31, 1903, in Philadelphia.

References: Obituary, *Boston Medical and Surgical Journal*, September 10, 1903, 304; Philadelphia city directories; Obituary, *Philadelphia Inquirer*, September 3, 1903; Polk, 1890, 1893, 1896, 1898, 1900, 1902.

Laura J. *ROSS* Wolcott (1826–1915)

Laura Ross, physician and suffragette, was the first woman doctor of medicine to practice in Wisconsin. Laura was born July 16, 1826, in Shapleigh, Maine, to James Ross and Lovey Huntress. She attended Horace Mann Normal School in Lexington, Massachusetts, and was subsequently a private student of Harvard science professors. She went to Female Medical College of Pennsylvania and received an MD degree in 1856. According to historian William Snow Miller, she was one of the first three women to have clinical training at the Philadelphia Hospital (Alms House). Formal education completed, she moved to Milwaukee, established an office, and practiced medicine there for the next thirty years (1857–87). The census of June 1860 records her on two occasions, nine days apart (once aged twenty-nine, once aged thirty-five, living at two different places) but both times denoting her a physician.

During 1867, Laura traveled abroad, visiting hospitals in England and France. In 1869, she married Erastus Bradley Wolcott, a man born in Western New York State and of a distinguished ancestry that included three governors of Connecticut, one of Massachusetts, and a signer of the Declaration of Independence. A widower, he had two surviving (of five) children by his first wife. Laura, already forty-three, had no children. Erastus, also a physician, received his MD degree in 1833 from the College of Physicians and Surgeons of the Western District of New York, known more familiarly as Fairfield, although he was already licensed to practice by the Yates County Medical Society in 1825. In 1836, he was commissioned as surgeon in the US Army, and it was during this time that he met and married his first wife. In 1839, he resigned his commission and moved to Milwaukee, where he went into practice. He was later surgeon general of Wisconsin.

After their marriage, Erastus and Laura practiced medicine together until he died in 1880, after which she gradually retired from practice, although she is still listed in the 1890 Polk medical directory as a practicing physician. Her practice had emphasized the care of women and children. She was also consulting physician for several institutions in Milwaukee: the Industrial School of Girls, the Convent of Notre Dame, St. Mary's Hospital, Passavant Hospital, Milwaukee Orphan Asylum, St. John's Home for Aged Women, and the county poorhouse and jail, where she cared for women.

As it was with most (probably all) early woman doctors, she was not readily received by her professional brethren. On January 21, 1869, with the backing of her soon-to-be husband, she was admitted to the Milwaukee Medical Society. It was not until later, in the 1870s, that women were more generally accepted into the formerly all-male medical societies. After the death of her husband, she returned on more than one occasion to study at Cambridge University and on the wards of the Paris hospitals, where, it is said, she attracted the attention and help of the Empress Eugenie.

Laura, like many other early woman doctors, was active in community affairs and especially in the woman's suffrage movement. She played a major role in organizing the first woman's suffrage convention in Wisconsin in 1869, as had Mary Wilhite (q.v.), in Indiana. Speakers included Susan B. Anthony, Elizabeth K. Stanton, and Mary A. Livermore. In later years, Laura had a statue of her husband, mounted on a horse, erected in a Milwaukee park. Laura died in Chicago, December 8, 1915, at the age of eighty-nine.

References: Obituary, *Chicago Daily Tribune,* December 9, 1915; Louis F. Frank, *The Medical History of Milwaukee, 1834–1914* (Milwaukee: Germania Publishing Co., 1915), 35–36; *Dictionary of American Medical Biography,* 2:817–18; William S. Miller, "Erastus Bradley Wolcott (1804–80)," *Wisconsin Medical Journal,* January 1931, 8–11; Dennis H. Phillips, "Women in Nineteenth Century Wisconsin Medicine," *Wisconsin Medical Journal* 71 (November 1972): 13–18; US census, 1860.

Anna M. *RUGGLES* Reed (b. 1838)

Anna Ruggles was born March 3, 1838, in Carmel, Penobscot County, Maine (another source says Calais, Maine), the eldest of six children (three girls, three boys) of James Ruggles and his wife Eunice S. Dennett. The locally prominent Ruggles family moved first to New York City about 1840 and on to Philadelphia by 1846. James Ruggles was a broker.

In 1855, the youngest Ruggles child, William, was born and died. By 1860, Anna and her younger brother Augustus were both at medical school, Anna at Penn Medical University, and Augustus at University of Pennsylvania. Also then living with the Ruggles family was another PMU medical student, Maria J. Dennett (q.v.). Both Anna and Maria graduated in 1861. It seems likely that Anna and Maria were cousins; Anna's mother was a Dennett. The 1860 census shows Maria living with the Ruggles family. Anna and Maria shared offices when they started practice in Philadelphia after graduating. In addition to Anna, Maria, and Augustus, one or two more of Anna's siblings became physicians—sister Amelia (PMU, 1863) and Myra (said to have attended PMU but no record of graduation). On March 12, 1863, Anna married Alfred Graham Reed, MD, also born in Carmel, and a fellow student at PMU (MD, 1862; also University of Pennsylvania, MD, 1868). They had no children.

Anna and Maria Dennett practiced medicine in Philadelphia for three or four years after graduating, sharing offices. Anna's name does not appear in Philadelphia directories as a physician after 1865. In the 1870 census she is listed as "keeping house." Her husband, Alfred, is listed regularly in the Butler and Polk directories until 1900. A brief notice in the *New York Times* in 1887 reports that Alfred sailed for Antwerp aboard the Red Star steamship *Noordland* and that he was author of a paper on the hot air treatment of rheumatism and gout. Whether Alfred and Anna were still together is not certain. Anna was still alive and living in Philadelphia, in 1908 (DAR directory). No death date has been determined.

References: Butler, 1974, 1877; Polk, 1886–98; Daughters of the American Revolution, *Directory of the National Society of the Daughters of the American Revolution* (Washington, DC, 1908); *New York Times*, May 29, 1887; US census, 1860, 1870.

Julia *RUMSEY* (b. ca. 1825–60)

Julia Rumsey was born about 1825. She matriculated at Eclectic Medical Institute in Cincinnati in the fall of 1852, coming there from the village of Avoca, located in New York State's Southern Tier. As will be seen in more detail below, she had to earn the money for her medical education. After her first term she took a term off and worked at a water-cure. She also borrowed money from one of her more prosperous classmates, Mary Malin Baily (q.v.), which she repaid in full.

Julia completed the medical requirements successfully and earned an MD degree in 1854. She practiced medicine for almost a decade in Tiffin, a town in north central Ohio, and was the first woman doctor in that community. In 1860, she was raising her orphaned twelve-year-old nephew. While on a vacation cruise on Lake Huron in August 1865, aboard the SS *Pewabie*, the ship collided with another, sank, and Dr. Rumsey was drowned. In October, her body was found, washed up on the Canadian shore.

A newspaper account of the accident contained the following obituary comment: Dr. Rumsey was "an accomplished and highly educated lady, with pleasing manners and gentle disposition. She had acquired a very large practice in this city . . . [and was] a benefactor to the poor" (*Seneca Advertiser*, October 26, 1865, 3). It is also mentioned that she was a zealous member of the Episcopal Church, a fact noteworthy because it was uncommon for female members of the more conservative denominations (e.g., Episcopal, Presbyterian, Roman Catholic) to become physicians at that time, Quakers and Methodists being those most often to enter the profession.

The following information about Julia Rumsey comes from the correspondence of medical classmate Mary Malin Baily (q.v.), presented here separately because of its length but in extenso because of its broader interest regarding the medical education of women: "Will live with another female student, introduced by Professor Buchanan. She is from Avoca, Steuben County, N.Y. where she studied with an allopath in Bath, N.Y., but she was unable to matriculate at the local medical school [probably Geneva or Buffalo]" (Mary to brother John, November 21, 1852). Mary and Julia attended the Unitarian Church.

> I have been fortunate in having a lady of the class with me, from the time I went to Mrs. Pinkham's until the present time who reads aloud for my benefit, which I very much prize—for we talk more upon [and] compare ideas of the subjects before us—A Miss Rumsey of Steuben Co., N.Y. attended the Winter Session, will again attend the approaching winter term, but her funds were exhausted for the time being and she is endeavoring to earn the means to do it. She takes charge of patients at these "Water-Cures" although an "Eclectic," but she has no responsibility in the matter, and it serves for clinical practice to a certain extent. She expects to locate for a physician, and if native bias and qualifications will ensure success in

this new pathway for woman, she is one who will reflect credit both on herself and her sex—if society is, as many think ready to sustain our sex in this more extended scope of duty—an advance certainly right and appropriate in every aspect—woman is a nurse—and why not be a scientific nurse as well as a blind nurse leading the blind, not to mention the thousand and one advantages that may be shed broadcast into a community by a more familiar knowledge of principles to be adopted either in the prevention or easy cure of besetting ills whether mental or physical—or both—the first causing the latter, or the latter the first—it is sometimes one and sometimes the other, as every one knows who pretends to look in the matter at all. (Mary to Aunt Sally, March 8, 1853)

I feel comfortable in knowing my guarantee for Miss Rumsey to Mrs. Meconkey is ended by a draft sent to Mrs. Meconkey a few days since, and this money Miss Rumsey has made by her practice since she and I graduated—besides being cheated out of as much more by her co-partner, but finding Miss Brown unfair, she closed partnership with her, and opened an office alone, in which she has succeeded so remarkably. On my guarantee for the money to Sarah Brinton Meconkey she obtained it to carry her through her Graduation—I risked; but I have more than ordinary gratification in having secured a profession to a deserving and energetic woman. (Mary to brother John, from Troy, New York, July 10, 1855)

To her cousin Sally, from Troy Female Seminary, September 7, 1855: Miss Rumsey paid her a visit during "this vacation." From Tiffin, Ohio, November 16, 1860: she is visiting Miss Rumsey and her twelve-year-old nephew, in Tiffin. To her brother John, from Troy Female Seminary, March 23, 1861: "Miss Rumsey performed this operation with entire success."

References: A. J. Baughman, *History of Seneca County Ohio* (Chicago: Lewis Publishing Co., 1911), 314; Daughters of the American Revolution, Dolly Todd Madison Chapter, *Ohio Early State and Local History* (Tiffin, Ohio, 1915), 60; *Seneca Advertiser* (Tiffin, Ohio), August 17, 1865; *Seneca Advertiser* (Tiffin, Ohio), October 26, 1865; Baily correspondence regarding J. Rumsey in the Evans family papers, 1709–1928, Library of Virginia, Richmond.

S

Sarah Whitman *SALISBURY* (1814–65)

Sarah Salisbury was born October 30 or 31, 1814, in Weymouth, Massachusetts, the fifth of nine children and eldest daughter of Abiah W.

and Patience Pratt Salisbury. Her father was a laborer with $1,550 in real estate, according to the 1850 census. Sarah, already worth $1,000 in 1850, graduated from New England Female Medical College in Boston, with an MD degree in 1856, and returned to Weymouth. She had been supported at medical school with a Massachusetts state scholarship from 1854 to 1856.

She probably practiced medicine there, but the evidence is conflicting. The *Progressive Annuals* for 1862, 1863, and 1864 list her as a physician in East Weymouth, but her name does not appear in the *Massachusetts Register* for 1858 or the *New England Business Directory* for 1860 in any Massachusetts community. It is not found in the Boston business directory for 1863–64. However, she was professor of chemistry, materia medica, and therapeutics at her alma mater from 1862 to 1864, and professor of anatomy in 1864–65. Sarah died in Weymouth, unmarried, on January 24, 1865, of pneumonia. Her death certificate gives her residences as Weymouth and East Boston.

References: *Boston Business and Co-partnership Directory*, 1863–64; Weymouth Historical Society, *History of Weymouth, Mass* (Boston, 1923), 4:608–9; *Massachusetts Register*, 1858; *New England Business Directory*, 1860; *Progressive Annual*, 1862, 1864; Weymouth, MA, town records, 1868.

Eveline Elizabeth *Moseley* Curtis SARGENT (1829–92)

Eveline Moseley was born March 26, 1829, in Franklinville, a community in Cattaraugus County in Western New York. The only daughter of Aaron Moseley and Eliza Sybil Sellon, she had an older brother, Alonzo. Nothing is known of her early education. About 1848, when she was nineteen, Eveline married Porter Daniel Curtis. They had one child, Elthera Esther Curtis, who was born in Watertown, Wisconsin, on May 20, 1849. Eveline and Daniel (as he was known) were divorced, probably about 1856. Soon thereafter, Eveline met and married Uzza Washington Sargent, of Sparta, Wisconsin, and the couple went together to New York City to attend lectures at the New York Hygeio-Therapeutic College. On March 29, 1861, they each graduated with an MD degree. Whether daughter Elthera went with them to New York is not clear. The Sargents returned to Sparta, where they practiced medicine and had three daughters. Fenora, the eldest, and Mary Uzza, the youngest, each became a physician. The middle daughter was a Chautauqua speaker and author. Elthera, the eldest, and half sister to the other three, also became a doctor. Mother Eveline was reputed to be the first water-cure doctor in Wisconsin.

Uzza, who had a twin brother name Uzzell, died September 22, 1867. Not long after this, Eveline, with three small children, and perhaps older daughter Elthera to help, moved to St. Louis, where they lived during most of the 1870s. Eveline is listed in St. Louis directories from 1870 through 1879 (no 1880 or 1881 directories are available), first as an electromagnetic physician (1871) and thereafter simply as a physician. Starting in 1875, her eldest daughter, Elthera Curtis, by then twenty-six years of age, joined her in practice. Elthera later moved to Los Angeles, where she died in 1914.

In the early 1880s, Eveline moved again, this time to San Antonio, Texas, where she is listed in local directories from 1883–84 to 1887–88, and Polk directories for 1886 and 1890, as a physician offering electric baths. In 1885 and 1887, her daughter Fenora practiced with her as a homoeopathic physician. Fenora had attended St. Louis College of Physicians and Surgeons and received an MD degree from that institution in 1882. Then she attended medical lectures at Boston University (successor to New England Female Medical College) and earned another MD degree in 1884. She later came back to Missouri, settled in the village of Cuba, married Jesse E. Sargent, and practiced medicine, as did her husband. She died in 1946.

Eveline's youngest daughter, Mary Uzza, went to Homoeopathic Medical College of Missouri, graduating with an MD degree in 1887, and practiced with her mother, who must have moved back to St. Louis, at least briefly. The 1890 Polk directory places them both at 3007 Easton Avenue, St. Louis, in 1890. Eveline died in San Antonio, December 24, 1892. Three of her four daughters had become physicians.

References: Descendants of Joseph Moseley website, http://www.genealogy.com/ftm/n/i/e/Walter-I-Nieber/GENE4-0001.html (accessed June 1, 2016); Polk, 1886, 1890; *Progressive Annual*, 1863, 1864; Aaron Sargent, *Sargent Genealogy* (Somerville, MA: Author, 1895); St. Louis city directories, 1870–79; San Antonio city directory, 1883/84–1887/88.

Martha Ann *Hayden* SAWIN (1815–59)

Martha Hayden was born May 30, 1815, in Marlboro, Massachusetts, to Isaac and Martha Hayden. She was the second of eight children and the eldest of six daughters. Little is known of her youth and education. At the age of twenty she married George H. Sawin, a fellow townsman who, in 1843, moved to Boston where he went into business as a merchant. The Sawins had no children. After Martha's death in 1859, George must have remarried. In 1863, $40,000 in debt, he declared bankruptcy, and two years later his wife and others were "committed for contempt of court" for refusing to tell what they had done with his property.

In 1849, Martha attended the newly organized (but as yet unchartered) Boston Female Medical College and, along with four other women, received a "certificate of qualification," presumably as a midwife. The Boston Female Medical College was not yet a bona fide medical school. The institution had been organized primarily through the efforts of Samuel Gregory. The faculty was composed of one professor, Dr. Enoch C. Rolfe, and the purpose was to train women as midwives so that modest mothers might have at childbed a competent alternative to the increasingly common male physician and his forceps.

With the opening of the Female Medical College of Pennsylvania, Martha enrolled in it and, after the required two courses, along with seven classmates, received a medical degree on December 30, 1851. She returned to Boston, established home and office (it may have already been her home) at 60 Temple Street in the middle of downtown, where she practiced medicine ("became a doctress" as her relative, Thomas Sawin, put it) for the seven and a half years until her death on August 30, 1859. The cause of her death is variously reported as scrofula (Boston) or cancer (Marlboro). She was listed as a practicing physician in the *Boston Almanacs* for 1854, 1856, and 1859. Historian Frederick C. Waite could find nothing "to indicate that her medical career displayed any outstanding capability or service" except that she was in the first graduating class of Female Medical College of Pennsylvania and was the first woman MD to practice in New England.

References: *Boston Almanac*, 1854, 1856, 1859; Thomas E. Sawin, *Sawin: Summary Notes concerning John Sawin, and His Posterity* (Wendell, MA: Author, 1866); Frederick C. Waite, "Dr. Martha (Hayden) Sawin," *New England Journal of Medicine* 205 (1931): 1053–55.

Lydia *SAYER* Hasbrouck (1827–1910)

Though she became a physician and practiced medicine for a year in Washington, DC, and at least a few years thereafter, Lydia Sayer was known as a reformer, especially of women's clothing, and in the matter of woman's rights, as well. Lydia Sayer was born December 20, 1827, on a farm near Bellvale, a hamlet in Orange County, New York, just north of the New Jersey border. Her parents were Benjamin Sayer and Rebecca Forshee. She received her basic education in the district school, Miss Galatian's Select School, and Central College in Elmira.

In 1849, when she was twenty-two, she adopted the "Bloomer" costume—knee-length skirt over trousers or bloomers—and, on applying to Miss Seward's Seminary in Rochester was refused admission because of her inappropriate dress. This might seem surprising considering the history of the school, a school that Miss Sarah Seward, herself a graduate of Troy Female Seminary, had opened in 1833. The school was very successful and quite liberal for the times. The mother of a student, upon visiting the school in 1837, wrote to her husband that the school was "well considered and very popular. . . . Rules are few & so judicious that the girls feel all the liberty they wish—there seems nothing like constraint." Just the place for Lydia. But, in 1841, Miss Seward married and turned the establishment over to her brother Jason, and the rules must have changed. In any case, the school declined, and Miss Sayer was so outraged that it was a turning point in her life. Displeased but not defeated she became from then on an activist in woman's dress reform. "As I left . . . I fairly bathed my soul in an agony of tears and silent prayers. . . . I registered a vow that I would stand or fall in the battle for women's physical, political and educational freedom and equality" (*Women of the Hudson Valley*).

After serving as a delegate to the Whole World's Temperance Convention at New York in 1853 the emphasis on water directed her attention to the relatively new and popular form of treatment—hydrotherapy. She attended and graduated from New York Hygeio-Therapeutic College in 1855, a school that emphasized water therapy, as well as proper diet and hygienic daily regimen. Then to Washington where she practiced medicine for a year and lectured on hygienic living in the surrounding towns (Perry). An English reporter who was visiting Washington asked a companion, upon encountering Dr. Sayer, "Who is this nice young gentlemanly-looking person who follows us?" "Oh, that is Miss Lydia Sayer, M.D., hydropathic physician and Bloomer,—a clever woman, let me tell you, and one of the *characters* of Washington. She is a frequent attendant at Congress, and this is about her usual position in the gallery of 'the House.'" Lydia was described as wearing a "suit of broadcloth, black pants, buttoned frock-coat, cloak with white collar over, and buff-coloured, low-crowned, broad-brimmed hat with black feather" (Henley).

Lydia's Washington stay was brief. John Whitbeck Hasbrouck, editor and publisher of the *Whig Press*, invited her to lecture in Middletown, New York. She accepted, apparently stayed, and became editor of Hasbrouck's new venture, *Sibyl*, a "review of the tastes, error, and fashions of society." Throughout its life this periodical emphasized dress reform, proclaiming "that unconfining clothing was at the core of women's struggle for equality and good health." It also offered articles and reviews of books on free love, not to mention diet, the benefit of baths, fresh air, and avoidance of alcohol and tobacco. When Lydia married Hasbrouck on July 27, 1856, she wore white satin bloomers and a white silk tunic and promised to "walk equally . . . through life [without] renouncing my individuality in yielding unto you the true wife's love and duty." The couple had three children and lived in an octagon stone house called "Sibyl Ridge" (Perry). A son, Sayer Hasbrouck, became a physician (MD, 1882, Boston University) and practiced in Providence, Rhode Island.

In March 1861, Lydia wrote to President Lincoln, seeking the job as postmaster of Middletown. That she was not appointed is not surprising. The letter is more a polemic on women's rights than a job application:

> May I a wife, mother, tax payer and hard working woman of America be heard, when I ask from you, a man of power a juster recognition of woman's individuality than has hitherto been shown her in the distribution of such offices as she is well fitted to fill? It is useless for me to remind an intelagent [*sic*] citizen of our progressive west of the growing spirit of discontent among the hard working *unrepresented tax paying* women of America in relation to the manner in which men arrogate to themselves all [power offices &c &c . . . I . . . will trust to you to right some of the injustice meted out to her at present.

In the house at Sybil Ridge Lydia established, for two or three years during the Civil War, a health spa—Sibyl Ridge Hygienic Retreat. There, patients could have baths and electromagnetic treatments, but the venture was not a success. It was off the main line and, unlike the most successful retreats, it did not emphasize diet and religious observance. It is not known whether Lydia cared for patients in later years. In the 1880 census she is listed as a physician, which would suggest she was in active practice. (The Hasbroucks were not found in the 1870 census, and the 1890 census was lost.) She was not, however, listed in the Butler medical directories (1874, 1877) or in the 1886 or 1890 Polk directories.

It is clear that Lydia's main focus was dress reform for women and, secondarily, achievement of greater rights for women generally. On several occasions she got herself into trouble by refusing to pay taxes, either because she was not allowed to vote, or, on another occasion, it was a road tax. In the first instance, the tax collector stole a pair of her bloomers and offered them for sale in lieu of payment. Lydia responded by calling the collector a "vulgar sneak" in the *Sibyl* and the collector withdrew his offer. The highway authorities were less forgiving. They required that she give several days labor on a road gang. Lydia opposed organized religion, contending that one's spiritual life was personal and private. In 1880, New York State passed a law allowing women to vote in school board elections and to run for positions on the boards. Lydia became the first woman on the Middletown school board. Dr. Hasbrouck died at Sybil Ridge, near Middletown, on August 24, 1910, at eighty-two.

Bibliography: Articles in *Sibyl* (1856–64), an eight-page reform periodical of which Dr. Hasbrouck was editor; With her husband, editor of a liberal newspaper *Liberal Sentinel* (1881–); Letter to President Abraham Lincoln, Middletown, March 8, 1861.

References: T. C. Henley, "A Glimpse of Uncle Sam's Managing Affairs," *New Monthly Magazine* (London) 108 (1856); Jean Thomas, s.v., "Lydia Sayer Hasbrouck," *Femilogue,* http://femilogue.blogspot.com/2012/12/0-false-18-pt-18-pt-0-0-false-false_20.html (accessed May 19, 2016); Hudson River Valley Heritage, "Dress Reformer: Lydia Sayer," *Women of the Hudson Valley,* http://omeka.hrvh.org/exhibits/show/women-of-the-hudson-valley/in-reform (accessed May 20, 2016); Dexter Perkins, "Letters Postmarked Rochester: 1817–1879," *Rochester Historical Society Publications,* 1943, 57–58; "Lydia Sayer Hasbrouck," *American National Biography,* 10:277–78; US census, 1850, 1860; *Who Was Who* (Chicago, 1968), 4:415.

Mary J. *SCARLETT* Dixon (1822–1900)

Mary Scarlett was born October 23, 1822, in Robeson Township, Berks County, Pennsylvania, the youngest of seven children. Her father was a farmer, and her parents both belonged to the Society of Friends. Her father died when she was four years old, and an older brother died not long after that, leaving the mother and six children on a relatively unproductive farm. According to Willard and Livermore, the Scarlett household was the only one in its neighborhood to take an active part in the 1830 agitation against slavery, becoming "the resort for anti-slavery lectures."

When Mary was sixteen, her mother died, and Mary started teaching in country schools. Except for a year and a half when she attended boarding school, she taught for seventeen years with the goal of saving enough to go to medical school. How this idea developed in her mind is not known. It would have been only in the later years of her teaching career that it was possible for a woman to become a doctor of medicine. Willard and Livermore state that she was told by one of the professors at the newly opened Female Medical College of Pennsylvania "that she was wanted" there.

Then thirty-three, she went to the school in 1855 and graduated with an MD degree in 1857. This was followed by an extra year of lectures. In her first year out of school, she lectured on hygiene in country towns and villages, perhaps to establish her name professionally. Her subsequent career was a combination of private practice, hospital practice, and professorial duties at her alma mater.

In 1859, she was appointed demonstrator of anatomy at Female Medical College of Pennsylvania and, three years later, professor of anatomy, as well. After a few years, she gave up the post as demonstrator but remained professor until 1881. The school had established a woman's hospital in Philadelphia, partly for the purpose of providing clinical training for its students. Women students were not welcome at other hospitals, whose medical staffs were exclusively male. Recent graduate Emeline H. Cleveland, MD (q.v.), on her return from postgraduate training in Paris hospitals, was appointed resident physician, and Dr. Scarlett became assistant physician, a position she held until 1865. After the death of Dr. Cleveland in 1868, Scarlett returned as resident physician, a position she held for three years. Thereafter, she was visiting physician to the institution. Throughout these years she was carrying on a private practice. It must have been a heavy load, leaving little time for outside activities. She did have a longtime interest in the temperance movement. On May 8, 1873, then fifty-one, she married G. Washington Dixon.

An interesting letter, written June 15, 1869, from Dr. Scarlett to Dr. Edwin Fussell, expresses some of the frustration and resentment then felt by woman doctors. (Dr. Fussell had been a founder of Female Medical College of Pennsylvania, professor, and, until three years earlier, dean of the school.)

> Thee will see by the Hospital Report that we have six attending physicians. . . . The laws require that one from each department of attending physicians shall visit as often as once a week. Some visit oftener and one (Dr. Hunt) does not come at all. He does not approve of the regulations, consequently he does not come to see us. The consulting physicians have their first consultation to hold. There was a time appointed for them to visit the Hospital, the ceremony of invitation was performed by some of the attending physicians, the house was cleaned from roof to cellar, the sheet and spreads were of snowy whiteness, the patients in their best attire, flowers bloomed for the occasion, the sun sent forth its most charming rays and—and three of the seven came. . . . I was disappointed. There was only one man

in the whole company that I cared specially to see here (Dr. Alfred Stille), and he did not come . . . a man combining native good sense with education and experience.

Dr. Scarlett also mentions that there are usually from eighteen to twenty-two patients in the hospital and "constantly" cases of interest—several patients with scarlet fever and one with dropsy. "I have been in the habit of giving calomel, Digitalis and Squill. One of our Doctors pronounces this bad practice. What is thy opinion?"

Toward the end of her life, Dr. Scarlett developed glaucoma and during her last three years was forced to give up practice because of it. She died January 28, 1900, and is buried at Fair Hill Cemetery, Philadelphia.

Bibliography: *Valedictory Address of Prof. M. J. Scarlett, before the Graduating Class of the Female Medical College, of Philadelphia, March 16, 1867* (Philadelphia: College, 1867).

References: Mary J. Scarlett, ALS, June 15, 1869, Philadelphia, to Edwin Fussell, in the Archives of the Medical College of Pennsylvania, at Drexel University College of Medicine, Philadelphia; US census, 1850, 1860, 1870; Frances E. Willard, *A Woman of the Century* (Buffalo: C. W. Moulton, 1893), 246; Woman's Medical College of Pennsylvania, Alumnae Association, *Transactions of the 25th Anniversary Meeting, May 17th and 18th, 1900* (Philadelphia, 1900), 24.

Finette E. *SCOTT* Seelye (1833–1914)

Finette Scott was born December 1833 in Brattleboro, Vermont, the second of three children of John M. Scott and his wife Chloa. John was a farmer. Finette had a brother, Edward, three years her senior, and a younger sister, Mary. Sometime in the 1840s, the family moved to Illinois, settling in Whiteside County near the Iowa border. As a young woman, Finette earned money by teaching and helped her siblings get an education. It was later written that she was highly esteemed as a young woman (Ingham, 321).

In the early 1850s, then twenty and a resident of Wheaton, Illinois, Finette matriculated at New York Hygeio-Therapeutic College (then known as New York Hydropathic and Physiological School and not yet chartered to grant MD degrees) and from which she received a diploma at the end of the school's second term in June 1854. (*WCJ* lists her as a graduate of the third term in May 1855.) She began practice in Litchfield, Connecticut. The *Water-Cure Journal*, however, reported

(August 1855, 38) that she "has put out her sign in Waterbury, Conn., where, we learn, she is already appreciated, and is doing a good business. She is also engaged in lecturing on the laws of health, as well as prescribing for the abnormalities of disease."

She soon moved to Cleveland as an assistant physician at the well-known Cleveland Water-Cure. The water-cure was opened in 1848 by Thomas Taylor Seelye, MD. Seelye, born in Connecticut, was an 1842 graduate of the New York College of Physicians and Surgeons. The water-cure was a three-story brick structure, built near a soft-water spring in a wooded glen, rural, well landscaped, with curving walks and drives. Treating female diseases and midwifery were its specialties. In June 1851, the cost was eight dollars a week for board, medical advice, and "ordinary" nursing. Hydropathy, diet, and exercise were the principal therapeutic modalities. It served 4,500 patients in its first eleven years and was probably the most successful water-cure west of those in Clifton Springs, Dansville, and Elmira, in Western New York.

In addition to Dr. Scott, at least two other early woman doctors worked at the Cleveland water-cure during the 1850s: Dr. Ellen Higgins (q.v.) and Dr. Cordelia Greene (q.v.). In 1846, Dr. Seelye had married Sarah Deming, and they had two daughters. Though a death date has not been found, it seems likely that Sarah died. Dr. Seelye soon married his assistant, Finette Scott. She bore him three more children: Sara E. (b. 1861), Thomas T. Jr. (b. 1864), and Finette Scott (b. 1868). Whether, or for how long, Finette continued to practice at the water-cure is not known. Her name is not listed in the Butler medical directories for 1874 or 1877, or in the 1886 Polk medical directory. Neither is her husband's name listed. The establishment prospered until after the Civil War, closed in 1868, became a Jewish orphanage in 1870. The site is now a metal scrapyard.

In the 1880s, the Seelyes built a winter home in Crescent City, Florida. An attractive structure that might be labeled southern Italianate in style, it had two-story arched verandas across the front façade. The Seelyes probably later came to live here full time. When Thomas died in 1890, he was buried in Palmetto Cemetery in Crescent City. By 1910, Finette, by then seventy-six, was living in New York City with her son, a divorced patent lawyer, her daughter Finette, whose occupation when she died in California in 1925 was listed as "retired traveler," her grandson, twelve-year-old Thomas, and a nurse. Finette died at eighty on January 29, 1914.

Of Dr. Finette's days in Cleveland, Mrs. Ingham wrote in her *Women of Cleveland and Their Work*: "She was the leading spirit among women in her quarter of Cleveland, helped, encouraged all young ladies who struggled with poverty in acquiring an education, especially, medical; she aided financially any who needed; established a sewing school, worked in Friendly Inns, was a fine housekeeper and good mother, and read a great deal of solid literature; was fond of the Greek poets. She was the center of reading and social circles."

References: *Cleveland Water Cure,* undated broadside signed T. T. Seelye, MD, at the Library of Congress; Patsy Gerstner, "The Medical Institutions of Cleveland: 1813–1910," in *Encyclopedia of Cleveland History* (Cleveland, 2002); Mrs. W. A. Ingham, *Women of Cleveland and Their Work* (Cleveland, 1893), 321–23; s.v. "Finette Scott SEELEY," Seeley Genealogical Society, http://www.seeley-society.net/vitals/vcaley49a.html (accessed May 20, 2016); US census 1850, 1870, 1880, 1900, 1910; *Water-Cure Journal,* August 1855, 38.

Cleora Augusta *Stevens* SEAMAN (1814–69)

Cleora Stevens was born June 9, 1814, in Middlebury, Vermont, a daughter of Levi Stevens and Lucy Boynton. Apparently frail in childhood, said to be the result of an unspecified accident during her infancy, she was schooled at home by a cousin, John Stevens, later founder of Denison College and its professor of Greek and Latin. The number of her siblings, if any, is not known.

In October 1832, then seventeen, Cleora married John Farmer Seaman of Rochester, New York. The couple settled in Cleveland, where they raised seven children and where Cleora was active in the community. She taught Sunday school and served as president of the Maternal Association. In 1852, she joined a group of women whose goal was to encourage young women to seek medical education. (It seems likely that Myra Merrick, who had graduated from Central Medical College in Rochester, New York, in 1852 and settled in Cleveland, was probably also a member of this group.)

In 1860, her children grown, Cleora, then forty-six, graduated with an MD degree from Western Homoeopathic College. Earlier that year the Seamans had given a party for the medical students at their home: "The entertainment was given by Mrs. Seaman, who is attending the course of lectures and will no doubt deservedly win the title of M.D. at Commencement, a title the intelligent and studious lady will certainly wear with graces as well as usefully" (*Cleveland Leader,* January 4, 1860).

In her practice, Dr. Seaman emphasized the treatment of chronic problems and favored the use of hydrotherapy and electrotherapy. She is said to have been the first to introduce the use of electric baths in the Midwest. At first, her services were free, but, as her practice grew, those who could afford to do so were asked to pay a small fee.

In 1867, she helped organize the Homoeopathic College for Women and was its president until her death two years later. The need for this school had come about when the other two medical schools in Cleveland, Western Reserve and Western Homoeopathic College, having previously accepted women as students, stopped doing so, probably because their enrollments of men were so high. The new woman's college served its purpose. In 1870, it merged with Western Homoeopathic College to become the Homoeopathic Hospital College of Cleveland. Judging from the Cleveland press in the 1860s, there was considerable support for the medical education of women. Cleora died July 10, 1869, in Providence, Rhode Island, probably on a trip. Her funeral was held in the First Baptist Church in Cleveland.

References: *National Cyclopaedia of American Biography*, vol. 23 (New York, 1933); *Cleveland Leader*, January 4, 1860, p. 2, col. 1; *Morning Leader* (Cleveland), May 3, 1860; *Cleveland Newspaper Digest*, 1860–70; Obituary, *Plain Dealer* (Cleveland), July 13, 1869; Funeral notice, *Plain Dealer*, July 16, 1869.

Anna E. SELLECK Olmsted

The biennial catalog of the New York Hygeio-Therapeutic College for 1858–59 lists as a medical student Mrs. Anne S. Selleck of High Bridge, Connecticut. The 1860–61 catalog lists Mrs. A. E. Olmsted, MD, from Greenwich, Connecticut, as a student. There is evidence that they were the same person. Mrs. Selleck, whose name was probably really Anna, kept an autograph book while she was attending the college in 1858. In it, her professors (O. W. May, M. L. Holbrook, and Levi Reuben) and thirty-one of her schoolmates, including thirteen women, entered inscriptions. Many of these have a heavily religious tone, and most of them reflect the missionary zeal with which the students regarded the health reforms their school espoused. In this book, Selleck is referred to as "Mrs." and as "Anna." One of the entries is addressed to "Anna Selleck," the others just to "Anna." This seems to establish Anna Selleck as owner of the book.

When the autograph book was purchased in 2000, a scrap of paper, tucked into the front, said the book had belonged to Anna Olmsted. So it seems likely that Anna Selleck, already married and probably a widow, married again about 1858, this time to a man named Olmsted. Who was Olmsted? A possible clue is an entry in the very back of the autograph book: "Ever yours in sympathy, Wm. H. Olmsted,

Poundridge 1858." It has not been possible to verify the obvious assumption that Wm. Olmsted became the new husband. Nothing further has been found regarding Anna Olmsted. The autograph book itself was bought by a book dealer in 1960 in Indianapolis from a family named Craig. Careful search of census reports, directories, and IRS tax rolls yielded no further data.

References: New York Hygeio-Therapeutic College, *Biennial Catalogue*, 1858–59, 1860–61; Anna Olmsted, autograph book kept by Anna Selleck, later Anna Olmsted, New York, 1858. (Edward G. Miner Library, University of Rochester)

Elizabeth G. *SHATTUCK* (1822–65)

Elizabeth Shattuck, known as Lizzie, was born October 21, 1822, in Dublin, New Hampshire, the third of nine children of Abraham Shattuck, a blacksmith (as was his father before him), and his second wife, Jerusha H. French. The Shattuck forebear had come to America in 1642. Jerusha died a few weeks after the birth of her last child, when Elizabeth was sixteen. Seven of the children lived to grow up. Elizabeth's siblings did useful things. One made his way from Dublin to Philadelphia. Another became headmaster of an academy in Phillipsburg, New Jersey. Still another became an educator in Colorado Territory. And still another went to sea on a whaler "to free the family from the shame of some indiscretion of his." Nothing is known of Elizabeth's childhood. She was living in Philadelphia in 1852 when she enrolled in the New England Female Medical College but later graduated from the Female Medical College of Pennsylvania in 1854 with an MD degree. Her senior thesis was entitled "An Inaugural Dissertation on Iodine."

It was Elizabeth's intention to go to Burma as a Baptist missionary. With this in mind, she sought hospital experience but was turned down by all the Philadelphia hospitals. Four years earlier, in 1851, Sarah Adamson had sought and received permission to work as a junior physician on the wards of the Philadelphia Almshouse at Blockley. This may have been achieved through the influence of her uncle Dr. Hiram Corson. But the governance of Blockley had changed, and, during the middle 1850s, political infighting was rife, so Elizabeth, after spending a third year at the medical school, settled for the position of head nurse of the women's wards at the Philadelphia Hospital at Blockley.

In 1858, she applied to the Baptist missionary board but was turned down because she was unmarried and would have no husband to protect her. She remained for the next seven years in her position at Blockley. In 1865, she was appointed professor of physiology and hygiene, and resident physician at Vassar College. Before she could assume this position, she came down with typhus during an epidemic in the Blockley wards. She died there on January 27, 1865.

As a result of the missionary board's refusal to accept single women for foreign service, in 1860, a group of Philadelphia Quaker women organized the Woman's Union Missionary Society, with more liberal rules for selecting candidates. Dr. Shattuck was the first woman to go to medical school with the intention of becoming a medical missionary. Many others would soon follow.

References: Gulielma F. Alsop, *History of the Woman's Medical College, 1850–1950* (Philadelphia: J. B. Lippincott, 1950); Rachel L. Bodley, *The College Story: Valedictory Address, Woman's Medical College of Pennsylvania, March 17, 1881* (Philadelphia, 1881), quoted in *Philadelphia Hospital Reports* (Philadelphia, 1890), 1:343; Lisa J. Pruitt, *A Looking Glass for Ladies* (Macon, GA: Mercer University Press, 2005), 136; Robert C. Shattuck, letters, December 31, 1979, and January 16, 1980, Littleton, CO, to the Medical College of Pennsylvania regarding the Shattuck family, now in the archives of the Medical College of Pennsylvania at Drexel University College of Medicine, Philadelphia; Frederick C. Waite, *History of the New England Female Medical College 1848–1874* (Boston, 1950).

Louisa *SHEPARD* Presley (1843–1901)

Louisa Shepard was born in August 1843 in Alabama, probably in Lafayette, a rural village in the east central part of the state. She was the third child and elder daughter (of six children) of Philip Madison Shepard and his wife Louisa Fielder. Her father, when twenty-one, started the study of medicine with Dr. John B. Boon of Social Circle, Georgia, to whom he was apprenticed for two or three years, and during which time he had two courses of lectures at the Medical College of Georgia in Augusta (org. 1829) and from which he received an MD degree in 1835. During those years he walked the 125 miles to and from Augusta each school season, was sick with malaria one summer, and continued practice with Dr. Boon. Soon, he married Louisa Fielder, a fellow townsman, and in 1837 their first child, John, was born.

The family moved one hundred miles westward, by wagon and horseback, to Lafayette, Alabama, where they stayed eight years, then spent a year in Wetumpka. In 1846, now with at least five of their six children born, the family moved to Dadeville, a village in east central Alabama, and here they settled. Philip had already showed interest in training young men for the medical profession and in performing dissections, and while he was in Wetumpka there had been an attempt to get a charter for a medical school (the first in Alabama). So, it is not surprising that, when he got to Dadeville, Philip conceived the idea of establishing a medical school.

In 1851, Philip sought and obtained a charter for Graefenberg Medical Institute. The school functioned for nine years (1852–61), had about fifty graduates and a faculty of one for the first three years (Dr. Shepard). All of Philip's children attended and are said to have graduated from the medical school, except his youngest child, Sarah, who though preparing for medicine died at age fourteen. The first three sons all became faculty members.

It is family tradition that Louisa received an MD degree from the school. Unfortunately, the school closed in 1861 after the elder Dr. Shepard died of sepsis resulting from a "dirty" dissection, and the school building burned down in 1876, with loss of all records. However, the fact that Louisa was only seventeen years old in 1861 is not certain proof she was not an MD. Her two older brothers were each eighteen when they received their degrees, and her younger brother, Orlando Tyler, graduated at seventeen and became, at that time, professor of obstetrics and diseases of women and children.

In any case, it is said that Louisa became a doctor and tried practicing medicine in Tallahoosa County, Alabama, but found great resistance to a woman practitioner. Sometime before 1870 she married William Henry Presley, a local farmer three years her junior. They had at least one child, Calvin, born 1869. Louisa is listed as "keeping house" in the 1870 census. The family moved sometime thereafter to southeastern Texas. No information has been found about her life there. Whether she practiced medicine or had more children is not presently known. She died in Beaumont, Texas, in 1901 and is buried in Spell Cemetery, Voth, Jefferson County, Texas. Though Louisa may not have practiced for any significant time period, and assuming she did receive a degree from Graefenberg, she is probably the only woman from the Deep South with a medical degree in the pre–Civil War era.

References: US census, 1870; Medical Association of the State of Alabama, *Transactions*, 1898, 162, 213, 214, 221 [listing fifty graduates from Graefenberg, six or seven of whom are still practicing in 1898]; Thomas Owens, *History of Alabama and Dictionary of Alabama Biography* (Chicago: S. J. Clarke Publishing Co., 1921), 1:665–66; Roy H. Turner, "Graefenberg, the Shepard Family's Medical School," *Annals of Medical History*, n.s., 5 (1923): 548–60; E. Bass, "Pioneer Women Doctors in the South," *Journal of the American Medical Women's Association* 2 (1948):

356–60; William P. Ingram, *A History of Tallapoosa County* (Birmingham, AL?, 1951), 44–51; Howard L. Holley, "Dr. Philip Madison Shepard and His Medical School," *De Historia Medicinae* [a publication of the local Alabama history of medicine society] 2 (February 1958): 1–5; T. Altes, "Philip Madison Shepard, 1812–1861," *Southern Medical Bulletin* 57 (1969): 64–69; J. A. Thompson, "Graefenberg Medical Institute," *Alabama Journal of Medical Science* 16 (1979): 350–52; W. Hugh Tucker, personal communication to the author [Tucker is a descendant of the Shepard family]; "Find a Grave Index, 1761–2012," *Ancestry.com.*

Phebe Ann *SHOTWELL* (b. 1834)

Phebe Ann Shotwell was born about 1834 in Galen, Wayne County, New York, the fourth of six children (one boy, five girls) of Samuel Shotwell and his wife Mercy Pound (sometimes Mary in census records). Samuel was born in New Jersey and Mercy in Ridgeway, a village in Canada West, on Lake Erie, ten miles west of Buffalo. In the early 1830s, the family was living in Elba, Genesee County, but soon moved eastward to Galen. Samuel's first wife, Phebe Laing, and infant daughter had died in the early 1820s. The son by this marriage, Joseph, died in Galen when he was fifteen. Nothing is known of Phebe's childhood or early education. Sometime between 1842 and the time of the 1850 census, the family moved west to Illinois and settled in the village of Rutland, LaSalle County, where Samuel and his son Benjamin were farmers. Benjamin's three youngest sisters, Phebe, Sarah, and Caroline were all in school.

Nine years later, in 1859, Phebe graduated from the New York Hygeio-Therapeutic College with an MD degree. She returned to the hamlet of Rutland. (The medical school catalog said she was from Ottawa, Illinois. Ottawa, the county seat, was also the postal address for Rutland.) Phebe continued to live with her parents in Rutland, according to the 1860 and 1870 census. The evidence that she was practicing medicine is that she paid the ten-dollar income tax levied on practicing physicians during the Civil War in both 1862–63 and 1865. She is also listed in the *Progressive Annual* for 1863 and 1864 as a practicing physician in Ottawa. According to the Shotwell genealogy, Phebe died, unmarried, in Illinois, at a date not yet found. The genealogy described her as a hydropathic physician who studied with Dr. Russell Trall.

References: *Progressive Annual,* 1863, 1864; Ambrose M. Shotwell, *Annals of Our Colonial Ancestors* (Lansing, MI: R. Smith & Co., 1895); US census, 1850, 1860, 1870; US Internal Revenue Service tax rolls, September 1862–November 1863, and 1865.

Salome Amy *SLOUT* Peterman (1822–91)

Salome Slout was born in February 1822, in Kingwood, Hunterdon County, New Jersey, the second of two children of Philip and Helena Slout. The Schlauts (as they were earlier) were among the original members of the German Reformed Church in Alexandria Township in Hunterdon County. Salome had an older brother (b. 1818), William, who had moved to East Bloomfield, New York, by 1850, and farther west to Marshall, Michigan, by 1860. Of Salome's childhood and early education no information has been found.

In the middle 1850s, Salome enrolled in Cincinnati's Eclectic College of Medicine. While there, she met and married fellow student Hiram Abiff Peterman, whose first wife, Lucinda Chapman, had just died (August 18, 1856), leaving Hiram with two small children. The new couple would have no children, and Hiram's children went to live with Lucinda's parents.

Hiram was already a doctor, having studied with Dr. Cyrus Thomson (son of Samuel Thomson, founder of the botanic medicine movement) in Geddes, near Syracuse, New York. He graduated from the Eclectic medical school at Syracuse, practiced medicine in Onondaga County and, later, in Weedsport, New York, just to the west in Cayuga County. His business card, with a Weedsport address, appeared in the October and November 1854 issues of the *Syracuse Medical & Surgical Journal.*

After graduation from Eclectic College of Medicine in 1857, Salome and Hiram probably moved at once to Michigan. The 1863 and 1864 issues of the *Progressive Annual* list a woman physician, A. L. Peterman, practicing in Nile, a community in southwest Michigan. (Though the initials are not correct, such errors were then common.) The couple is known to have settled in Marshall, Michigan, at least by August 27, 1864, when Hiram enlisted in the Ninth Michigan Infantry, Company H. He served in the Tennessee theater and, at forty-two, was one of the oldest men in his unit.

Both Salome and Hiram became established practitioners in Marshall, Salome as a homoeopath, Hiram as a Regular. The 1869–70 Marshall business directory lists both Salome and Hiram in the "physicians & surgeons" category: Mrs. S. A. Peterman (Eclectic), office and residence on State Street; Hiram A. Peterman, proprietor and manufacturer of the "Michigan Ague Cure" medicine, office and residence on State Street. Hiram is also listed as an oculist and as a medicine manufacturer. In addition to the ague cure, Hiram also sold Peterman's Family Medicine and Peterman's Cough Elixir. There were probably others. An 1876 analysis of the ague cure reported that "each bottle contains five fluid ounces of a red, syrupy liquid, with much resinous sediment, a very bitter taste, and odor of cinchona. Contains an alcoholic extract of the bark, with chinoidin as the chief medicinal agent, and with a little sulphuric acid and syrup. Cost, complete, not over 25 cents per bottle; price at wholesale, 60 cents."

Tuberculosis was apparently a special interest of the two doctors. In the *Portrait and Biographical Album of Calhoun County* (1891) is written, "The Drs. Peterman do not claim to cure consumption in its last stages, but have determined the fact that in earlier stages it is curable, and had they done nothing else in medicine would be entitled to gratitude and respect. They have become well known in this part of the county and their reputation is rapidly extending."

Hiram was a Mason, a member of the Knights Templar, and both were Universalists and Prohibitionists. Salome died September 6, 1891, at the age of sixty-nine. Hiram married a third wife, Hannah M. Paye, the following year. Hiram died at home at eighty-four, with senile debility and a fractured hip on February 26, 1906. He and Salome are buried in Oakridge Cemetery in Marshall.

References: Butler, 1874, 1877; *Calhoun County Business Directory for 1869–70* (Battle Creek, MI: E. G. Rust, 1869); *History of Calhoun County, Michigan* (Philadelphia: L. H. Everts Co., 1877); *Plat Map of Marshall, Michigan* (n.p., 1873); *Portrait and Biographical Album of Calhoun County, Michigan* (Chicago: Chapman Bros., 1891), 409–10; *Syracuse Medical & Surgical Journal*, October–November 1854; US census, 1880.

C. L. SMALLEY

Mrs. C. L. Smalley was already practicing as a hydropathic and hygienic physician in Ohio after her first year (1854–55) at New York Hygeio-Therapeutic College (then called the New York Hydropathic & Physiological School). She was also referred to as MD even though the school was not yet chartered by the state and she had finished but one course at the school. The August 1855 issue of the *Water-Cure Journal* reported that she "is now at Garrettsville, Ohio. . . . She is thoroughly prepared to lecture as well as to practice, and is about to make her debut in professional life at Painesville, Ohio, where she and our cause has [*sic*] warm friends" (38). In the December 17, 1855, the *Painesville Telegraph* she advertised her professional services at her residence on High Street ("first door west of the steam mill") and informed the public that she gave special attention to diseases of women and children. In the April 1857 *Water-Cure Journal*, she is reported to be "a female physician" at the Jamestown Water-Cure in Western New York. The July issue of the journal relates that she had visited New York City, that she has had two years' experience as a hygienic physician, and that she might soon attend the winter term of the school (by then the New York Hygeio-Therapeutic College). In the meantime, she returned to her position at the Jamestown institution (*WCJ*, February 1858).

On April 13, 1858, Dr. Smalley received an MD degree from the recently chartered college and apparently stayed on in some capacity at Dr. Trall's hydropathic institution that was associated with the college. Things may not have gone well. The March 1859 issue of the *Water-Cure Journal* reports that Dr. Smalley had "quit" Dr. Trall's employment and was advertising for a job as medical department manager at a water-cure. In the June 30, 1859, issue of the *New York Daily Tribune*, Mrs. C. L. Smalley, MD, is said to be resident physician at Bergen Heights Water-Cure in New Jersey. This was said to be only a half hour from New York by ferry to Hoboken or Jersey City and thence by stage, which stopped at the door. About her subsequent career no information has been found.

References: *Painesville Telegraph* (OH), December 17, 1855; *Water-Cure Journal*, August 1855, April 1857, February 1858, March 1859; Harry B. Weiss, *The Great American Water-Cure Craze* (Trenton, NJ, 1967), 186.

Mary E. *SMITH* Wilder (b. ca. 1828–92)

Mary Smith was born, probably in Mayville, Chautauqua County, in Western New York, about 1828. No specific date or place has been identified. Her father, William Smith, had been born in Barre, Massachusetts, immigrated to Oneida County, New York, in 1808, and a few years later removed to Mayville, where he opened a law office. In 1821, he was appointed county surrogate by Governor DeWitt Clinton, a post he held until 1840. He and two others started the *Mayville Sentinel* in 1834. The maiden name of Mary's mother, Charlotte, is not known, though census records say that she was foreign born. Mary had a younger brother, William, who died at two and a half. No details of her early education are known. When she matriculated at medical school, she listed Buffalo as her home.

On June 2, 1852, Mary graduated from Syracuse Medical College with a medical degree. She started practice in Syracuse and is listed as a physician in both the Syracuse business directory and the Ormsby Syracuse directory for 1853. She boarded at 14 Greene Street, and an advertisement in the Ormsby directory said that she would "remain a season in this city" and that she gave special attention to midwifery and the like. By June of that year, however, the *Syracuse Standard* wrote of her as formerly of Syracuse, now a student at Female Medical College of Pennsylvania in Philadelphia, a school from which she graduated in 1855 with a second MD degree. She apparently returned to Syracuse and resumed practice, with an office at Going's Block, 32 Lemon.

On December 28 of that year, she married Alexander Wilder, MD, the eighth of ten children of a local farming family, who had himself graduated from Syracuse Medical College in 1850, been on the editorial staffs of two Syracuse newspapers, and was then working for the State Department of Public Instruction. The couple soon moved to New York City, in 1856 it is said, though it is not until 1863 (possibly 1862) that Wilder's name appears in New York directories, listed as a notary. From 1858 to 1871 he was an editor of the *New York Evening Post.* He was elected an alderman in 1872 but found the work distasteful, preferring a behind-the-scenes role in political life.

Meantime, the couple bought a substantial house at 222 West Thirty-Fourth Street. It seems unlikely that Mary practiced medicine after moving to New York. Her name is not found in city directories or medical directories, and evidence suggests that she was well off (either by inheritance or from her husband or both) and that she liked the social life. The marriage, which had been based probably on intellectual attraction, fell apart in the middle 1870s. Alexander was intent on his professional work. He moved to New Jersey and lived the rest of his life in the household of Dr. Anna Nivison (sister of Samantha Nivison [q.v.]). His accomplishments included nineteen years (1876–95) as secretary of the Eclectic Medical Society of the State of New York, during which time he edited the organization's *Transactions* (1870–72). He also served as its president. A prolific writer, among his twenty publications were "Plea for the Collegiate Education of Women" (1876), *A History of Medicine* (1902), and several volumes on philosophical and religious subjects.

The 1870 census shows the couple still living together, Alexander with $10,000 in personal property, Mary with $25,000 in real estate and $10,000 in personal property. City directories show Alexander living at 222 West 34th as late as 1873 (and perhaps later) but not in 1879. In his biographical tribute to Wilder, protégé Robert A. Gunn writes:

> There was one event of Dr. Wilder's life on which he was extremely sensitive, and of which he never spoke. During his most prosperous days, while connected with the *Evening Post,* he had accumulated a considerable sum of money. At this time he married a cousin, and bought a handsome home on West Thirty-Fourth Street, New York City. The union did not prove congenial, though his wife had great admiration for his intellect. He was a close student and constant worker, while she was fond of society and wanted constant excite-

ment. Other interests and pleasures soon occupied her and she became discontented and irritable. One day, while in a passion, she said to him, "I wish you would go away and never come back." "Do you mean it," he asked? "Yes," she replied, "I mean every word of it, and you know I do." "Very well," he replied, and left the house. He went to Albany that day, and on his return he wrote her a note, saying if she meant what she said at their last interview to please send his clothes, and he would send for his books in a few days. They never met again, but when he sent for his books he also sent her a transfer of the house and all it contained. [It would seem, from the 1870 census data, that Mary already had title to the house.]

It has not been possible to find any trace of Mary in New York. Probably, she spent the rest of her life in the house at 222 West Thirty-Fourth Street but did not practice medicine. She died of pneumonia at the home of her niece, Mary E. Colie, in Buffalo, on March 2, 1892. Her funeral was held at Trinity Chapel on Delaware Avenue, but the church records list her as a resident of New York, and she is buried in Cypress Hills Cemetery in Brooklyn. Neither notices of her death in Buffalo newspapers nor the Trinity Church register notes her as a physician. Recognition of her death published in the proceedings of the Alumnae Association of the Woman's Medical College of Pennsylvania does not shed light on her later years: "There passed away in Buffalo, N.Y., after a life of great usefulness, Dr. Mary C. Smith Wilder, one of the earlier graduates of the Woman's Medical College, and a woman of great brilliance of mind and wonderful character."

References: *Buffalo City Directory*, 1892; *Buffalo Daily Courier*, March 3, 1892, p. 6, col. 5, March 4, 1892, 6; Robert A. Gunn, "Alexander Wilder, M.D., F.A.S., His Life and Work," *American Medical Journal* 36 (1908): 451–83; New Jersey census for 1895; Obituary of A. Wilder, *New York Tribune*, September 20, 1908; *Ormsby's Syracuse City Directory*, 1853, 203; *Syracuse Business Directory & New York State Gazetteer*, 1853; *Trow's New York City Directory*, 1863–1884/85; US census, 1859, 1870, 1880, 1900; Woman's Medical College of Pennsylvania, *Report of Proceedings of the Eighteenth Annual Meeting of the Alumnae Association of the Woman's Medical College of Pennsylvania May 4 and 5, 1893* (Philadelphia, 1893); Andrew W. Young, *History of Chautauqua County, New York* (Buffalo: Matthews & Warren, 1875).

Rebecca Lippett *Brooks* SMITH (1837–1910)

Rebecca Brooks was born September 28, 1837, in Union Valley in Central New York's Cortland County, the daughter of Alfred Brooks and his wife, Nancy Greene. The Brookses had been married for fifteen years and Nancy was forty years old at the time, so Rebecca was probably one of the couple's youngest children if, in fact, they had more than one child.

Rebecca's obituary states that prior to her twenty-first birthday she married. Her husband was William R. Smith Jr., also a resident of Union Valley. Together, they entered the Eclectic Medical College of New York (actually, it was the New York Hygeio-Therapeutic College), and both received their medical degrees in March 1859. Later, in 1877, Rebecca attended the New York Free Medical College for Women (actually the New York Medical College and Hospital for Women) founded in 1863 by Dr. Clemence Lozier (q.v.).

Rebecca and William returned to Cortland County and established their practices in Freetown. Sometime thereafter, they moved to Troy, New York, where, in 1874, they both contracted typhoid fever, and William died. Rebecca moved to Utica, where she practiced medicine before moving to Syracuse in 1894, where she continued to practice. "Despite her advanced age [she was then seventy-three], she had practiced medicine actively," according to her obituary.

She died, unexpectedly, at her home at 223 West Fayette Street on Sunday evening, December 11, 1910. She had taken ill the Wednesday before with what she thought was "the grippe." She was confined to her bed "but believed that she was fully able to take care of herself. Early last evening her heart weakened and death came suddenly."

References: Obituary, *JAMA* 56 (1911): 133; Obituary, *Post-Standard* (Syracuse, NY), December 12, 1910, 7:2.

Sarah *SMIZER* (1826–1914)

Sarah Smizer was born in Ohio in August 1826. Nothing has been found about her parents, childhood, or early education. Sarah graduated with an MD degree from the Eclectic Medical Institute, Cincinnati, in 1854. At that time she was a resident of Ashland, Ohio, a community near Mansfield. She practiced medicine for many years in southwest Ohio, never married, and lived with her younger physician brother and, later, her nephew. She was still alive at the time of the 1910 census.

The only information found about Sarah comes from census data. In 1860, she was living with her younger brother, Dr. Wesley Smizer (MD, 1857, Eclectic Medical Institute), his wife Elizabeth, and their two small boys. The family lived in Sycamore, a township in Hamilton County (where Cincinnati is located). Both Sarah and her brother are denoted "physician" in the census.

In 1870, the situation is similar except that Sarah's occupation is now listed as "helps in house." But in the 1880 census, Sarah, still living in her brother's house, is again listed as a "physician." By 1900 the family has moved to Sharonville, another community in Hamilton County. Both Wesley and Sarah, now seventy-two and seventy-three, respectively, are listed as "physicians." Wesley's wife, Elizabeth, had died that year. The two sons, Charles and Stanley, are now twenty-one and nineteen and still at home. Though only Wesley is listed in Polk's 1886 medical directory and neither is listed in the 1890 edition, both Wesley and Sarah are found as physicians in the 1893 and 1896 editions. Only Wesley is listed in the 1898, 1900, and 1902 editions of Polk. Wesley died in 1903.

By 1910, then eighty-four, Sarah was still alive but no longer practicing medicine and appeared to be living with the widow of one of her nephews, Louise Smizer. Sarah died in 1914 at age eighty-eight and is buried in Spring Grove Cemetery, Cincinnati, with Wesley and Elizabeth. Though she seems to have practiced medicine for a substantial period, the amount and degree of that practice are not known.

References: Polk, 1886, 1890, 1893, 1896, 1898, 1900, 1902; US census, 1860, 1870, 1880, 1900, 1910.

Elizabeth *Phillips* SOMERBY Bartlett (d. 1890)

No information has been found about the date or place of Elizabeth's birth or family. The 1850 Massachusetts census lists Elizabeth Phillips as living in Suffolk County, Massachusetts, where Boston and Chelsea are located. In 1861, now married to a "fancy painter" with whom she had a daughter, Elizabeth Somerby of Chelsea, Massachusetts, graduated from New England Female Medical College. She had been a Massachusetts state scholar from that town.

The 1867 *Massachusetts Register* and the 1868 Chelsea city directory list her as a practicing physician. Mr. Somerby died in 1871. By 1878, Dr. Somerby had married the Rev. William S. Bartlett (1809–83). In seven Chelsea directories published between 1868 and 1890, Elizabeth Bartlett is listed as a physician in Chelsea, Massachusetts, living first at 111 Broadway, and from the late 1870s at 154 Park Street. As was so common at the period, her office was in her house. Dr. Bartlett died August 1, 1890, having outlived two husbands, and practiced medicine in Chelsea for twenty-nine years.

References: *The Chelsea Directory*, 1868, 1870, 1872; *The Chelsea and Revere Directory*, 1876, 1878, 1880; *Chelsea, Revere and Winthrop Directory*, 1890; US census, 1850.

Rachel T. *SPEAKMAN* (b. ca. 1828–1915)

Rachel Speakman was born about 1828 in Chester, Pennsylvania, to Thomas Speakman and Dinah Pierce. No information has been found about her family, childhood, or early education except that she had a sister. At eighteen, she left home.

When Henry Foster opened his water-cure at Clifton Springs in Western New York in 1856, Rachel, then twenty-eight, was one of two women among the six physicians on the staff. She did not yet have a medical degree but would soon attend the Female Medical College of Pennsylvania and graduate in 1861, a doctor of medicine. The title of her dissertation was "A Disquisition on Physiology." Another source, not verified, says she had an 1863 MD degree from Cleveland Homoeopathic College. She may have remained at or returned to Clifton Springs, because she is listed as becoming a member of the Ontario County Medical Association on February 28, 1863.

Three issues of the *Progressive Annual* (often inaccurate) list her as a practicing physician at 126 Second Avenue, New York, in 1862, 1863, and 1864. In the middle 1870s she must have been a physician in Battle Creek, Michigan (perhaps at the Western Health Reform Institute, which had been established there in 1866 by Seventh Day Adventists and which came under the leadership of James Harvey Kellogg in 1876). While in Battle Creek, Rachel was preceptor of a medical student: Sarah Jane Allen of Charlotte, Michigan, a graduate of Holyoke Seminary in Kalamazoo, who "studied medicine under Rachel T. Speakman of Battle Creek" (King).

In 1884, Rachel became resident physician and professor of hygiene and physiology at Wellesley College in Massachusetts, a post she held for ten years until her retirement. An 1888 issue of the *Wellesley Courant* announced one of her lectures: "Dr. Speakman spoke to the freshman class about restoring the nervous system in a practical way."

While at Wellesley she became interested in Christian Science, united with the Mother Church in 1894, studied in the class of 1898 with Mrs. Eddy, and in 1900 completed a course in obstetrics given by her nephew, Dr. Alfred E. Baker, becoming thereafter C.S.B. (Bachelor of Christian Science?). She apparently returned to Wellesley as resident physician in 1903. In later years, she lived in her house in Brookline, Massachusetts, with her sister, Hannah Baker.

Dr. Speakman suffered increasingly from valvular heart disease during the last two years of her life, which she treated with Christian Science methods. She died March 30, 1915, at eighty-seven and was cremated. One of her obituaries records that she was identified with women's educational movements at Female Medical College of

Pennsylvania and Wellesley. At Wellesley "she played a revolutionary part in introducing new methods in teaching hygiene" (*North American*).

References: Lewis C. Aldrich, *History of Ontario County, New York* (Syracuse, NY: D. Mason & Co., 1893); Obituary, *JAMA* 64 (1915): 1343; Laura B. White Baker, letter dated April 2, 1915, Auburndale, MA, to Mary Caswell, Wellesley College Archives; Obituary, *Evening Transcript* (Boston), April 1, 1915; Clifton Springs Water Cure, *Report of the Address and Sermon at the Dedication of the Clifton Springs Water-Cure Held July 25, 1856* (Rochester, NY: Daily Democrat, 1856); William H. King, *History of Homoeopathy and Its Institutions in America* (New York: Lewis Publishing Co., 1905); Massachusetts Death Register, Brookline, 1915, 8:104; Obituary, *North American* (Philadelphia), April 21, 1915; *Progressive Annual,* 1862–64; Lucia C. Warren, letter dated March 18, 1922, Boston, to Mary Caswell, Wellesley College Archives; *Wellesley Courant* 1888, no. 5, 1.

Annie M. *STAMBACH* Galvin (1838–72)

Annie Stambach was born July 10, 1838. She came from a Quaker background, but the names of her parents and information about her childhood and education have not been found. From early in life she showed interest in the subject of women's education and resented the fact that colleges did not accept women as students. She also became identified with the antislavery movement.

At the age of sixteen she entered Penn Medical University in Philadelphia, where she studied for almost three years and earned an MD degree with honor in 1857. Thence to New York City, where she studied for three months with Dr. Carroll Dunham, a prominent homoeopath. Presumably, though it is not documented, she practiced medicine thereafter.

On June 29, 1865, then twenty-seven, she married Edward Ilsley Galvin, a Unitarian minister in Brookfield, Massachusetts. After her marriage she did not practice formally but "was often consulted by those who wished to avail themselves of her knowledge, and had not a few patients, especially among the poor." From Brookfield, the Reverend Mr. Galvin moved to a parish in Peabody, and it was in that town that Annie became much involved in the newly organized Essex County Woman Suffrage Association, an involvement that led to her presidency of that organization.

Dr. Galvin developed tuberculosis, went with her father to St. Augustine, Florida, and in the summer of 1870, to Nassau with her husband. She did not improve, returned to her father's home, and steadily worsened. A final trip for her health was made to Aiken, South Carolina, where she died, April 14, 1872, at the age of thirty-three. The Galvins had one son, Carroll D., named after Dr. Dunham, Annie's preceptor.

Dr. Galvin practiced medicine for only a brief time, and that informally. Her greater contribution may have been as a reformer. The Proceedings of the Pennsylvania Yearly Meeting of Progressive Friends record her considerable involvement in that organization's activities from 1860 until her death twelve years later. The group met each June in Longwood, Pennsylvania. Annie was one of twenty-one signatories at the founding. She served for several years on the committee to revise and edit the annual minutes, was one of two clerks for two years, and after marrying and moving to Massachusetts, wrote letters describing how much she missed daily involvement with the organization. She did, apparently, attend each annual meeting. The organization attracted prominent reformers such as Lucretia Mott to its ranks. Its members wrote letters to politicians, including President Lincoln, about the many issues in which they were interested: equal rights, temperance, prison reform, woman suffrage, the Indian question, religion in common schools (they were against it), tobacco, public and private charity, rights of children, peace, kindness to animals, and the labor question. The names of three other early woman doctors of medicine appear in these minutes: Maria J. Dennett, MD (q.v.), Sarah A. Entriken, MD (who served on a committee to raise funds for educating freed blacks; q.v.), and Mary E. Breed, MD (q.v.).

References: Obituary, *Proceedings of the Pennsylvania Yearly Meeting of Progressive Friends*, 1860–72 (New York: Baker and Godwin, 1872), 12.

Juliet Hall *Worth* STILLMAN Severance (1833–1919)

Juliet Worth was born July 1, 1833, in DeRuyter, a village near Cazenovia in Central New York State. She was the second of six children of Walter Folger Worth and his second wife, Catherine Stillman. Juliet's father was a Quaker, a native of Nantucket, and a cousin of Lucretia Mott. By his first wife he had fathered eleven children (1811–28). Her mother lived to be ninety-three, with faculties intact. Juliet's older brother died two months before she was born, but there would have been at least four or five half siblings under fourteen living in the home.

At thirteen, Juliet started school in DeRuyter, attending the local seminary in the winter and, from the age of fourteen, teaching school in the summer. Apparently in delicate health as a child, it is said that she studied "hygienic methods of treatment," grew stronger, and, in her twenties, studied medicine with a local physician for three years. On September 18, 1852, then nineteen years old, she married John Dwight Stillman, six years her senior and a native of Chenango, New York, who would, himself, become a physician. They had three children, a girl and two boys. Two of them became actors and the third, a musician.

By 1855, the family had moved to DeWitt, Clinton County, Iowa, as part of a group of Seventh-Day Baptists. There Juliet established herself as a hydropathist (*WCJ*). Soon, she attended lectures at the New York Hygeio-Therapeutic College and received an MD degree in 1858. Following graduation from medical school, Juliet returned to DeWitt, where she established her practice.

In 1862, John left Juliet, attended Chicago's Rush Medical College, from which he received an MD degree in 1865, remarried (1869), and moved to St. Louis. Juliet moved to Whitewater, Wisconsin, in 1862, and, after divorcing Stillman, met and married Anson B. Severance. Juliet would spend the rest of her life in the Midwest practicing medicine and working for social reform. She became very interested in Spiritualism. Relatively little is known about her practice. She favored hygienic methods and vegetarianism, and employed psychic modalities, though the extent to which her interest in Spiritualism influenced her professional work is not clear. She is said to have always willingly provided care for those who were unable to pay her.

From the time she started teaching school at fourteen, she was an active worker for the rights of women and a supporter of the antislavery and temperance movements. After starting practice, she became a freethinker and a devotee of Spiritualism. Whitewater was a national center of the Spiritualist movement and of mystic experimentation. Here, "her views on religion, health and politics found a receptive audience, and soon she had a flourishing medical practice" (*Wisconsin State Journal*, August 20, 2008).

After the Civil War she and her husband moved to Milwaukee, where Juliet practiced medicine and Anson ran a dancing school. Louis Frank, in his *Medical History of Milwaukee*, says that she practiced medicine there from 1872 until 1891. She also became involved in the nascent labor movement—serving as an officer in the Knights of Labor and a delegate to several national conventions of the Union Labor Party. At one of these conventions, she proposed a plank for women's suffrage in the party's platform. Active in many other organizations, she was president several times of the State Associations of Spiritualism in Illinois, Wisconsin, and Minnesota. In 1880, she was elected a vice president of the Liberal League, a national organization of free-thinkers. At the sixth national convention, held in St. Louis in 1882, in the absence of the president and first vice president, she assumed the chair. Needless to say, she had ceased to be a practicing Baptist. Of all of her activities, it was her work for the emancipation of women that was her major accomplishment and the work at which she remained active until the end of her life.

In an 1869 article published in *Universe*, a progressive Chicago newspaper, she expressed the following views on marriage:

> Marriage should be a soul-union, not a curse . . . not a merging of one life into another, but . . . two individuals uniting their lives for mutual good and for the good of humanity—it may be in reproduction, or it may be in giving birth to higher, nobler ideas, and outworking them in noble deeds and grand achievements. . . . There is not a child in a hundred that is begotten with the consent of the mother. As the present marriage system makes the man the owner of woman—her legal master—she is expected to submit to his gratification . . . When the marriage system is what it should be, and woman controls in these matters, instead of man. . . . Restellism [the reference is to Madame Restell, a well-known New York abortionist of the time] shall cease, because there will be no demand for it.

Years later, in 1886, Dr. Severance addressed a different aspect of woman's life. In an article in the *Wisconsin Agricultural Society Journal*, she expressed the view that the farm wife was just as important to the success of the farm as the farmer himself and hence should have equal access to the money and to opportunities for education. Women, she wrote, should be taught proper methods of raising children, and they should be educated for "enlightened motherhood." This would lead to "salvation from evils that fill our penitentiaries, our asylums, our dram-shops and brothels." Juliet lived to be eighty-six. In 1891, she left her husband and moved to Chicago "to live among anarchists, free thinkers, and sex radicals," and, in her final years after retirement, she lived with her actress daughter Lillian at 27 West Forty-Sixth Street in New York. She died in September 1919, probably on the 3rd of the month.

Bibliography: "Hints on Dress," *Banner of Light*, January 23, 1865.

References: Ann Braude, *Radical Spirits: Women's Rights and Spiritualism in Nineteenth-Century America* (Bloomington: Indiana University Press, 2001); Louis Frederick Frank, *The Medical History of Milwaukee 1834–1914* (Milwaukee: Germania Publishing Co., 1915); Amanda Frisken, *Victoria Woodhull's Sexual Revolution* (Philadelphia: University of Pennsylvania Press, 2004), 168n45, 47; Obituary, *New York Times,* September 4, 1919, 13; Francis D. Stillman Jr., *The Stillman Family: Descendants of Mr. George Stillman of Wethersfield, Connecticut and Dr. George Stillman, of Westerly, Rhode Island* (Greenburg, PA: Author, 1989); *The Universe* (Chicago), August 28, 1869; *Water-Cure Journal,* August 1855, 92; Frances E. Willard, *A Woman of the Century* (Buffalo: C. W. Moulton, 1893); Wisconsin Agricultural Society, *Transactions,* 1886, vol. 24; "Odd Wisconsin Archive: Juliet Severance, Radical Victorian," Wisconsin Historical Society, *Wisconsin State Journal,* March 21, 2006; "Odd Wisconsin: Activist Gave Working Women Free Medical Care," Wisconsin Historical Society, *Wisconsin State Journal,* August 20, 2008; Wisconsin Historical Society, *Dictionary of Wisconsin History,* "Juliet Severance, Radical Victorian: A Good Mother, a Good Friend, and a Good Woman," http://www.wisconsinhistory.org/Content.aspx?dsNav=Ny: True,Ro:0,N:4294963828-4294963805&dsNavOnly=N:1099&dsRecor dDetails=R:CS259&dsDimensionSearch=D:Juliet+Severance,Dxm:All, Dxp:3&dsCompoundDimensionSearch=D:Juliet+Severance,Dxm:All, Dxp:3 (accessed June 1, 2016).

Eliza Leavitt *Ingersoll* STONE (1832–1913)

Eliza Ingersoll was born in Greenfield, Massachusetts, August 7, 1832, daughter of C. J. J. Ingersoll and Eliza Hubbard Leavitt. When she was twenty-three, she married Dr. Joshua Stone, then of St. Johnsbury, Vermont, though born in Greenfield. The couple settled in Greenfield, where Joshua "soon established a good practice for the new school of medicine" (Thompson). Joshua died September 1, 1859, at the age of thirty-five. Eliza enrolled forthwith at the New England Female Medical College in Boston and, in 1861, received her own medical degree.

It appears that she practiced medicine in Greenfield thereafter. This assumption is based on three pieces of evidence: The 1868 and 1875 editions of the *New England Business Directory* list her as a practicing physician in Greenfield, as does Pettet's 1877–78 *Homoeopathic Directory of North America.* The Greenfield directories for 1885 and 1887 list her as a homoeopath. The Greenfield directories for 1880, 1892, and 1897 do not list her at all. She is not listed in Cleave's Homoeopathic directory, the Butler medical directories for 1874 and 1877, the 1886 Polk directory, or the American Institute of Homoeopathy registry, 1893.

Eliza, then eighty-one, a widow, and living in the Brattleboro (Vermont) Home for the Aged, died December 2, 1913, of chronic interstitial nephritis and a stroke. She is buried in the Federal Street Cemetery in Greenfield, Massachusetts, where she had practiced medicine from 1861 to 1885.

References: *Greenfield City Directory*, 1885, 1887; Massachusetts Vital Records; J. Pettet, *The North American Homoeopathic Directory for 1877–78* (Cleveland: Robison, Savage & Co., 1878); *New England Business Directory*, 1868, 1875; Francis M. Thompson, *History of Greenfield Shire Town of Franklin County Massachusetts* (Greenfield, MA: T. Morey & Son, 1904), 773.

T

Elizabeth *TAYLOR* (b. 1827)

Elizabeth Taylor was born in 1827, probably in Pitcher, Chenango County, in Central New York State, to George Taylor, a farmer, and his wife, Anna Ensign. Elizabeth was the eldest of five children, one girl and four boys. George Taylor's father and mother had come from Connecticut in 1803. Nothing is known of Elizabeth's childhood and early education.

As a student at New England Female Medical College in Boston during 1856–57 and 1858–59, Elizabeth was supported by a Wade scholarship, a scholarship given to those who were not residents of Massachusetts and, hence, not eligible for a state scholarship. She graduated in 1859 and returned to Pitcher. The 1860 census lists her as practicing there as an "allopathic physician." Her name is also listed as a practicing physician in the *Progressive Annuals* for 1862, 1863, and 1864. Elizabeth's name is not found in the 1870 or 1880 census. Nor is it in the 1874 or 1877 Butler medical directory or the 1886 Polk medical directory. Whether this is because she married or died is an unresolved question.

References: US census, 1850, 1860, 1870, 1880; *Progressive Annual*, 1862, 1863, and 1864.

Eliza L. *Smyth* THOMAS (1830–64)

Eliza Thomas, who became the first woman doctor in Stark County, Ohio, was born in Willoughby, Ohio, on November 26, 1830. We have no information about her parents, siblings, or early schooling. In 1852, she became the second of G. Kersey Thomas's three wives. Thomas was born in York County, Pennsylvania in 1818 of Quaker parents, came to Salem, Ohio, as a young man, and started the study of medicine with Dr. Benjamin Stanton when he was eighteen. He married Rebecca Shaw when he was twenty-two, settled in Marlborough, Ohio, where he started practice, and had a daughter, Josephine Elizabeth Thomas, in 1843. Rebecca died in 1849.

Kersey Thomas was thirty-four when he married Eliza, then twenty-two and a teacher in Marlborough Union School. After she was married, Eliza started the study of medicine with her husband as preceptor. In the middle 1850s, they both went to Philadelphia for formal training at a medical college. Kersey is said to have graduated in 1857, but his name does not appear as a graduate of any Philadelphia school, including those now extinct. Eliza received an MD degree from Female Medical College of Pennsylvania in 1855. The couple had a son, George M., and a daughter, Ona Marie, born during these years.

The family returned to Ohio and settled in Alliance, where they both practiced medicine. Kersey emphasized surgery; Eliza did obstetrical work primarily. It was the opinion of the editor of the *Stark County History* that "her practice would compare favorably with the general run of male practitioners." They must have been moderately successful: the 1860 census lists their household as having real estate worth $1,500 and personal property worth $1,500. In 1862, Kersey was appointed surgeon of the 104th Ohio Volunteer Infantry, but in December of that same year he came home on a gurney, prostrated with paralysis, and resigned his commission.

Eliza died at the age of thirty-three on January 1, 1864, of pyaemia resulting from an abrasion on her hand incurred while delivering a stillborn fetus. Kersey apparently recovered from his paralysis. In 1868, he married Mrs. Rosanna Milner but died soon thereafter. At the time of his death, he was serving as surgeon for both of the railroads that passed through Alliance. In his will, he left his body to a friend who was professor at Charity Hospital Medical College in Cleveland "for the purpose of public dissection."

References: Ohio Genealogical Society, Stark County Chapter, *Cemetery Inscriptions, Stark County, Ohio* (n.p., 1982), vol. 1; William H. Perrin, *History of Stark County* (Chicago: Baskin & Battey, 1881), 278, 282; Kersey G. Thomas, Will, 1866; US census, 1860.

Lovina Dolly *Bacon* THOMAS (1820–94)

Lovina Bacon was born in 1820 or 1821 in New York State, probably in Watertown, the daughter of Deacon Isaac Bacon and Eleanor Schull.

Nothing has been found regarding her childhood or early education. On August 30, 1842, then living in Watertown, New York, Lovina married Avery Thomas, a native of the Watertown area. Avery had considered becoming a minister, but poor health redirected him to the drug, paint, and oil business, and he "carried on a general painting business in Watertown." The couple had five children: Isaiah, Eleanor, Frank, Marie, and Hattie. Isaiah enlisted in the army during the Civil War while still a minor and caught "camp fever" (probably typhus). His mother, according to Thomas genealogy, "procured passes through the lines and succeeded in getting him home, where he died July 9, 1863, aged nineteen." Daughter Eleanor married Judge James Linden and had four children, the only grandchildren Lovina would have. Frank graduated from Hahnemann Medical College in Philadelphia in March 1871 and, after residency at Albany Homoeopathic Hospital, practiced in Dayton, Ohio, where he, unmarried, lived with his two younger maiden sisters.

In 1857, her children then aged fourteen to five, Lovina graduated with an MD degree from Penn Medical University in Philadelphia. Though she was the only woman in her family, at least at that time, to become a physician, her husband had a brother, a cousin, and a cousin-in-law who were doctors, and there were four more doctors in the next family generation, including Lovina's son, Frank William. Amos Russell Thomas, MD, who married Lovina's sister, Elizabeth, had graduated from the Eclectic school in Syracuse in 1854, where he would have been a classmate of Minerva Jane Averell (q.v.) and Dolly Ann Porter (q.v.). He was professor of anatomy at PMU from 1856 to 1866, when Lovina was a student there. He later became professor of anatomy at Hahnemann Medical College in Philadelphia (1867–94) and was dean of the school from 1874 to 1894. All of these things may have influenced Lovina in deciding to become a physician.

After graduating, Lovina went into practice in Watertown. She is listed in the 1859–60 *Watertown Directory* as a practicing physician. She also advertised in the *New York Reformer* (Watertown) from July 30, 1857, almost weekly, until September 8, 1859: "Mrs. L. D. Thomas, M.D. Practicing physician for the treatment of women and children. Calls from town or country, adjacent villages promptly attended to. Office and residence—49 State Street corner of High Street, Watertown."

In September 1859, the family moved to Dayton, Ohio, where husband Avery continued in the paint and painting business, and Lovina in practicing medicine. She is listed as a physician in Dayton directories for 1860–61, 1862–63, and 1864–65.

The family moved again in 1866, to Hammonton, New Jersey, a community about thirty-five miles southeast of Philadelphia, where Avery had purchased a fruit farm. It is reported that his health improved while there, but he returned to Dayton after a year, to take charge of one of the largest varnish manufactories in the United States, a position he held at least until 1891. (The 1870 census of Dayton shows Avery living alone in a boarding house.) He died March 31, 1897. Lovina, presumably with the children, stayed in Hammonton. The girls at the time of the census were fifteen, eighteen, and twenty-one, all unmarried, and Frank, twenty-one, was about to matriculate at Hahnemann Medical College in Philadelphia, where his uncle was professor of anatomy.

Sometime in the 1870s, Lovina probably moved back to Dayton, but she is never thereafter listed as a physician. Son Frank, now a doctor, returned to Dayton in 1872, where he practiced until his untimely accidental death by explosion in 1891. (He was making a house call on a patient who was cleaning a carpet with gasoline, which was ignited by a fire in the adjacent room.) Lovina died September 1, 1894, in Devon, Pennsylvania, probably while visiting her sister and brother-in-law, Amos, who lived there. She is buried with her husband in Dayton's Woodland Cemetery.

References: *New York Reformer* (Watertown), July 30, 1857–September 8, 1859; *Dayton (OH) City Directories*, 1860–61, 1862–63, 1864–65; Death notice, *Dayton (OH) Journal*, September 5, 1894, 1; A. R. Thomas, *Genealogical Records and Sketches of the Descendants of William Thomas of Hardwick, Mass.* (Philadelphia and London, 1891); US census, 1850 (Watertown), 1860, 1870, 1880 (Dayton); *Watertown (NY) Directory*, 1859–60.

Mary Frame *Myers* THOMAS (1816–88)

Born December 28, 1816, at the home of her maternal grandparents in Bucks County, Pennsylvania, Mary Myers was the younger daughter of schoolteacher Samuel Myers and his wife Mary Frame. Both parents were Friends and were descended from early settlers of southeast Pennsylvania. Mary's mother died when she was an infant. Her father married again, in 1818, and five more daughters and two sons were born. Two of the daughters, Hannah E. Myers Longshore (q.v.) and Jane Viola Myers (q.v.), became physicians.

The family lived in Silver Spring, a Quaker community in Maryland, and later moved to Washington, where Mary's father was active in abolitionist activities. In 1833, they moved to a farm near New Lisbon,

Ohio, another Quaker community. Mary's early education was a combination of homeschooling and attendance at district public schools.

At twenty-three, she married Owen Thomas, moved to Salem, Ohio, and during the next nine years, bore three daughters. The family moved to near Fort Wayne, Indiana, where Mrs. Thomas began the study of medicine with her husband, who had already studied medicine with a physician preceptor and started practice. It required "the most vigorous discipline of my mind and systematic arrangement of time [so that children and husband would not] suffer for any comforts a wife and mother owed them" (*Woman's Journal*, 1888). "In September 1853, having by steady sewing provided her family with clothes for six months in advance and having arranged for her children's care" (all three under thirteen), she enrolled at Penn Medical University in Philadelphia, where her younger half sister, Hannah, was demonstrator in anatomy. Soon called home by the sickness, and ultimate death, of her eldest child, she attended medical lectures at Western Reserve, where her husband was a student, during the winter of 1853–54. She resumed her studies at Penn Medical University in the spring of 1856 and graduated in July. Later that year the family moved to Richmond, Indiana, where Mary and her husband would practice medicine henceforth. During the Civil War, Mary worked for the Sanitary Commission and, "by direction of Gov. Oliver P. Morton, carried supplies to the front by steamer; on the return trip she nursed soldiers wounded in the battle of Vicksburg. She later served as an assistant physician with her husband, an army contract surgeon, in a hospital for refugees in Nashville, Tenn" (Phillips). After the war Mary practiced medicine for the next twenty years until her death. She is listed in the Butler directories for 1874 and 1877 and the Polk directory for 1886. Her husband became a dentist.

In addition to her practice, Mary was active in public health affairs, professional affairs, and in various social reform movements. She was city physician, working especially among the black citizens. She served for eight years on the local board of health and even longer on the board of the Home for Friendless Girls, a group she helped to organize. After being rejected twice, she was elected to membership in the Wayne County Medical Society in 1875, became its president in 1887, and in 1876 was the first woman to be regularly admitted to the Indiana State Medical Society. In 1877, she represented both societies at the national American Medical Association convention. A Methodist, she was an ardent supporter of the temperance movement. She was very active in support of woman's suffrage and in 1859 petitioned the Indiana General Assembly to amend the state constitution so that women had property rights and the vote. She spoke frequently at national suffrage conventions and in 1880 was president of the American Woman Suffrage Association.

Mary Myers Thomas died of dysentery in Richmond on August 19, 1888, after a period of poor health—a "faithful worker in everything that aimed to better the human race" (Medical Society obituary). Her funeral was held in the Methodist Church, and, as she had asked, her six pall bearers were members of the Good Templars, the Woman's Christian Temperance Union, and the African Methodist Episcopal Church. She was buried in Maple Hill Cemetery in Hartford, Michigan, where her older daughter lived. Her younger daughter, a graduate of Cornell and professor of Greek, became the fourth president of Wellesley College.

Bibliography: "The Influence of the Medical Colleges of the Regular School, of Indianapolis, on the Medical Education of Women of the State," *Transactions of the Indiana State Medical Society*, 1883, 228–38.

References: Florence M. Adkinson, "The Mother of Women," *Woman's Journal*, September 29, 1888, 307–8; Obituary, *JAMA* 11 (1888): 538–39; Obituary, *Transactions of the Indiana State Medical Society*, 1889, 210; *Notable American Women 1607–1950*, 3:450–51.

Martha Nichols *Spalding* THURSTON (b. 1801)

Martha Spalding was born September 24, 1801, in Compton, Quebec, the second of eight children (five girls, three boys) and eldest daughter of Joseph Spalding and his wife, Mary Elkins. Both parents were natives of New Hampshire. The eldest child, a boy, and youngest, a girl, were born in Pomfret, Connecticut, the others in Compton. The family seems to have been a mobile one. The father died in Dubuque, Iowa; one daughter in Salem, Iowa; another in India; some grandchildren were born in Wisconsin. Martha would move to San Francisco.

Nothing is known of Martha's early education. She had become a Freewill Baptist speaker, and, in 1830, at the age of twenty-nine, she married Nathaniel Thurston, a man five years her junior and the seventh of twelve children of Oliver Thurston, a farmer in Freedom, New Hampshire, and his wife, Austress Cross. Nathaniel studied medicine until "fitted to practice" but then had a call to preach as a Free Baptist minister in Dover, New Hampshire, and later in Lowell, Massachusetts. In Lowell, in 1834, he founded the Free Baptist Church and erected a $20,000 church building for which his congregation was unable to pay and had to vacate. Nathaniel was indicted and convicted of "cheating," but the superior court set aside the verdict, saying that Thurston was an honest man but naïve in matters of business.

Martha enrolled at New England Female Medical College in Boston and graduated with an MD degree in 1854. The couple moved to San Francisco, where they practiced medicine and where they remained the rest of their lives. Martha is listed in the *Progressive Annual* for 1862, 1863, and 1864 as a physician practicing in San Francisco, but not in the Butler or Polk directories (1874–1900).

That she was an active practitioner in the 1850s is documented. The *Daily Alta California* for January 1, 1855, carried the following ad: "Dr. N. H. Thurston and Martha N. Thurston, M.D., Physicians to Women and Children, Office at Hillman's Temperance House, Davis St., (2 rooms)." In the February 1855 *California Farmer and Journal of Useful Sciences* was the following: "Dr. Thurston, Office, Room No. 20, Hillman's Temperance House, No. 80 Davis Street, San Francisco Cal., Mrs. T., Physician for Women and Children."

In December 1856, Dr. Thurston had a thirty-five-year-old patient, a recently married schoolteacher, Mrs. Mary Hodges, who had stenosis of the vagina and an unconsummated marriage. She referred her to the prominent San Francisco surgeon, Dr. Elias S. Cooper, a man in whom she had great professional confidence. Dr. Cooper, with Dr. Thurston as assistant, corrected the problem—a vaginal opening "the size of a quill." But he found other vaginal abnormalities such as a general thickening or fibrosis of the vaginal walls and advised the patient not to get pregnant. However, she did. Dr. Cooper tried to avoid further involvement in the case, but Mrs. Hodges would not let him go, and the reluctant Dr. Cooper performed a caesarean section on November 11, 1857, using chloroform anesthesia. It was known, prior to the operation, that the fetus (which weighed 11.5 pounds) was dead, but it was thought that there was a twin—Dr. Cooper's assistant claimed to have heard a second fetal heartbeat—and this was the reason for taking the risk of what was the first caesarean section done on the West Coast in which the mother survived. It turned out that the second "fetus" was a full bladder, about which the assistant, when questioned, had falsely assured Dr. Cooper he had successfully catheterized moments before. The patient survived, had a long convalescence, and sued Dr. Cooper for malpractice. The details of the affair may be found in *Transactions of the Medical Society of the State of California.*

The Thurstons can be traced through the 1860s. In the 1861 San Francisco directory, Nathaniel is listed as a physician and Martha as a "female physician." The next year Martha is listed as a midwife and physician, and in 1865 simply as "physician." Nathaniel may have retired; his occupational entry for that year says "vegetable garden."

However, the following year, 1866, when Nathaniel registered to vote, he was again denoted a physician. Nathaniel died in 1866 at sixty. Martha is described as a widow in the 1868 directory. The year 1871 is the last Martha's name is found in San Francisco directories, so she probably died in the early 1870s.

References: *California Farmer and Journal of Useful Sciences,* various issues, February–March 1855; *Daily Alta California,* January 1, 1855, p. 1, col. 3; *Transactions of the Medical Society of the State of California* (Sacramento, CA, February 11–13, 1857); San Francisco voter registry, 1866; San Francisco city directory, 1861, 1862, 1864, 1865, 1868, 1869, 1873; *San Francisco Evening Bulletin,* September 22, 1866 [Nathaniel's death]; Samuel J. Spalding, *A Genealogical History of Edward Spalding, of Massachusetts Bay, and His Descendants* (Boston, 1872), 175; Brown Thurston, *Thurston Genealogies,* 2nd ed. (Portland, ME, 1892), 124; US census, 1860.

U

Catherine Josephine *UNDERWOOD* Jewell (1834–73)

Catherine Underwood was born June 11, 1834, in Williamson, Wayne County, New York, the third of eight children of Daniel Underwood and his wife Chloe Durfee. The Underwoods were liberal Quakers. Daniel, a tanner, was characterized as an "easygoing, happy dispositioned, fun-loving man" without much ambition. His wife, Chloe, was "industry personified." In 1849, after the birth (and death) of their last child, the family moved to nearby Clyde, and in 1851, to Palmyra, both larger villages in Wayne County. In 1854, the family left New York State and moved to Morris, Illinois, and in 1868, on to Lake City, Minnesota, where they settled permanently.

In 1859, Catherine graduated from the Female Medical College of Pennsylvania. Somewhat puzzling is the fact that she was listed as a resident of New York State when she graduated, though her family was then living in Illinois. She had very thorough training, having spent four years at the medical school and had an additional year of postgraduate experience at the New York Infirmary for Women with the Blackwell sisters. At medical school she is reputed to have been "a dear friend and almost constant companion of Dr. Ann Preston" (q.v.; Hanaford).

Catherine proceeded to set up practice in Bloomington, Illinois, after graduation. While living in Bloomington she married Dr. Phineas

Anson Jewell, a medical graduate of the University of Michigan. Like Catherine, Phineas was a native of Western New York, having been born in Steuben County. Moving to Ann Arbor, where her husband then had his medical practice, she established a practice of her own.

In 1867, it became apparent that Catherine had developed tuberculosis, and the couple (they had no children) moved to Lake City, Minnesota, hoping for better health. Here, Catherine, Phineas, and Catherine's younger brother, Joseph Merritt Underwood, established the Jewell Nursery, a business that continued for more than a century. Whether Catherine continued to practice medicine in Lake City is not known. One would suspect not, considering her poor health. However, she is listed in the Lake City directory for 1873 as a practicing physician. (There is an "E. Jewell," not otherwise identified, in Lake City, Minnesota, in the 1874 and 1877 editions of Butler's medical directories.)

Catherine was described as "a handsome woman with dark eyes and hair." She was also known for her unselfishness. She died March 30, 1873, in Illinois, where she had gone for the winter in hopes of regaining her health. Said her obituary, "It is with profound sorrow that we learn of the death of this truly noble, estimable and gifted woman. . . . [She had a] life of usefulness . . . well known to every member of this community." The obituary also mentions the mental energy and cheerful hope so characteristic of her nature.

References: Butler, 1874, 1877; Phebe H. Hanaford, *Daughters of America; or, Women of the Century* (Augusta, ME, 1883); Jewell Nursery Service, *Jewell Scattergun* 20, no. 10 (November 1924); *Lake City City Directory*, 1873; Obituary in an unidentified Lake City, MN, newspaper dated April 4, 1873; Lucien M. Underwood, *The Underwood Families in America* (Lancaster, PA, 1913), 2:420.

V

Elizabeth Josephine *VAILE* (1832–73)

At least two generations of the Vaile family had lived in Winhall, Vermont. Among the ten persons in Elizabeth's parental generation who survived to adulthood, two were lawyers and one a physician. Elizabeth, born in Winhall April 11, 1832, was the fifth of nine children, five males and four females. Her parents, Harvey Vaile and Elizabeth Sprague, moved about 1835 to Kendall, in Orleans County, New York, where they and two of their daughters spent the rest of their lives. Four other siblings went to Missouri or Texas.

Elizabeth grew up in Orleans County, New York, graduated from New England Female Medical College on March 3, 1858, and practiced medicine in Albion, New York, until her premature death on July 29, 1873. A listing in the *Orleans County Directory* for 1869 locates her office upstairs in the Harrington Block on Canal Street. An inventory of her estate (valued at $7,000) includes thirty volumes of medical books, eleven volumes of medical journals, medicines worth forty dollars, an operating table valued at one dollar, and forty dollars in surgical instruments. She is buried in Mt. Albion Cemetery with her parents and sister Fidelia Montgomery.

Josephine's sister Sarah, three years her senior, went to New England Female Medical College in Boston but left after one year to marry John Quincy Brooks, younger brother of Rachel Brooks Gleason (q.v.), to the displeasure of her younger brother, Merrick, who wanted her to become a physician. Also, it is said, the Vaile family thought that Sarah was marrying "a bit" beneath her. In any case, *her* daughter Rachel Gleason Brooks *did* become a physician, practiced in Buffalo, and cared for her aged aunt and uncle, Rachel and Silas, who had run the Elmira Water-Cure.

References: Rachel G. Brooks, *This Is Your Inheritance: A History of the Chemung County, N.Y. Branch of the Brooks Family* (Watkins Glen, NY: Century House, 1963); *Orleans County Directory*, 1869; Dr. Vaile's will and inventory of her estate, Orleans County Clerk's Office, Albion, NY.

Emily A. *VARNEY* Brownell (1824–1905)

Emily Varney was born February 23, 1824, in Danville, Vermont, one of ten children of a locally prominent family of North Danville, a community in Vermont's Northeast Kingdom known earlier as Varney's Mills, and where the Varney family had operated the larger of the two local grist mills. Little is known of Emily's childhood. There is evidence that she attended Danville Phillips Academy as a student and probably later taught there.

When she was twenty-eight, she attended Syracuse Medical College for one session (1852–53), then went to the medical school at Worcester (MA) Academy (1853), and eventually received an MD degree from the Female Medical College of Pennsylvania on March 10, 1855. While at Worcester, Dr. Hatfield Halsted, of motorpathy and water-cure fame, was her preceptor. At medical school in Philadelphia, she was the first woman allowed to attend the clinics of Jefferson Medical College.

She returned to Danville, probably the second woman doctor of medicine in Vermont (after Marenda Randall), and spent the next eighteen years practicing medicine in various villages in the Northeast Kingdom. Directories place her in Danville (1862–63), St. Johnsbury (1864–69), Lyndon (1870–71), and Concord (1872–74). There appears to be a lag in updating directory entries: a November 28, 1862, newspaper notes that "Miss Emily Varnell, M.D., late of North Danville, moved to St. Johnsbury, where she [is] located as a physician." St. Johnsbury was the largest community in the area and was probably better able to support her practice. There is also an advertisement for her professional services in that same newspaper.

About 1870, Dr. Varney married H. M. Brownell (1828–1909), of Lyndon, Vermont, variously described as a physician or as a veterinary surgeon. The exact date of the marriage or whether there were progeny is not known. Since she was still referred to as Miss Varney in 1862, when she would have been thirty-eight years old, it seems unlikely that she had children.

The Brownells moved to California in 1873. Though several sources put the date at 1875, Emily registered in California as a physician on December 6, 1873. The Brownells lived in Oakland, where other members of the Varney family had located before them. Emily continued to practice medicine. She is listed as a practitioner in each Polk medical directory from 1886 through 1898, and in the 1901 edition of the official California register of physicians and surgeons. She was registered as a regular physician on December 6, 1876. About 1898, she retired and moved to Hayward, California. She had practiced medicine for forty-three years, eighteen in Vermont and twenty-five in California. Dr. Brownell died February 11, 1905. She and her husband are buried in the Varney plot in Oakland.

References: *Thirteenth Edition of the Official Register and Directory of Physicians and Surgeons in the State of California* (San Francisco, January 1901); Claire D. Johnson, *"I See by the Paper . . .": An Informal History of St. Johnsbury* (St. Johnsbury, VT, 1983); John W. King, "Early Women Physicians in Vermont," *Bulletin of the History of Medicine* 25 (1951): 432; *Walton's Vermont Directory*; Woman's Medical College of Pennsylvania, *Transactions of the 31st Annual Meeting of the Alumnae Association* (Philadelphia, 1906), 34–35.

Eliza de la VERGNE (ca. 1830–90)

Eliza de la Vergne was born in New York about 1830. The names of her parents and details of her childhood are not known. Sometime before 1855, she married Silas K. de la Vergne, a confectioner by trade. On April 14, 1855, she received a diploma from New York

Hygeio-Therapeutic College, a school whose therapeutics were based on hydropathy as well as healthful diet and regimen. The school was not yet chartered by the state and therefore not authorized to award the degree doctor of medicine. However, it did offer three months of formal training, probably had a curriculum not unlike that provided after the charter (April 1857), and these early graduates were recognized in the community as doctors of medicine. Eliza's graduation thesis—"Infants: Their Improper Nursing and Medication"—was read at commencement and was cited some years later by Seventh Day Adventist Ellen G. White in her book *Health; or, How to Live* (172).

Between 1857 and 1870, Eliza bore at least five children: Charles E. (ca. 1857), Ida B. (ca. 1860), Florence M. (ca. 1863), Frank R. (1867), and Louisa A. (1870). During this period she was practicing medicine in Brooklyn, an activity probably made possible by the presence of household help. The 1860 census lists three "servants" among the six non–family members living in the household; the 1880 census lists one servant.

In the early years, Dr. de la Vergne was located at 258 Pacific Street and in later years at 393 Adelphi. Evidence that she was practicing medicine includes, in the early years, professional advertisements in the *Water-Cure Journal* (1855) and later in the *Herald of Health* (1863) and the *Phrenological Journal* (1865). In 1865, she is listed on the Internal Revenue Service tax rolls, taxed as a physician. The 1870 census denotes her an MD, and the 1889 census, a physician. She is listed as a practicing physician in the 1886 Polk medical directory and in the 1887–88 *Business Directory of Brooklyn*.

Eliza probably was in practice for thirty-five years, from 1855 to 1890. She died at home, July 12, 1890, at fifty-nine. Her elder son, Charles, became a physician. He earned an MD at Long Island College Hospital Medical School in 1878 and practiced in Brooklyn.

References: *Herald of Health* (January–February 1863): 3, 51; *Lain's Business Directory of Brooklyn, 1887–88* (Brooklyn, NY, 1887); New York Death Index (1862–1948) website, search.ancestry.com/search/db.aspx?dbid=9131; Obituary, *New York Times*, July 14, 1890; *Phrenological Journal & Life Illustrated* 41–42 (1865); Polk, 1886, 1890, 1893; US census, 1860, 1870, 1889; US Internal Revenue Service tax rolls, 1865; *Water-Cure Journal*, July 1855.

W

Hannah Maria *Woodward* WALCOTT Butterfield (1816–1911)

Hannah Woodward was born in Boston circa May 10, 1816, daughter of Elisha Woodward and his wife, Irish-born Hannah English. The younger Hannah was married in Stow, Massachusetts, on April 21, 1832, to Lewis Walcott, a truckman twelve years her senior. In 1866, Mr. Walcott was a saloon keeper at 126 Canton (according to the 1866 Boston almanac); later, he is described as a "teamster and provision merchant." Hannah's brother-in-law, George H. Walcott, a clerk, and his wife Mary F. Walcott, lived with the family. Lewis and Hannah had two children, Lewis, born about 1835, and George Henry, born 1837. Hannah later adopted her son George's two children, George and Chastine. After Lewis died on July 12, 1873, in Boston, Hannah married John Butterfield.

In 1855, Hannah graduated from New England Female Medical College in Boston, where she had been supported by a scholarship from the state during the year just passed. She is listed in Boston almanacs as a physician from 1855 until 1905, at 101 Pleasant Street in Charlestown from 1858 to 1875, at 161 Pleasant Street from 1879 to 1893, and at 4 Winchester Street in Boston from 1898 to 1902. Her name is also found in the Polk medical directories from 1886 to 1902. Hannah died at her home at 70 Dudley Street in Boston, of bronchopneumonia, on May 3, 1911, at the age of ninety-four years, eleven months, twenty-four days. She is buried in Mt. Auburn Cemetery. Hannah appears to have practiced medicine in Charlestown, probably midwifery and diseases of women and children, for almost forty years.

References: Death certificate, City of Boston, filed May 6, 1911; *Boston Almanacs*; Arthur S. Walcott, *The Walcott Book* (Salem, MA, 1925), 123.

Mary Edwards *WALKER* Miller (1832–1919)

There is a considerable amount written about Mary Edwards Walker, some of it factual, some of it fictional. It is not entirely clear whether Dr. Walker was a reformer upon whom unreasonable public opprobrium and ridicule were heaped or whether she was an eccentric woman who liked to draw attention to herself. The answer is probably a little of both.

Mary Edwards was born on Bunker Hill Road in Oswego Township, New York, on November 26, 1832, the fifth of five daughters of Alvah Walker and his wife, Vesta Whitcomb. The Walkers' firstborn, a son, died in infancy. After Mary, another son, Alvah H., was born. The Walkers, pioneers in the Oswego area, each traced ancestry to Plymouth Colony. The elder Alvah's father died when Alvah was thirteen. Alvah left school, learned the trade of carpenter, and helped support his mother and five sisters until his mother remarried. At nineteen, he left home in central Massachusetts, worked his way across New York, down the Ohio and Mississippi Valleys to New Orleans, returning to Boston by sea. Back home, he married Vesta Whitcomb, moved to Syracuse, raised a family, and found plenty of work as a carpenter. Early on, he was sick a lot. An avid reader, he studied the Scriptures and medical books and evolved into a minister and physician as well as being a farmer and a carpenter. After ten years the family moved to a farm near Oswego, where Mary was born.

Mary's father believed that tight clothing was bad for a woman's health. He also thought that women should be educated and encouraged to enter the professions. With the help of neighbors, he built a schoolhouse on the farm, the first school in the area. His five daughters all received common school instruction in the little schoolhouse. At least three of them, including Mary, went on to Falley Seminary in nearby Fulton. The eldest daughter was licensed to teach at eighteen. Mary taught in nearby Minetto for several years. In December 1853, then twenty-one years old, Mary matriculated at Syracuse Medical College and, after two winter terms and one spring term, graduated on February 22, 1855, with an MD degree. She was the only woman in her class to graduate that year, though there were seven female students at the winter session of 1853–54, and four females at the spring session of 1854. Mary gave the opening address at commencement. Her total college costs had been $185; room and board was about $1.50 a week.

Dr. Walker started practice in Columbus, Ohio, where a paternal aunt lived. After a year of meager success, she moved back to Rome, New York, where she practiced medicine for the next four years and where, on December 19, 1855, she married medical school classmate Albert E. Walker, who was also practicing in Rome. It was not a conventional marriage. Mary, from later schooldays, had taken to wearing bloomers and, later, men's pants and frockcoat. She would dress this way the rest of her life, and her costume came to define her more than her profession. The wedding was performed not by the local Methodist minister but by a well-known liberal Unitarian and abolitionist. The bride was in pants and dress coat. The bride did not promise to "obey," and she retained her maiden name. The marriage was apparently a happy one at first, and the two practiced medicine together. But it seems that Miller's eye was inclined to wander, and divorce soon followed, though Albert had told Mary that she "might have the same privileges." After the two parted, Miller left town (and died not long thereafter). Mary practiced alone. Between March and August 1860 she grossed $108 (excluding accounts outstanding) but had expenses of $140: $63 for rent and board, $40 for clothes, $35 for offices expenses (which included $7.69 for medicine, $2 for a sign, and $9.63 for a portrait and frames for a picture and for her diploma).

With the coming of the Civil War, Mary applied for a commission as army surgeon but was turned down. She went to Washington, anyway, in October 1861, and volunteered to serve as a nurse, working in the hospital being established in the elegant but as yet unfinished Patent Office, becoming assistant to Dr. J. N. Green, the surgeon in charge. She called on the surgeon general, again seeking the position of assistant surgeon, a request refused again. During these years, "she was a hospital administrator, therapist, counselor, amanuensis, expediter and confessor" (Snyder). She accompanied sick and wounded soldiers to their homes. On one such trip, at Ravenna, Ohio, she stayed long enough to give a lecture to benefit the Soldier's Aid Society. On another occasion, she persuaded a clergyman to provide checkerboards to the several hospitals around Washington. She visited the deserters' prison, interviewed prisoners, including a sixteen-year-old boy who, apparently, had gone to see his dying mother. Dr. Walker interceded successfully on behalf of the boy with Secretary of War Stanton (Snyder). During this time she also found time to attend the New York Hygeio-Therapeutic College, a medical school operated by the famous hydropathist Russell Trall, graduating April 1, 1862. Her thesis was entitled "The Secessionist."

From Mary's later recollections it sounds as if she moved from hospital to hospital in Washington, sometimes helping, sometimes causing trouble, sometimes going to New York or home to Oswego, all of which, since she had no military status, she was at liberty to do. Her work was pro bono. We do know that she cared for casualties after the Battle of Chickamauga in September 1863. In January 1864, she was finally commissioned as an assistant surgeon, replacing a man who had died unexpectedly from an overdose of morphine, and was assigned to the Fifty-Second Ohio Volunteers. In the history of that regiment, written by Nixon B. Stewart and published in 1900, Stewart, a sergeant in the war but by then a minister, provided one of the few firsthand, albeit retrospective, accounts of Mary's activities:

She had the rank of 1st Lieutenant and was dressed just like any other officer. The uniform was dark blue and the trousers had a stripe of gold lace down the side. She wore curls, so that everybody would know she was a woman. She was thirty-two years of age. . . . In form she was slender and rather frail looking in body. The men seemed to hate her, and she did little or nothing for the sick of the regiment. She began to practice in her profession among the citizens in the surrounding country. Every day she would pass out of the picket line, attending the sick. All this time many of the boys believed her to be a spy. [Factual documentation of this is not available, and Dr. Walker does not seem to have mentioned it.] On April 10, 1864 rebel cavalry took her prisoner and she was sent to Richmond, where she was a prisoner in Libby for four months.

After her exchange (for a male First Lieutenant), she revisited the regiment. "We believe she was honest and sincere in her views, posing as a reformer, yet the majority of the men in the regiment believed she was out of her place in the army, and have so treated her since the war."

In 1866, Congress awarded her a Medal of Honor for what was described as care for the "dental, obstetrical, surgical and medical distresses" of the local farmers and their families whom she had attended after Chickamauga. It is claimed that this was the only Medal of Honor ever given to a woman. The award, in those days, did not have the significance it later did. In 1917, the Medal of Honor Board deleted the names of 911 medal recipients (including Dr. Walker) for reasons explained in *Wikipedia*'s entry on Walker. The medals were not recalled, however, and Mary wore her medal daily for the rest of her life. It was formally restored by President Carter in 1977.

Mary's wartime experiences may have been the high point of her life. "As a Civil War celebrity Dr. Walker enjoyed brief fame in the immediate postwar years." After the war she continued to work for dress reform (a cause then waning in popularity), for woman's suffrage (though she rejected the suffrage amendment, in the belief that the Constitution already granted women the right to vote, an opinion that alienated her from the movement), and for other feminist causes generally. She made lecture tours in England and in the American Midwest. She sought, and received, a pension for her military service. She worked, briefly, in the mail room at the Pension Office in Washington but, accused of insubordination, was soon discharged. She wore only man's costume. In the 1870s, she wrote two books, the autobiographical *HIT* (1871) and *Science of Immortality* (1878).

Around 1890, she retired to the family farm in Oswego, where she would spend the remaining thirty years of her life, alone and poor. It does not appear that she practiced medicine after her army days.

She was criticized for her costume—not so much that she wore pants but that she copied male dress so precisely. There were also unfavorable reports as to her professional ability. A board of medical officers who examined her at Chattanooga during the war called her medically ignorant and thought it "doubtful whether she has pursued the study of medicine" and reported that her practical knowledge of diseases and remedies was "not much greater than [that of] most housewives." Her alma mater saw it differently. At the time of her capture, it was reported in the *Herald of Health*, house organ of her second medical school, that "the 'rebs' . . . have secured a prize in this 'female surgeon,' and the best they can do for themselves, so far as the fair prisoner is concerned, is to employ her in her professional capacity. As she is a graduate of the New York Hygeio-Therapeutic College, we can endorse her competency."

In spite of her eccentricities and questioned professional competence, she was the first (and probably only) woman physician to serve as an officer in the Union army (though, according to Stewart, her name does not appear on the regimental roster of the Fifty-Second Ohio Volunteer Infantry, nor does it appear on the official published list of army medical officers). This may be explained by the apparent fact that she was not a commissioned officer but rather a contract acting assistant surgeon (civilian), US Army (*Wikipedia*). Whatever her status in the Union army, she shares with Orie Moon (q.v.), who had a similar position in the Confederate army, the honor of being pioneer women in the military.

Bibliography: *HIT: Essays on Women's Rights* (New York: American News Co. 1871); *Unmasked; or, the Science of Immortality* (Philadelphia, 1878); *Statement on Woman's Suffrage at the Hearings before the Committee on the Judiciary, House of Representatives, Sixty-Second Congress, Second Session, February 14, 1912* (Washington, DC: Government Printing Office, 1912).

References: *American Medical and Surgical Journal* 7 (1855): 148–50; *Dictionary of American Medical Biography* 2 (1984): 771–72; *Notable American Women 1607–1950*, 3:532–33; Mercedes Graf, *A Woman of Honor: Dr. Mary E. Walker and the Civil War* (Gettysburg, PA: Thomas Publications, 2001); *Herald of Health*, June 1864, 227; Carla Johnson, *Civil War Doctor: The Story of Mary Walker* (Greensboro, NC: Morgan Reynolds Publishing Co., 2007); Obituary, *Oswego Daily Palladium*, February 22, 1919; Funeral notice, *Oswego Daily Palladium*, February 24, 1919; Obituary, *Brooklyn Eagle*, February 26, 1919; Linda Poynter, "Life of Mary Edwards Walker, M.D.," undated, unpublished manuscript in the Archives of the Woman's Medical College of Pennsylvania at Drexel University College of Medicine, Philadelphia; Jane E. Shultz, *Women at the Front: Hospital Workers in Civil War America* (Chapel Hill, NC, 2004); Charles M. Snyder, *Dr. Mary Walker* (New York, 1974); Nixon B. Stewart, *Dan McCook's Regiment, 52 O.V.I.* (n.p.: Author, 1900), 81–82; *Syracuse Medical and Surgical Journal* 6 (1854): 190–91; John B. Taylor, "Recollections of Mary Edwards Walker," 1944, handwritten manuscript in the archives of the Female Medical College of Pennsylvania at Drexel University Medical College, Philadelphia; Dale L. Walker, *Mary Edwards Walker: Above and Beyond* (New York: Forge Books, 2005); *Water-Cure Journal*, May 1862, 109; *Water-Cure Journal*, June 1864, 227; "Mary Edwards Walker," *Wikipedia*, January 12, 2013; Frances E. Willard, *A Woman of the Century* (Buffalo, 1893); Helen B. Woodward, "The Right to Wear Pants: Dr. Mary Walker," in *The Bold Women* (New York, 1953).

Sarah Elizabeth *Nichols* WARFIELD Walker (1819–96)

Sarah Elizabeth Nichols was born in Reading, Massachusetts, on April 19, 1819. Her father, Job Nichols, married Betsy Temple, October 20, 1818. Sarah, the eldest, was followed by five more children, three of whom lived to adulthood. In the early 1840s, Sarah married a painter named Elijah B. Warfield of Holliston. They had three children: William V. (1845), Frank A. (1846), and Abijah Baker (May 9, 1849). Two days before the birth of Abijah, the father died of typhus fever.

Sarah, now a widow, with three children aged six to ten, went to New England Female Medical College in Boston, where she held a state scholarship from 1855 through 1858, and from which she received the degree of doctor of medicine in that latter year. She is listed in Boston directories as a physician in 1858, 1859, and 1860, sharing office space with Mary Jenks (q.v.). The *Progressive Annuals* for 1863 and 1864 also place her as a physician in Boston. She must have moved thereafter to Holliston, Massachusetts, where the *Massachusetts Register* for 1867 locates her. According to her obituary in the *Boston Transcript*, she practiced medicine in Holliston for thirty years and was prominent in Woman's Relief Corps work.

On February 4, 1867, she married Deacon Timothy Walker (b. ca. 1802) of Holliston, a second marriage for both. (One source says it was her third marriage.) She apparently continued using the name Warfield professionally. (Her youngest son was then seventeen, so it seems likely it was to provide name recognition for her patients.) She is listed under the Warfield name, as a physician, in Holliston directories for 1875, 1878, 1882–83, and 1884–85. In 1889 and 1891 directories she is listed as Mrs. Timothy Walker but no longer as a physician. She probably practiced in Holliston from the early 1860s to 1888. Sarah died in Brockton, following a stroke, on February 22, 1896.

References: Boston city directory, 1858, 1859, 1860; Obituary, *Boston Transcript*, February 24, 1896, p. 5, col. 4; Holliston city directory, 1875, 1878, 1882–83, 1884–85, 1889, 1891; *Massachusetts Register*, 1867; Massachusetts Vital Records; *Progressive Annual*, 1863, 1864; Reading Vital Records (MA).

Rachel M. *Bewley* WATSON (1814–95)

Rachel Bewley was born May 1, 1814, in Wrightstown, Bucks County, Pennsylvania, daughter of Amos Bewley and his wife, Mary Price. Except that she was raised in the Quaker tradition, nothing is known of her background, parents, childhood, or early education. In the mid-1830s she married Theodore Watson, a woodworker. They had four children: Nathan, Anna Mary, Matilda, and Sarah. Only Nathan and Matilda lived to adulthood. During this period, Rachel was active in the antislavery movement, and, like fellow Quaker Phebe M. Way (q.v.), she attended an Anti-Slavery Convention of Women in 1838, held May 15–18 in Philadelphia.

In the fall of 1850, not long after the birth of Sarah, the family moved to Salem, Ohio, where Rachel and her husband would live the rest of their lives. Anna Mary and Sarah both died before 1856, events that may have motivated Rachel to become a physician. She attended Penn Medical University in Philadelphia, received an MD degree in 1857, and returned to Salem, where she practiced medicine for more than thirty years. The 1877 Butler medical directory and the 1886 Polk medical directory each list her as a practicing physician. (In spite of this and as was then often the case with woman physicians, the 1860 US census lists her as having no occupation, and the 1870 census says she was "keeping house.")

In 1868, she published a book entitled *The Family Physician;* a thousand copies were printed. The volume was dedicated to Philadelphia botanic pharmacist Aaron Comfort (grandson of prominent Quaker John Woolman), who may have provided some financial support for Rachel's medical education. Dr. Watson refers to herself as a "grateful friend" of Comfort. Though Dr. Watson was not a botanic physician, she did use botanic remedies and also quoted botanic doctors in her book: Samuel Thomson, Wooster Beach, John W. Comfort, and Morris Mattson, and several letters supporting botanic practice written by Benjamin Waterhouse, Harvard's first professor of medicine.

The book describes "simple remedies, easily obtained, for the cure of disease in all its forms" and is intended "to diffuse information in regard to attendance upon the sick; how to cook for them, and to prepare drinks, poultices, etc., and how to guard against infection from contagious diseases. It gives the symptoms of fevers, with the best and simplest remedies for their cure. It also treats of the various diseases of children, of cholera in all its forms, with infallible remedies if timely and perseveringly applied." Among the remedies she describes (and for which she provides the formula) is Balm of Gilead. "I obtained this recipe twenty years ago [1848] and can recommend it as valuable; it was at that time manufactured by a lady in Rochester, New York, who, by its sale, had provided a comfortable home for herself and her family."

Dr. Watson also felt strongly about educating people, the young especially, about the anatomy and physiology of their bodies and promoted the use of anatomical manikins for instruction in every high school, college, and university. "No young man, or woman, should be considered as properly instructed, who is not made familiar with the practical anatomy and physiology which can be taught with the aid of the manikin . . . an ingenious piece of French mechanism." Dr. Watson died July 9, 1895, at the age of eighty-one.

Bibliography: *What Every Family Wants: The Family Physician, Containing Simple Remedies, Easily Obtained, for the Cure of Disease in All Its Forms* (Salem, OH, 1868); *The Life of My Family; or, The Log-House in the Wilderness* (New York, 1871).

References: Butler, 1877; Atwater catalog, #3724; Horace Mack, *History of Columbiana County, Ohio, Illustrations and Biographical Sketches* (Philadelphia: D. W. Ensign & Co., 1879), 43; Polk, 1886; US census, 1850, 1860, 1870, 1880.

Phebe M. *WAY* (b. ca. 1814–76)

Phebe Way was born about 1814, probably in Chester County, Pennsylvania. Nothing has been found about her parents, background, childhood, or early education. She was a Quaker.

In 1850, age thirty-six, she was then living at home in Pennsburg, Chester County, with her widowed mother, Susana, and her older brother, Israel. During those early years she was active in the antislavery movement and in 1838 attended an antislavery convention of women, held in Philadelphia, as a delegate from Kennett, Chester County (as did fellow Quaker, Rachel M. Watson [q.v.] then of Middletown, Bucks County).

Several years later Phebe enrolled in the Female Medical College of Pennsylvania and graduated with the school's first class in December 1851. Her whereabouts during the next five years are not known, but she may have been practicing medicine in Philadelphia. In 1857, she was listed as a physician at 27 North Twelfth Street, was at 123 North Fifteenth Street the next year, and at 36 North Sixteenth Street, in 1859, 1860, and 1861, in both the general and the classified sections of the city directory for those years. An 1862 directory places her at 1510 Cherry St., Philadelphia. She must have returned later that year to Kennett Square, where on September 1 she was taxed ten dollars as a practicing physician.

The 1870 census describes her as a resident of Kennett, a "gentlewoman" with $2,000 in personal property, living with the family of Thomas and Mary Marshall and their three teenage children. There is no mention of professional status. Phebe died April 6, 1876, at sixty-two, still living with the Marshalls. Her death notice in *Friends' Intelligencer* describes her as "M.D."

References: *Friends' Intelligencer* 76 (1876): 170; *McElroy's Philadelphia City Directory*, 1857, 1858, 1859, 1860, 1861; US census, 1850, 1870; US Internal Revenue Service tax rolls, Kennett Square, PA, September 1, 1862.

Sarah Abigail *Sheldon* WETHERBEE (1819–70)

Sarah Sheldon was born April 27, 1819, in Pittsford, Vermont, the second daughter of Jacob Sheldon and his wife, Joanna. Nothing is known of her childhood or early education. On January 3, 1837, not quite eighteen, she married Isaac Josiah Wetherbee, a young man two years her senior, from South Reading, a village thirty miles east of Pittsford, across the mountains. Wetherbee's father was a prominent Free Baptist clergyman and abolitionist and Isaac himself studied for the ministry and was ordained in 1841 but withdrew from it five years later because of "poor health." The couple had one child, a son, who died at three days.

Isaac, who had always been mechanically inclined, turned to dentistry, attended Baltimore College of Dental Surgery (then the only dental school in the country), graduated in 1850 with a DDS, and established a practice in Boston. The 1850 census shows the Wetherbees living in adjacent Charlestown. Also in the house were two dental students, aged sixteen and eighteen, and a domestic.

What Sarah was doing in Boston during the 1850s is not known—probably keeping house. Toward the end of the decade she enrolled in New England Female Medical College where she had scholarship support from the Commonwealth from 1855 through 1859. In 1859, then forty, she graduated with an MD degree. Whether she practiced medicine thereafter is uncertain. Her name is not listed as a physician in various Boston business directories for the 1860s (1860, 1863–64, 1866, 1867, 1868) or in *Boston Almanacs* (1860, 1861, 1864, 1867, 1868, 1869). She is listed as a practicing physician in Boston in the *Progressive Annuals* for 1863 and 1864, but that publication was often a listing of medical school graduates rather than an on-the-ground determination. According to the 1860 census, the couple was living in a Boston hotel with eighty-five unrelated people.

Sarah died at the age of fifty-one in Boston, December 27, 1870, with some kind of ovarian problem. During the 1860s, Isaac was founding president of the Boston Dental Institute. In 1868 he founded and for fifteen years was president of Boston Dental College and professor of dental science and operative dentistry.

References: Boston city directory; *Boston Almanac*; Richard Herndon, *Men of Progress: One Thousand Biographical Sketches and Portraits of Leaders in Business and Professional Life in the Commonwealth of Massachusetts* (Boston, 1896), 270–71; US census, 1850, 1860.

Rebecca B. WHEELER (b. ca. 1807)

The earliest information about Rebecca Wheeler is her graduation from Syracuse Medical College on March 17, 1852. At that time she was forty-five years old and was married to Charles Wheeler, a farmer five years her senior and with personal wealth of $800. The 1860 census shows her living in the Third Ward of Rochester, New York, with her husband and an eighteen-year-old daughter, Marietta. Rebecca is there denoted a "physician." For thirty years after her graduation she practiced medicine in Rochester. Notable is the fact that, during that period, she lived at no less than eleven different addresses located in all parts of the city, sometimes moving every year. The Rochester city directory for 1880 lists her as a physician at 111 Mount Hope Avenue. No death date or obituary has been found for Dr. Wheeler. The last year she is listed in Rochester directories is 1883.

References: Rochester city directory, 1860 et seq.; US census, 1860.

Rebecca S. WHITNEY (b. ca. 1826)

Reliable information about Dr. Whitney has been found only for the six-year period 1858–64. The 1860 federal census places Rebecca S. Whitney in the town of Adams, in western Massachusetts, living with the family of Samuel C. Woodward. Woodward was cashier in a local bank. Whitney is described as a thirty-four-year-old physician, born in Maine. She had graduated with an MD degree from Penn Medical University earlier that year and had been a student at the New England Female Medical College in 1858. When she matriculated at the Pennsylvania medical school, she gave Lawrence, Massachusetts, as her place of residence, and this is supported by the fact that she was listed in the 1859 Lawrence city directory as "Mrs. Rebecca S. Whitney, house, Turnpike, cr Tremont." This establishes that she was married. She was probably a widow.

She did not stay in Adams for long, moving soon to Boston. The 1862 Boston directory lists "Rebecca S. Whitney, widow, boards at 20 Dwight." The directory for the following year is more helpful. It lists "Rebecca S. Whitney, Mrs., M.D., boards 38 Summer" and also lists her in the classified section under "female physicians."

Rebecca seems to have soon moved again. In the Lowell city directory for 1864–65, Dr. Whitney is listed as a physician with home and office at 45 Chestnut St. But the 1867 Boston directory has her back at 38 Summer. The Boston almanac, which listed her at 38 Summer in 1864, does not include her name in the 1867, 1868, or 1869 editions. So the Boston directory information may just be outdated data carried over from an earlier edition.

No verified information about her subsequent career has been found. Did she remarry? There was a Rebecca S. Whitney who married William H. Chase in Boston on July 13, 1863. This Rebecca was the daughter of Jonathan and Olive Perkins, was born in Maine, but born several (eight) years earlier than "our" Rebecca was born, based on 1860 census data. The most likely explanation is that widow Whitney became a physician to support herself, remarried, and may or may not have continued to practice thereafter. But this is only speculation.

References: *Boston Almanac,* 1864, 1867, 1868, 1869; *Boston City Directory,* 1862, 1865; *Lawrence City Directory,* 1859; *Lowell City Directory,* 1864–65; United States census, 1860; Frederick C. Waite, *History of the New England Female Medical College 1848–1874* (Boston, 1950), 125. Harold J. Abrahams, *Extinct Medical Schools of Nineteenth-Century Philadelphia* (Philadelphia, 1966).

Elizabeth Jane *WILEY* Warren Corbett (1833–1916)

Elizabeth Wiley was born July 10, 1833, in Kent, Indiana, the eldest of seven children (three girls, four boys) of Preston Pritchard Wiley, a preacher in the Christian Church and early abolitionist in southern Indiana, and his wife Lucinda Weir Maxwell. Elizabeth later wrote of her father: "Though not a college-bred man, [he] was a deep student, a mathematician, an historian, and above all a philologist, and woe be unto us if we made a lapse in English!" One of Elizabeth's younger brothers, Harvey Washington Wiley, would become the force behind the US Food and Drug Act in 1906.

The family lived on a farm and grew almost all they ate. They sold eggs and butter to buy sugar and other things for the table. The family was Presbyterian, the parents strict, obedience was required, as was Sabbath observance, wrote Harvey Wiley in his autobiography. Elizabeth, being the eldest, helped raise the other children. When she was eleven, her mother sick, she took care of her infant brother, Harvey. She improvised a nursing bottle from an empty flask, a cork, and a quill with its end wrapped in linen, and with this fed Harvey with pure cow's milk until he outgrew his babyhood. As a result, she became, according to her obituary in the *New York Times*, "the foster mother of the pure food law."

The girls all taught school to earn money for higher education, but none of them would be able to finish. Elizabeth was turned down by nearby Hanover College. Elizabeth later recalled that the request that she be admitted there was unprecedented and the president of the college, a good friend of her father's, said, "Do you want your daughter to come here and recite with these men?" "Why, yes; she would not hurt the men." "Is she prepared to enter college? Does she read Greek?" "Yes, she reads Greek very well." "Well, there is something the matter with a girl who reads Greek and she cannot enter here." So, off to Antioch she went, away from home and her father's tutelage. But only for a year.

> At as early an age as fourteen, I decided to study medicine. The terrible experience of having my mother pass through a siege of typhoid (treated with calomel to the degree of salivation until she picked out all her beautiful teeth and laid them in my hand), was enough to decide me to find a better way of treating fevers—if there was one—than the mercurial method employed at that time. But how and where in the "wild and woolly West," was a problem that seemed beyond me. My father at this time subscribed for the *Phrenological* and *Water Cure Journals*, in which were advertised the Hygeio-Therapeutic College in New York which admitted women. This appealed to me,

and so it was arranged that I go to New York, in company with an uncle, Anderson Maxwell, who was en route to California with his family. I took the course and received my degree [MD, March 29, 1859] and, incidentally, learned something more efficacious in the treatment of fevers than calomel for medicine and 'sheepnanny tea' for drink and nourishment.

I went home, gave my invalid mother a course of treatment which completely restored her health, much to the disgruntlement of the village doctor, who always employed the "calomel and tea." My mother lived, a la the fairies, "happily ever after," unto eighty-six years, and died of the old peoples' friend—pneumonia (Corbett).

Soon, Elizabeth moved to San Francisco, where she would practice medicine for the next forty or forty-five years. Later that year (1859) she married Colonel L. W. Warren, with whom she had a daughter, Bertia. Whether Col. Warren died or the couple was divorced is not determined. On March 7, 1867, Elizabeth married Samuel J. Corbett, MD, of San Francisco. They had two sons. On two occasions during the next forty years Elizabeth went to Europe, in 1879 to study medicine in Vienna ("clinical work as the guest of Billroth, the famous surgeon") and Paris, and in 1900 to see her son, Harvey Wiley Corbett, an architect, graduate from the École des Beaux Arts in Paris. On the earlier trip she and her brother Harvey met in Paris and attended the World Exposition, and on the way home she stopped in Ann Arbor, "with letters to some of the professors, especially one to Professor Vaughn, into whose laboratory I went for 'brushing up' in chemistry, and after a three months' course, I asked for an examination and the privilege of presenting a thesis, for a degree. This was granted in spite of considerable opposition on the part of the students because of the limited time I had spent in that particular college. I received my degree [MD, 1879, University of Michigan] and returned to California, where I continued my practice until 1900" (ibid.).

After the San Francisco earthquake of 1906, Elizabeth moved to New York to live with her architect son. While there she was made an honorary member of the New York State Women's Medical Association and of the American Medical Association. "But allow me to say, in closing," she wrote, "that the only distinction I ever really attained was as the *originator of the Pure Food Law*, in that at the age of eleven, I brought up my distinguished brother, Doctor Harvey W. Wiley on a bottle, and I fed him *pure milk*!!"

At the age of eighty-two, she was still "hale and hearty; can walk five miles without fatigue and am as delighted with a new idea as I was at fourteen." Dr. Corbett died in June 1916 at Tacoma Sanitarium in Washington, DC.

References: Elizabeth W. Corbett, "Autobiographical Sketch," *Maxwell History and Genealogy*, by Florence W. Houston et al. (Indianapolis, ca. 1915), 72–73; Obituary, *New York Times*, June 7, 1916; Polk, 1886 et seq.; Harvey W. Wiley, *An Autobiography* (Indianapolis, 1930); Personal communication from James Harvey Young, March 24, 1989.

Olive A. *WILLIAMS* Maxson (b. ca. 1834)

Olive Williams was born in Ohio about 1834. No information has been found about her parents, childhood, or early education. When she matriculated at the New York Hygeio-Therapeutic College, she was a resident of Deerfield, Portage County, Ohio. In 1861, she and her medical school classmate, Daniel H. Maxson, graduated with MD degrees and were married at the commencement ceremony. After Dr. Russell Trall had conferred the degrees, then "to the surprise of nearly all persons present, Dr. David H. Maxson, of Petersburg, N.Y., and Dr. Olive A. Williams, of Deerfield, Ohio, arose, joined hands, and united in holy wedlock. On concluding the marriage ceremony, and in congratulating the happy pair on this result of the acquaintance they had formed and matured during the school term, Dr. Trall referred them to the beautiful motto on the diploma which had just been awarded them . . . 'a sound mind in a sound body.' The applause which followed the wedding episode was long and loud."

As was often the case with graduates of the medical school they attended, the young couple started work at a water-cure establishment, sort of an internship, in this case at the Octagon Water-Cure in Petersburg, Rensselaer County, New York. The following years they had moved to another such establishment in Alliance, Stark County, Ohio. During the Civil War, Daniel served in the 115th Ohio Infantry, apparently as a foot soldier. He is not listed in the official roster of regimental surgeons and assistant surgeons during the War of the Rebellion.

After the war, the couple moved to Nebraska, at least by 1867, when their son Horace was born, and remained there. The 1870 census places them in Table Rock, Pawnee County, Nebraska, where Daniel was a "farmer" and Olive was "keeping house." Daniel had holdings of $1,500 in real estate and $250 in personal property. In the 1880 census they were located in Humboldt, Nebraska. Daniel is denoted a "physician" and Olive as "keeping house." The 1885 state census finds them still in Humboldt, Daniel is again said to be a farmer, and Olive is keeping house. The 1900 federal census omits Daniel, who has presumably died, and Olive was living with her son, Horace (a.k.a. D. H.). He was a dealer in either hogs or hay (illegible).

It has not been possible to determine whether, or to what extent, the two Maxsons practiced medicine. The fact that the census consistently (one exception) failed to describe them as physicians is not reliable in deciding this question. Census data are notoriously inaccurate, and during the late nineteenth century women definitely known to be practicing medicine were often said to be "keeping house." No death date has been found for Olive. She was last known to be alive in 1900, when she would have been sixty-six years old. Daniel died sometime between 1888, when he filed a claim as an invalid Civil War veteran, and 1893, when Olive, as his widow, renewed the claim.

References: Nebraska State census, 1885; US census, 1870, 1880, 1900; *Water-Cure Journal*, May 1861, June 1862, 123–24; *Water-Cure World* (Brattleboro, VT, May 1861), 36.

Savina Leah *Fogle* WILLIAMS (1825–1910)

Savina Williams practiced medicine in Columbus, Ohio, for a decade and for forty years in Clarence, Iowa. She was born Savina Fogle, October 27, 1825, in Strasburg Township, Lancaster County, Pennsylvania. The family moved to Ohio in 1835 and lived in Columbus. In 1851, Savina was married to Isaiah Williams, a Methodist minister who, two years later, graduated from Eclectic Medical Institute in Cincinnati, gave up the ministry, and practiced medicine and dentistry thereafter. He did this, it is written, because of his poor health! (Thirty years later Isaiah studied law and was admitted to the bar.) The Williamses had four children, one son and three daughters.

In 1858, Savina, having attended at least two courses at the Eclectic College of Medicine in Cincinnati, earned her own MD degree. In 1869, leaving her brother and two sisters behind in Columbus, Savina and her family (all six of them) moved to Clarence, Cedar County, Iowa, a village of only several hundred, where both husband and wife practiced medicine thereafter. Several medical directories list them as practicing physicians. Savina is listed as a homoeopathic physician in Pettet's 1878–78 homoeopathic directory. King reports that both husband and wife were homoeopaths from the 1850s. The 1877 Butler medical directory and the 1886 Polk medical directory each includes them, as do the 1878–79 and 1880–81 medical and surgical directories of Iowa.

Both Savina and Isaiah were active in the Methodist church, both having joined in their youthful years. Isaiah was a great reader—science, philosophy, history, and current events—and they were both interested in various reform movements, especially temperance. Savina died December 13, 1910, at eighty-five, her husband having gone almost five years earlier. "Her mind was clear and strong to the last, she being conscious when her translation came . . . she drifted away to an unknown land."

References: Butler, 1877; Obituary for Isaiah, *Clarence Sun,* January 11, 1906; Obituary, *Clarence Sun,* December 15, 1910, p. 4, col. 6; William H. King, *History of Homoeopathy and Its Institutions in America* (New York, 1905), 1:387; *Medical and Surgical Directory of the State of Iowa for 1878 and 1879; Medical and Surgical Directory of the State of Iowa for 1880 and 1881; North American Homoeopathic Directory for 1877–78*; Polk, 1886.

Adaline Melinda *WILLIS* Weed (1837–1910)

Adaline Willis and her husband-to-be, Gideon Allen Weed, were class-mates at New York Hygeio-Therapeutic College. They spent the fifty years following their marriage working together professionally on the West Coast. When Gideon died, in 1905, it was front-page news. When Adaline died, five years later, her obituary was fourteen lines on page 12 that did not mention that she was a doctor.

Born in Illinois in 1837, Adaline grew up in Marion, Iowa. Her father and mother had been born in South Carolina and Kentucky, respectively, so her background was Southern. She had an older sis-ter and brother. In the 1850 census her mother, Ann, is listed but not her father, who had probably died. The family was of moderate means. They held $1,500 in real estate. Adaline's eighteen-year old brother, Stephen, and a forty-five-year-old hired hand ran the family farm. Adaline herself would later be described as "a lady of education and refinement."

In the spring of 1857, Adaline received an MD degree from the New York Hygeio-Therapeutic College and returned to Marion, Iowa, where, it was reported in the *Water-Cure Journal,* she was "preparing to talk to the people in that vicinity. As she is the youngest graduate of our late class, we recommend the doctors to try their hands at an argu-ment with her on any medical topic they please. . . . She is not yet out of her teens, so they need not be afraid."

The following year, she married former classmate Gideon Allen Weed. Weed, who came from Jersey City, was of New England ancestry and had grandfathers who had fought in the Revolution. The wedding was quite an event. It took place in the school's lecture hall. All the professors and students were invited to see the couple unite "hands, hearts, fortunes, and *diplomas* in the place and among the associations where they had so faithfully studied the laws of life."

In 1858, the young couple set out for the West Coast aboard the *Star of the West*, crossed Panama, arrived at Sacramento February 14, rested for ten days, and moved on to Salem, capital of Oregon Territory. The trip had taken twenty-five days as far as Sacramento. They stayed in Salem for two years, after which they returned to Sacramento. While in Oregon, Adaline later wrote to the *Water-Cure Journal*:

> we traveled much of the time, visited the principal towns and villages, and lectured upon hygiene and hydropathy in all parts with a good degree of success. We had good practice, too, and as many patients as we could accommodate in our house. We hope our labors there have smoothed the way for those who may come after us. We know our teachings aroused some to *think* for themselves of the true causes of diseases and rational medication. On our second tour it was very encouraging to meet a person here and there who had put into practice our teachings; to find a young man who had been induced by our admonition to free himself from the use of tobacco; to hear a mother say she had ceased to feed her little ones on pork and grease, tea and coffee; and to find the wholesome Graham loaf on the table, where bakers' bread or soda-biscuit had ever been before . . . Yes . . . this was *pay*.

This passage makes clear how much the graduates from the New York Hygeio-Therapeutic College were teachers, reformers, and missionaries rather than pharmaceutical dispensers. The couple worked as a team. "Mrs. Weed does the principal lecturing, while her husband makes the arrangements and does the outdoor work."

In April 1860, back in the San Francisco area, the Weeds planned to travel and lecture in California for the next year or so, staying for a couple of days to a week in each place, looking for a suitable site to set up a hydropathic establishment. The discovery of silver in western Nevada (the Comstock Lode) in 1859 led to a change in their plans, and they spent the next eight or nine years at various communities in mining country around the Virginia City–Lake Tahoe area; six years in Washoe City; two years at Crystal Peak, Nevada; and a year in Truckee, California. Gideon practiced medicine in these mining towns. Whether Adaline was practicing or lecturing has not been determined. During the Civil War, Gideon was commissioned as a surgeon, with rank of major, on the staff of Brig. Gen. Slingerland of the Nevada State Militia. Internal Revenue Service tax assessments for December 1863 and May 1865 list him as paying a tax as a physician and on his income as well; Adaline was not so taxed.

In the spring of 1870, the Weeds left mining country and moved to Vallejo, California, across the bay from San Francisco. That same spring, Gideon received his second MD degree, this one from Rush Medical College in Chicago, and the couple's first child, Benjamin, was born. The following year, the family moved to Seattle, then a community of about one thousand people, and settled. In 1872, a daughter, Mabel, was born. Both children would later attend the University of California. Benjamin would go on to teach at the Junior College in Ross, California. Mabel, a social worker, never married, but had a lifelong companion, Bertha Wright, who shared with her the raising of three adopted children.

In Seattle both Weeds became prominent citizens. Adaline was not listed as a physician in the 1874 or 1877 Butler or the 1886 Polk medical directories; Gideon was in all three. (In 1874, there were only forty physicians in the territory.) Gideon practiced medicine, Adaline was probably occupied with raising the children. In 1874, they established a private infirmary, and Adaline almost certainly would have been involved in that project.

In 1876, Gideon was elected mayor of Seattle, an office he held capably for two terms. He was connected with a hospital established for the indigent sick of the county, and he was a regent of the Territorial University for ten years. He was an organizer (1873) of the Territorial Medical Society and, after its reorganization in 1879, its first president. Though retiring and modest, he was interested in politics, was a fighter for causes, and with other citizens successfully defied the greed of the railroad in its attempt to "treat the territory and its people as its property." He was an abolitionist and, later, a Prohibitionist. Adaline was "well-known throughout our city, and has always been foremost in religion, philanthropic and moral reform work. Her influence upon the social life of our city has been pronounced and in every way beneficial." During the almost quarter century the Weeds lived in Seattle, the town grew to fifty thousand inhabitants. The Weeds had prospered, not by medical practice but by investing in real estate.

In 1895, the Weeds retired and moved back to California to live in Berkeley with their daughter Mabel. Gideon, having been an invalid for some years, died in April 1905. Adaline died September 9, 1910. Her role as practicing physician had long since ended. Her brief obituary in the *Seattle Times* did not even mention her professional standing but said, simply, "During her residence here [she] was well known for her many works of charity."

References: Butler, 1874, 1877; Frederic J. Grant, *History of Seattle, Washington* (New York, 1891); H. K. Hines, *An Illustrated History of the State of Washington* (Chicago: Lewis, 1895), 878; Rockwell D. Hunt, *California and Californians*, vol. 3 (Chicago: Lewis, 1932); Polk, 1886; Gideon's obituary, *Seattle Post Intelligencer*, April 23, 1905; Obituary, *Seattle Post Intelligencer*, September 11, 1910; Obituary, *Seattle Sunday Times*, September 11, 1910; Margaret Strachan, "Early-Day Mansions, No. 47—Dr. G. A. Weed," *Seattle Times*, July 22, 1945; US census, 1850, 1880, 1900, 1910; US Internal Revenue Service tax assessment lists, Washoe City, Nevada, December 1863 and May 1865; Washington Territorial census, 1885; *Water-Cure Journal* 24 (July 1857): 15; *Water-Cure Journal* 24 (November 1857): 107; *Water-Cure Journal* 30 (September 1860): 42; Adaline Weed, "Water-Cure Travels on the Pacific Coast," *Water-Cure Journal* 31 (1861): 40.

Eliza E. L. WILLIS (b. ca. 1815)

Eliza E. L. Willis was born in New York State about 1815. Her maiden name and information about her parents, childhood, and early education are lacking. Sometime after 1840, she married John Ellis (b. ca. 1818). In the 1840s, they were living in Leroy, in Western New York, had two children, John F. (b. May 1846) and Fannie E. (b. ca. 1848). Young John died on August 30, 1848, to be followed eight days later by his father. They are buried in Myrtle Street Cemetery. Eliza was probably a native of Leroy, because she later mentions that several other members of her family were sick at the time, suggesting something like cholera or diphtheria. The 1850 census show Eliza and "Fanny" still living in Leroy.

Eliza soon entered Syracuse Medical College, an Eclectic school, and received an MD degree in April 1852. She was class valedictorian and, in her valedictory address, "Medical Education of Women," she provided some clues to her motivation for becoming a doctor:

> The necessity of having a class of educated women who are properly qualified to take care of the sick, has been deeply impressed on my mind in a manner that can never be forgotten.—While my husband was lying on a sickbed which proved to him the bed of death, my little son was taken with the same disease. I was obliged to leave the bed-side of my husband to attend upon the dying hours of my child; at the same time there were three other of my family on the sick-bed. O! what would I not have given then for a nurse that I could trust with my loved ones. But such could not be found; no price could procure them. But with much effort the Physician procured a *man nurse* whom he declared superior to any woman in the country. I shall never forget the morning after my little son breathed his last, when I returned to the bed-side of my husband to see how he fared.—His first exclamation was "O! how glad I am that you have come; you don't know what care I have had." The Doctor then came in and said

very exultingly, "Good morning, Mr. Willis, how do you like your new nurse, don't you find him first rate." "Ah! Doctor, said he looking up with a most ironical *smile*, These men may do very well to nurse sick *cows* and *horses*, but give me a woman to nurse me what little time I have to stay."

Sometime between graduation and the following August, Mrs. Ellis may have married Dr. E. S. Strong, for in the August 1852 issue of the *American Medical & Surgical Journal* is written, "the Saratoga Analytic Institute and Infirmary . . . owned by Dr. E. S. Strong and his lady, Mrs. E. L. Strong, M.D., a graduate of Syracuse Medical College." This can hardly be anyone other than Eliza. At the institute, in addition to water treatment, other remedies were used that were "innocent and efficient in their action." The institute must have lasted at least a few years, in competition with the more famous Saratoga Water Cure operated by Nathan Bedortha. In M. L. North's book, *Analysis of Saratoga Waters; also of Sharon, Avon, Virginia, and the Mineral Waters of the United States*, is the following description: "Dr. E. S. Strong, and his wife, also a regular physician, have an institution at Saratoga for treatment of female complaints and weaknesses, on the plan of the celebrated Dr. Hamilton of Rochester."

Whether Mrs. E. L. Strong, MD, was, in fact, Eliza Willis cannot presently be confirmed. If she was, the couple must have parted ways, and Eliza assumed her former name. The 1860 census shows Eliza Willis and Fanny living in the Fourth San Francisco District, with F. Snell, a twenty-three-year-old male clerk, and O. Snell, a sixteen-year-old druggist whose personal worth was $7,000. The 1870 census has Eliza, now fifty-six, listed as a physician in San Jose. She was said to have $400 in personal property. Presumably, she was practicing medicine there. No death date for Eliza has been found. She does not appear as Eliza Willis in the 1880 census and may, by then, have remarried or died.

Bibliography: Mrs. E. L. Willis, "Female Medical Education," *American Medical & Surgical Journal* (Syracuse), September 1851, 181–83; Eliza L. Willis, MD, "Valedictory Address, Syracuse Medical College," *Religious Recorder*, 1852(?), Edward G. Miner Library, University of Rochester, photocopy, place of publication and exact date of this newspaper has not been determined.

References: *American Medical & Surgical Journal* (Syracuse), August 1852, 191; Cooley's, *Tombstone Inscriptions from Abandoned Genesee County Cemeteries* (Batavia, NY, 1952); M. L. North, *Analysis of Saratoga Waters*, 6th ed. (Saratoga Springs, NY, 1855), 68; US census, 1850, 1860, 1870.

Phila *Osgood* WILMARTH (1806–59)

Phila was an Osgood of Wendell, Massachusetts, the fourth of five children of Joseph Osgood and Sarah Graves. Mr. Osgood was a farmer who, for that day, was considered prosperous. Phila was born November 21, 1806, in Wendell. She would have no more than a common school education. She did not become a doctor of medicine until she was forty-nine years old and was able to practice for only four and a half years before her death, a practice that was primarily obstetrics. Like many of her female colleagues, she had lost her husband and two of her four children before entering medical school.

In 1830, a Dr. Butler Wilmarth from nearby Montague, Massachusetts, had been called to see Phila's sick father. One thing led to another, and, a year later, she and Dr. Wilmarth were married. Phila was twenty-four, Butler thirty-two. Phila was described as "unassuming, modest, retiring, amiable, gentle, and Christian." They set up housekeeping in the easternmost (and least fashionable) part of Montague, where Butler had built a one-and-a-half story house for them. Here they stayed for three or four years. Wilmarth's practice grew, especially in surrounding towns, and around 1834 they moved to nearby Leverett. Between 1831 and 1841 they had four children, but only two survived infancy.

Butler was the illegitimate son of Peggy Coleman and, at the age of two, was bound out by the village selectmen to Amos Wilmarth of Rowe, Massachusetts, until he was twenty-one. Wilmarth adopted the boy. For a while, Butler taught school in Montague. At the age of twenty-three he apprenticed himself to Dr. William F. Selden of Amherst and later worked with Dr. Brigham of Greenfield, but he never took lectures at a medical school or obtained a license.

In 1844, Butler and Phila joined the Hopedale Community, a utopian experiment at Milford, Massachusetts, that hoped to amalgamate religion with industry. From that community, ill health sent Butler to the water-cure at New Lebanon, New York in 1847, where he seemed to benefit and whose methods he subsequently embraced. He returned to Hopedale intending to establish a water-cure infirmary. He was able to raise sufficient capital, refitted a large house owned by the community, and opened the institution in September 1850 under the management of the two Wilmarths. Patients were charged four to five dollars a week, plus laundry. It failed to prosper. In the spring of 1851, Dr. Wilmarth took charge of the water-cure at New Graefenburg, New York, and moved there with his family. From here, on February 2, 1852, he wrote to Dr. J. H. Hero, with whom he would soon open a water-cure at Westborough, Massachusetts: "If the Lord will, my wife and [daughter]

Phila will soon leave here—Phila for Hopedale School, and my wife for a higher school, viz., 'The Boston Female Medical College.'" Phila did enroll in the New England Female Medical College in 1852 but did not graduate from that school.

Wilmarth had been elected president of the Hydropathic Association of Physicians and Surgeons in 1851. On May 6, 1853, still president and on his way to the annual meeting in New York City, Butler Wilmarth was drowned when the train in which he was riding encountered an open drawbridge and sank in the Connecticut River. Phila, then forty-seven, was left with a twenty-one-year-old son and a twelve-year-old daughter. Two years later, probably with the help of the Hopedale Community in caring for young Phila, and apparently with financial help from the railroad, she graduated with an MD degree from the Female Medical College of Pennsylvania. Returning to Hopedale, she advertised that she "was prepared to attend the problems of the women of the surrounding towns." For the next four and a half years until her death, she practiced obstetrics. Phila died, at fifty-three, on August 14, 1859.

References: Adin Ballou, *History of Hopedale Community, from Its Inception to Its Virtual Submergence in the Hopedale Parish* (Lowell, MA, 1897), 204–6; William H. Fish, *Memoir of Butler Wilmarth, M.D.* (Boston, 1854); Ira Osgood, *Osgood Genealogy* (Salem, MA, n.d.); Edward Spann, *Hopedale: From Commune to Company Town 1840–1920* (Columbus, Ohio, 1992), 60–61.

Angeline M. *Lockwood* WILSON Moore (1837–1905)

Angeline M. Lockwood was born in May 1837 in Lafayette, Indiana, daughter of Rufus Lockwood and his wife Harriet. Her father, "a lawyer of wealth and prominence," was lost on the ill-fated ship *Central America* on which he was returning with his family from California, where he had visited his friend and client, Gen. John C. Fremont. Angeline had two sisters and a brother.

Of her education nothing is known. She married McK. Wilson, of Crawfordsville, Indiana. The marriage was short lived, the family fortune was lost, and Angeline decided to go medical school. She attended and graduated in 1859 with an MD degree from Penn Medical University in Philadelphia. She probably went from there to St. Louis; at least, that is where the *Progressive Annuals* for 1863 and 1864 locate her. In July 1865, she paid the IRS tax on physicians and was then living in Decatur, Illinois. But she must have soon moved to Chicago, where she studied at Hahnemann Medical College and Hospital and practiced medicine until after the Great Fire in 1871, when she moved to Terre Haute, Indiana, and lived the rest of her life.

In Terre Haute, according to her obituary:

> she built up a splendid practice in the city, numbering among her patients the most prominent families in the city, whose men as well as the women employed her exclusively. She was not only a skillful practitioner but a wonderful nurse. In those early days there were no trained nurses. When she had a serious case she stayed right with it day and night until the danger was passed. . . . She not only cured her patients but accumulated money and established herself in society, entertaining with a generous hospitality and becoming the center of the merry throng, with her wit and general information.
>
> On June 14, 1884, she married Thaddeus S. Moore, a job printer. It was "the best thing she ever did," she is quoted as saying. During the last ten years of her life, she was an invalid, bedridden, and cared for by her husband and adopted stepdaughter, Agnes Parker Moore. She died February 6, 1906, and is buried at Highland Cemetery. Though she attended the First Congregational Church, "she never made any especial profession of church religion." Angeline was a woman "of more than ordinary interest . . . her deeds of kindness, her influence for good can not be numbered."

References: Butler, 1874; Illinois State Archives, June 14, 1884 [Wilson and Moore married in Cook County]; Polk, 1886, 1890, 1893, 1896; *Progressive Annual*, 1863, 1864; *Terre Haute City Directory*, 1874, 1890, 1892; Obituary, *Terre Haute Saturday Spectator*, February 11, 1905; US census, 1900; US Internal Revenue Service tax list for Decatur, IL, July 1865.

Phebe *WILSON* (b. ca. 1815–90)

Phebe Wilson was born about 1815 in Pennsylvania, probably at Old Kennett. Nothing is known about her background, parents, childhood, or early education except that she was a Quaker. In the mid-1850s, she matriculated at the Female Medical College of Pennsylvania and graduated with an MD degree in 1857 at the age of forty-two. The *Progressive Annual* for 1864 lists her as a practicing physician in Kennett Square. In the 1870 US census she was still in Kennett Square, was practicing as a physician, held $1,400 in real estate and $1,000 in personal wealth, and lived with Hannah G. Pennock, a fifty-four-year-old "gentlewoman." She was in Kennett Square at the time of the 1880 census but then living with her sister-in-law, Ellen Wilson, sixty, and her two grown children (a carpenter and a seamstress), and a second sister-in-law, Lydia Wilson. Then sixty-five, Phebe was listed as a "doctor." The 1886 Polk medical directory places her in Hamorton, Pennsylvania, a village of 175 in Chester County. Dr. Phebe died August 17, 1890, in Wilmington, Delaware, in her seventy-sixth year and was buried in Old Kennett. She probably practiced medicine in Chester County, Pennsylvania, for thirty years.

References: *Friends' Intelligencer and Journal* 47 (1890): 553; Polk, 1886; US census, 1870, 1880.

Martha *Butterworth* WITHAM (1834–1915)

Martha Butterworth was born in Ohio in 1834. Nothing is known of her background, parents, childhood, or early education. In 1856, then twenty-two, she married Charles Emerson Witham. Witham, born in Maine in 1830, had graduated with an MD degree from Eclectic Medical Institute in Cincinnati that same year. Three years later, in 1859, Martha became a doctor of medicine, with a degree from Cincinnati's other Eclectic medical school, the Eclectic College of Medicine. The Withams did not have children.

Subsequent knowledge of the couple comes entirely from census data. In 1860, they were in Maineville, Ohio, a village about twenty miles northeast of Cincinnati. Charles must have been doing reasonably well. He is listed as having $2,000 in real estate and $4,000 in personal property. Sometime before 1870, the Withams moved to Wilton Junction, Iowa, a village twenty miles west of Davenport. Charles continued to prosper, by then having $6,000 in real estate and $20,000 in personal property. Martha herself is listed as having $1,500 in real estate and $6,000 in personal property. This makes it likely that she was practicing medicine. However, though the census reports for 1860, 1870, 1880, 1900, and 1910 all denote Charles "phys. & surg.," or "gen. pract.," Martha is listed as "keeping house" or has no designation. Such labels were common practice in the late nineteenth century and are often encountered in connection with those definitely known to be in practice.

The Withams remained in Wilton until 1886. That year they moved to Lawrence, Kansas, a community larger than Wilton Junction, located twenty-five miles east of Topeka, forty miles west of Kansas City, Missouri, and home of the University of Kansas. They remained there the rest of their lives. Charles is listed as a practicing physician in every Polk medical directory from 1886 through 1902 and in American Medical Association directories for 1906, 1909 (he is no longer in practice), and 1912. Both Charles and Martha are listed in the 1915 Kansas State census. No death dates have been found. Whether Martha practiced medicine cannot be determined with certainty. Most likely, she did.

References: *American Medical Directory*, 1906, 1909, 1912; Kansas State census, 1915; Polk, 1886, 1890, 1893, 1896, 1898, 1900, 1902; US census, 1860, 1870, 1880, 1900, 1910.

Lamoille WITHERBY (b. ca. 1806–81)

Lamoille Witherby was born about 1806 in Williston, Vermont. We have no knowledge of her maiden name, her parents, background, or early education. Sometime before 1847 she married Silas Charles Witherby. Their son, Charles E. Witherby, was born in 1847. After the fall session, the following year, Silas graduated from Castleton Medical College. He must have practiced in Vermont for a while: the *History of Colchester* records that Dr. L. F. Burdick, the oldest practitioner in Colchester, had studied medicine with Dr. Witherby, then in Westford, Vermont, before himself graduating from Castleton Medical College in 1852. In 1854, seven-year-old Charles died. The Witherbys must have had at least one other son.

Sometime between 1852 and 1860, the Witherbys moved to the Canton, New York, area, where Silas continued to practice. He is listed in the 1860 census as a physician in Canton, owning $500 in real estate and $100 in personal property. Lamoille attended the New England Female Medical College in Boston, graduated with an MD degree in 1861, and started her own practice in Canton. Four years later, Silas died (June 6, 1865) and was buried in Essex Common Burial Ground, Essex, Vermont, where, in another plot, his parents and son are also buried. Sometime thereafter, Lamoille moved to San Francisco. Her name appears in San Francisco directories regularly from 1868 through 1881 as a physician. In the ten directories consulted, covering a period of fifteen years, she is listed at five different addresses. Lamoille died July 31, 1881, in San Francisco, at the age of seventy-six. Her funeral was held at the home of her son, Daniel S. Witherby, a broker.

References: Lists of burials in Essex Common Burial Ground, Essex, Vermont; W. S. Rann, *History of Chittenden County, Vermont* (Syracuse: D. Mason & Co., 1886), 553–68; San Francisco city directory, 1868, 1869, 1871, 1872, 1874, 1875, 1876, 1879, 1880, 1881; Death notice, *San Francisco Morning Call*, August 2, 1881, p. 4, col. 5; US census, 1860.

Mary Ellen *WOLFE* (1835–60)

Mary Ellen Wolfe was born January 27, 1835, in Lewisburg, Pennsylvania, daughter of Samuel Wolfe and Catherine Lawshe and sister of Charles S. Wolfe. She attended the Female Institute that had been recently (1853) organized in Lewisburg. In her late teens, she enrolled at Penn Medical University, an Eclectic school in Philadelphia, and graduated with an MD degree in 1856, when she was twenty-one years old. Unfortunately, she contracted tuberculosis, from which she died on November 15, 1860. Curiously, her listing in the 1860 census labels her as "insane."

She was said to have been "foremost in the battle to win the right to vote," so she may have been able to practice medicine during the three or four years between her graduation and her death. She is listed as a practicing physician in the 1864 *Progressive Annual*, which suggests two things: one, she did practice medicine, at least for a while, and, two, there is a lag in the data found in the *Progressive Annual*.

A photograph of her and one of her medical school lecture tickets is shown in the Union County history "Silhouettes" (8). Dr. Wolfe's niece, Mary Moore Wolfe, attended and graduated from Bucknell (1896) and University of Michigan Medical School (1899), and was a psychiatrist at Norristown (PA) State Hospital, Women's Division.

References: Lois Kalp, *Silhouettes: The Historic, Memorable and Notable Women of Union County, Pennsylvania 1785–1985* (Lewisburg, PA, 1985); Tombstone in the Lewisburg Cemetery provides birth and death dates.

Olive Chesilla *Arnold* WOOD (b. ca. 1820–86?)

Olive Arnold was born about 1820, probably in Herkimer County in Central New York's Mohawk River Valley. Nothing has been found about her background, childhood, or early education. She was one of nine children (four girls and five boys) of George Arnold and his wife. On August 25, 1847, Olive married William W. Wood, a local farmer, in Fairfield, New York. They had two children, Elena (b. ca. 1847) and Annie D. (or Annice), born about 1852.

The 1850 census shows the Wood family living with Olive's eighty-year-old father. The mother was not listed and had probably died. There was also a two-month-old male child, Orsman, that must have died before the 1860 census. By 1860, the family had moved to nearly Utica, where William was listed as being a millwright and Olive a physician. Olive had attended and graduated from the New York Hygeio-Therapeutic College with an MD degree in 1859. She is listed in Utica directories for 1861–62 and 1863–64. On August 4, 1864, she served as recording secretary for a temperance mass meeting in nearby Eatonville.

Sometime between 1864 and 1878 William died, and Olive and Annie moved to Atchison City, Kansas. The 1880 census lists Olive as a widow and a physician, Annie as a schoolteacher. Hoyne (1881) records her as a homoeopath in Atchison, and the 1880 Atchison city directory has an advertisement for "Mrs. O. C. Wood, M.D., Homoeopathic physician, 426 Commercial Street (upstairs). Residence west side Sixth Street, 2d door above Parallel." Office hours were 9–11 a.m. and 2–5 p.m. The 1880 census also showed a twenty-four-year-old boarder, Robert F. Fitzpatrick, living with the Woods; he was a schoolteacher. On August 11, 1880, Robert and Annie were married by the rector of Trinity Church.

By 1883, Olive had moved to Topeka and was living there alone. A city directory lists her that year and also in 1885–86 as a physician, as does the Kansas State census for 1885. Olive's whereabouts subsequent to 1885 and the date of her death are unknown. She was not in the 1887–88 Topeka directory, the 1890 census data were lost, and the 1900 census does not list her. She probably died about 1886.

References: George Arnold's will, probated September 1, 1856, recorded K/244, Town of Fairfield, NY; *Hoyne's Annual Directory of Homoeopathic Physicians in the State of Illinois, for the Year 1881* (Chicago, 1881); Kansas State census, 1885; Marriage notice, *Mohawk Currier* (New York), September 2, 1847; *Oneida Weekly Herald* (New York), August 20, 1864; US census, 1850, 1860, 1880, 1900; Utica city directory, 1861–62, 1863–64.

Zelinda *WOOD* Watkins (b. ca. 1833–96)

Zelinda Wood was born February 17, 1833, though her place of birth and the names of her parents have yet to be identified. Nor is there information about her early education. When Zelinda attended Penn Medical University in Philadelphia, she was recorded as a resident of Pennsylvania, was already married to a Mr. Wood, and had a daughter, Hattie, born in 1852. Possibly Mr. Wood had died, and, as a widow, she was seeking a livelihood. After graduation, in 1860, she went to the Grand Ligne Mission, a Baptist organization proselytizing in Roman Catholic Quebec. She is located there in 1863 and 1864 editions of *Progressive Annual* as a practicing physician. How long she remained at that work is not known.

About 1870, she met and married the Rev. Benjamin Utter Watkins, father of four grown children by a previous marriage, and went to live with him in Pearl Lake Place in southwest Minnesota, just north of the Iowa border, where she practiced medicine and helped run the farm. Later, probably about 1884 when his son-in-law Datus bought the farm in Pearl Lake, Zelinda and Benjamin moved to Cameron, Missouri. Watkins had relatives there and was called to ministry at a local church. He died in Cameron, March 15, 1892, at the age of eighty-one. In the fall of 1895 Zelinda moved to Des Moines, and, the following spring, she had surgery for a large fibroid and died the next day, April 24, 1896. She is buried in Woodland Cemetery, Des Moines.

One of her stepchildren, writing about the family, said of Zelinda:

> She was a woman who in early life, through much energy and exertion, had obtained a good education; she had studied French and prepared herself to be a teacher, as well as taking her medical degree. She went as a missionary teacher and physician to the French provinces of Canada under a Baptist Mission Board. She was of a courageous and independent character, ready for emergencies. When our father married her, she was a widow with one child, a daughter. After their marriage, father returned to Minnesota and settled down again at Pearl Lake Place. Here he spent some years among the quiet scenes of rural life. Father passed much time in his study and with the pen. He wrote for the Original Essay columns of a church paper, *The Christian Standard*, for years, while his wife looked after the household and practiced medicine as opportunity offered.

The farm was run with hired help.

One of Zelinda's stepsons, J. R. Watkins, established the well-known J. R. Watkins Medical Company, which operated well into the twentieth century. Zelinda's obituary relates that she spoke several languages, was noted for her good works, "especially in the interests of home and foreign missions . . . was a skilled physician and practiced with success . . . and was personally acquainted with many of the leading men and women in the Christian church throughout the Union."

References: Obituary, *Daily Observer* (Cameron, MO), April 25, 1896; Julia W. Frost, *Annals of Our Ancestors* (Chicago: Privately printed, 1913) [photograph of Z.W.W.]; *Progressive Annual*, 1863, 1864.

Mary *WRIGHT* Pierson (1824–1900)

Mary Wright was born December 26, 1824, in Eagleville, a village in what is now Ashtabula County, in northeast Ohio. She was the youngest of thirteen surviving children (ten girls, three boys) of Moses Wright Jr., nine of whom were born to his second wife, Esther Hurd.

The Wrights had come from Connecticut, where they had played a prominent role. Moses's father, Moses Sr., built the first house in Goshen, was a deacon in the Congregational Church in Colebrook, and fought in the Revolutionary army. His son, Moses Jr., was a selectman at Colebrook (1799–1806) and representative in the legislature in 1806. But misfortune befell the younger Moses's family. Moses Jr. lost his wife, stillborn twin boys, and, in 1804, his daughter Anna. In 1803, he married Esther Hurd. In 1807, he went to Ohio, where he bought two hundred acres near Eagleville, and in 1808 the whole family moved west. Four surviving daughters by his first wife and two by the second made the trip in a covered wagon drawn by oxen. It was another sixteen years before Mary was born; by then her oldest half sister, Clarissy, was thirty-three. Mary's closest siblings were her brothers Seth and Alvin, six and four years her senior.

Mary attended a one-room school and later went to Oberlin College for seven years while she taught school in Austinburg. Once finished, the male students received baccalaureate degrees; Mary was given a four-year literary certificate. From there, she went on to the American Medical College in Cincinnati, where she was required to sit sequestered behind a glass-bead curtain during biology lectures. The school soon failed and was assimilated into the Eclectic Medical Institute (from which women graduated between 1853 and 1857, but not in the years immediately following). Mary went to New England Female Medical College in Boston, graduated with an MD degree in 1858, and returned to Eagleville to set up in practice.

On May 8, 1859, then thirty-five, Mary married Julius Egbert Pierson, a local farmer ten years her senior. The couple moved to nearby Kirtland, where they would settle, and raised a family of four. Family tradition holds that Mary practiced medicine for a time, but available evidence suggests that this was not a full-time profession. Her name appears in none of the standard medical directories of the period. In both the 1870 and 1900 census lists, she is listed as a housekeeper, not as a physician.

But whether she practiced or not, she made a contribution of another kind to the medical profession: her eldest son, Egbert Alvin Pierson, became progenitor of physicians. Mary's grandson, Marshall Pierson, became the first ear, nose, and throat specialist in Akron, Ohio; her great-grandson, Marshall Pierson Jr., practiced medicine in Cuyahoga Falls (1947–96); her great-great-granddaughter, Susan Pierson, was a neurologist in Hyannis, Massachusetts; and great-great-great grandson, Joseph Pierson, recently graduated from Ohio State

Medical School and is in an anesthesiology residency program in Chicago. Mary's husband, Julius, died September 20, 1885, in Kirtland. Mary died there March 17, 1900.

References: Untitled, undated newspaper clipping in the Genealogical Collection, Geneva Public Library (OH) regarding family of Moses Wright; Two-page typewritten article titled "Wright Genealogy" at the Geneva Public Library; Two-page typewritten article titled "Moses Wright" at the Geneva Public Library; Mark J. Price, "Local History: Amazing Women," *Beacon Journal* (Akron, OH), March 2, 2009; US census, 1850, 1860, 1870.

Y

Margaret G. *YOUNG* Coleman (1822–1904)

Margaret Young was the first woman doctor of medicine in north central Pennsylvania. She was born in Glasgow, Scotland, in April 1822, the eldest daughter, second child of John Young and Mary Anderson. The family immigrated to New York in June 1827. Her father, a practical geologist, worked first in public works in Rhode Island, then went to Pennsylvania where he managed two different iron works and a coal company, eventually settling on a farm in Tioga County, Pennsylvania. Margaret had an academic education at schools in Elmira and Canandaigua, in Western New York, and soon began a career as teacher at rural schools in Lycoming and Tioga Counties, at the villages of Blossburg, Ralston, Jackson, and Block House. Later, she worked as a governess on a plantation in the South.

In 1849, when she was twenty-seven, two brothers and a sister died of typhoid fever, "because of improper treatment, as [Margaret] fully believed. She resolved to study medicine." She read medicine for two years, attended lectures at Penn Medical University for three years, and graduated with an MD degree in 1858 when she was thirty-six years old. Thereafter, she settled in Williamsport where she practiced medicine for more than forty years, specializing in women's diseases.

On June 14, 1864, then forty-two, she married German immigrant Joseph Coleman, aged twenty-six. He worked as a carpenter, groom, livery man, and grocer. The couple had one son, Albert, born in 1866 when Margaret was forty-three. The family lived in an Italianate-style "mansion" at 20 High Street (later #406), where they offered rooms to out-of-town patients. The establishment had a Hoffman electrotherapeutic bath cabinet in which Dr. Coleman gave "Russian, Turkish, electro-vapor, and electro-medicated baths." The 1870 census lists an apparently unrelated child, six years older than Albert, living with the family.

About 1877, Margaret moved to Ocean Grove, New Jersey, a seaside resort, religious center, and early feminist enclave, where she established a spa at Block House. Here she offered first-class accommodations and treatment with electro-therapeutic baths. Apparently not a successful venture, she was back in Williamsport living with Joseph by the time of the 1880 census. The couple was soon living apart again.

Husband Joseph died of tetanus in 1894. Son Albert, who had attended medical school in Washington but did not finish, took over management of the family grocery store at the corner of Sherman and Sheridan Streets. Margaret sold the house on High Street and moved in with Albert. Later, they rented rooms at 812 Washington Street, where Albert died, in August 1900 at the age of thirty-four. Margaret died four years later on January 9, 1904. She had been a member of the Second Presbyterian Church.

References: Judith Gouldin, *Williamsport Sun-Gazette*, August 10, 2014; John Meginness, *History of Lycoming County, Pennsylvania* (Chicago, 1892), 801.

Sarah H. YOUNG (b. ca. 1822)

Sarah was born about 1822, in New Hampshire. Names of parents and first name of Mr. Young, her husband, are not known. Sarah, already married, received an MD degree from Penn Medical University in Philadelphia in 1856. She was a resident of Lowell, Massachusetts, at the time. Though her name is not found in the 1857 or 1858 *Massachusetts Register*s, she is listed as a physician in Lowell directories for 1860 and 1861, as well as the *Massachusetts Business Directory* for 1860. Her name is not listed in the 1867 *Massachusetts Register*, the 1868 *Massachusetts Business Directory*, or the 1869 *Massachusetts Register and Business Directory*. There is a Sarah Young, widow, listed in Lowell in 1865.

Sarah was a signatory to the Articles of Association for an Old Ladies' Home in Lowell on April 20, 1862 (along with Rachel Allyn, MD; q.v.). *Progressive Annuals* for 1862, 1863, and 1864 place her as a physician in San Francisco. There is a Sarah Young listed in the 1860 census of San Francisco, but this conflicts with the Lowell directory data. Also, no vocation is given. *Progressive Annual* data are frequently outdated. This leads to a reasonable speculation that Sarah may have gone to San Francisco immediately after graduation from medical school, stayed until after the 1860 census, at which time she returned to Lowell. Sometime after 1865, Sarah must have remarried, moved, or died.

References: California State census, 1860; Lowell, MA, city directory, 1860 and 1861; *Massachusetts Register*, 1867; *New England Business Directory*, 1860; *New England Business Directory*, 1868; *Progressive Annual*, 1862, 1863, 1864.

Z

Marie Elizabeth *ZAKRZEWSKA* (1829–1902)

Marie Zakrzewska (pronounced Zakchefska) was born in Berlin on September 6, 1829, the eldest of seven children (four girls, one boy, two early deaths) of Martin Ludwig Zakrzewski (*sic*) and his wife Caroline Fredericke. The Zakrzewski grandparents had migrated from Poland to Prussia in the eighteenth century after the invasion of Poland by Russia and the pre-emption of the family's property. The family forsook Roman Catholicism for the Lutheran Church but retained the liberal political sentiments of Polish republicanism. Martin Ludwig worked his way up to junior officer in the Prussian army, a post that opened to him a place in the civil service. His wife, said to have gypsy ancestry, was a midwife and carried on a long family tradition of being healers.

Marie herself became a midwife, following in her mother's footsteps. After training at Berlin's Charité hospital, she became for six months head midwife at that institution. Even at this early time in Berlin, the thought of establishing her own hospital for women and children was on her mind. But the fact that women in the United States could now become doctors of medicine attracted her. A close friend is reported to have told her that "in America women will now become physicians like men; this shows that only in a republic can it be proved that science has no sex" (Tuchman).

And so, in 1853, with her parents' consent, accompanied by her younger sister Anna (at her father's insistence), she sailed for New York. Her plan to attend the Female Medical College of Pennsylvania may have been aborted by her lack of facility with English, a great problem for her at first. At her boarding house she "never conversed with anyone . . . not even asked for anything at the table; but was supplied like a mute" (ibid.). Instead, she enrolled at the medical department of Western Reserve College in Cleveland. There, she had the good fortune to be sponsored first by Caroline Severance and, later, by Amory

Mayo, pastor of the Unitarian Church. These people introduced her to social activities—the abolition, temperance, woman's rights, and woman's suffrage movements—movements to which she was, at first, resistant. With the removal of the Severances to Boston, Marie moved in with her classmate, Sarah Ann Chadwick (q.v.).

Marie did well in medical school. In 1855, her mother and two sisters were immigrating to the United States, but the mother died en route and was buried at sea. In March 1856, Marie graduated with an MD degree, and returned to New York City, where she worked with the Blackwell sisters in establishing the New York Infirmary for Women and Children, which opened in 1857. Two years later she moved to Boston, where she would spend the rest of her life.

At least one of Marie's reasons for leaving New York was to organize her own hospital; in New York she would always be second in command. In Boston, after a three-year stint as director of the new clinical department at the New England Female Medical College, she established the New England Hospital for Women and Children. She remained its director for twenty-five years and was significantly involved in the years after her retirement.

Dr. Zakrzewska died May 12, 1902. Three days later, her friends gathered at the hospital to hear one of the directors read some words Marie had written three months earlier in anticipation of her departure. Over the years of her life, others spoke of her "magnetism," of her "fearless courage and persuasive tongue." Friend William Lloyd Garrison, prominent abolitionist and journalist, wrote that she was "a woman of decided opinions and the frankest speech, a circumstance which gave zest and animation to any group in which she mingled." In the words of her excellent biographer, Arleen Tuchman, Dr. Zakrzewska thought "too much sympathy and compassion confused one's ability to reason, thus making it impossible to provide good medical care."

Bibliography: *Introductory Lecture, Delivered Wednesday, November 2, before the New England Female Medical College at the Opening Term of 1859–60* (Boston, 1859); *A Practical Illustration of "Woman's Right to Labor"; or, A Letter from Marie E. Zakrzewska, M.D.* (Boston, 1860); "Report of 187 Cases of Midwifery in Private Practice," *Boston Medical & Surgical Journal* 121 (1889): 557–60.

References: *Notable American Women 1607–1950*, 3:702–4; Virginia G. Drachman, *Hospital with a Heart* (Ithaca, NY, 1984); *Dictionary of American Medical Biography*, 2:834; R. M. Morantz-Sanchez, *Sympathy and Science* (New York, 1985); *New England Hospital: For Women and Children,*

Marie Elizabeth Zakrzewska; A Memoir (Boston, 1903); Arleen M. Tuchman, *Science Has No Sex* (Chapel Hill, NC, 2006), 3, 53, 73; Agnes C. Vietor, *A Woman's Quest* (New York, 1924).

Eliza J. *ZIMMERMAN* Burnside (1831–1915)

Eliza Zimmerman was born August 23, 1831, in New Windsor, Maryland, the eldest of at least four children (three girls and a boy) of John and Hannah Zimmerman. The family moved to Tiffin, Ohio, when Eliza was still a child, and it was there that she attended public schools. In 1858, she enrolled at the Female Medical College of Pennsylvania, and, after three annual courses, she graduated in 1860 with an MD degree. Later that same year, on June 19, she married Thomas J. Burnside, for many years a teacher at Pennsylvania Institute for the Deaf and Dumb in Philadelphia. Eliza practiced medicine in Philadelphia from the time of her graduation until about 1908, a total of forty-eight years. Her name is found regularly in Philadelphia, Butler, and Polk directories as a physician. The couple had no children. After her husband's death in 1897, she continued to practice for about ten more years and then retired to her childhood home in Tiffin, where she lived with her younger sister, Ruth Arnold. Dr. Zimmerman-Burnside, as she was known, died May 28, 1915, at eighty-three. She is buried in Tiffin's Greenlawn Cemetery.

References: Butler, 1874, 1877; *Medical and Dental Directory of Pennsylvania, New Jersey and Delaware, 1907–08*; Philadelphia city directory; Polk, 1886 et seq.; *Progressive Annual*, 1864; Obituary, *Tiffin Daily Tribune*, May 28, 1915; Women's Medical College of Pennsylvania, *Transactions of the Forty-First Annual Meeting of the Alumnae Association, June 1 and 2, 1916* (Philadelphia, 1916), 34.

Appendix A

CHRONOLOGICAL LIST OF GRADUATES
AND THE SCHOOLS THEY ATTENDED

Note: Surnames at graduation are in uppercase. Maiden surnames, when known, are in italics. An *x* preceding a name signifies that no information has been found about that person. An asterisk preceding a name signifies that the medical school attended then had a limited or no charter. A question mark before a name means that documentation of graduation has not been confirmed.

Year Graduated	Name	Institution
1849 January 24	*BLACKWELL*, Elizabeth	Geneva Medical Institution
1850 June 5	FOWLER, Lydia *Folger*	Central Medical College
1851 February 20	*ADAMSON* Dolley, Sarah Read	Central Medical College
1851 February 20	GLEASON, Rachel *Brooks*	Central Medical College
1851 March 6	GLEASON, Margaretta *Baldwin*	Syracuse Medical College
1851 December 6	**AUSTIN*, Harriet Newell	American Hydropathic Institute (see also 1859)
1851 December 30	*ELLIS*, Susanna H.	Female Medical College of Pennsylvania
1851 December 30	HUNT, Angenette A. *Payne*	Female Medical College of Pennsylvania
1851 December 30	*LONGSHORE* Potts, Anna Mary	Female Medical College of Pennsylvania
1851 December 30	LONGSHORE, Hannah E. *Myers*	Female Medical College of Pennsylvania
1851 December 30	MITCHELL, Frances G.	Female Medical College of Pennsylvania

(continued)

Year Graduated	Name	Institution
1851 December 30	*PRESTON*, Ann	Female Medical College of Pennsylvania
1851 December 30	SAWIN, Martha Ann *Hayden*	Female Medical College of Pennsylvania
1851 December 30	*WAY*, Phoebe M.	Female Medical College of Pennsylvania
1852	? McQUIGG, Eliza Jane *Hall*	Syracuse Medical College
1852 February 19	*BRONSON*, Permilia R.	Central Medical College
1852 February 19	DOUD, Lettice *Hyde*	Central Medical College
1852 February 19	xSAWYER, Mary A.	Central Medical College
1852 February 28	x*COOK*, Helen	Western College of Homoeopathic Medicine
1852 March 3	CLARK Binney, Nancy E. *Talbot*	Western Reserve University
1852 March 17	HANCHETT, Mary E. *Baum*	Syracuse Medical College
1852 March 17	WHEELER, Rebecca B.	Syracuse Medical College
1852 March 17	WILLIS, Eliza L.	Syracuse Medical College
1852 May 27	MERRICK, Myra K. *King*	Central Medical College
1852 June 2	*SMITH* Wilder, Mary E.	Syracuse Medical College
1852 June 23	HALL, Lucinda Susanna *Capen*	Worcester Medical Institution
1853 March	BAKER, Clemence S. *Harned* Lozier	Syracuse Medical College
1853 March 27	ADAMS, Charlotte G.	Female Medical College of Pennsylvania
1853 March 27	ANDERSON, Anna N. *Smith*	Female Medical College of Pennsylvania
1853 March 27	BEVERLY, Julia A. *Bridgeham*	Female Medical College of Pennsylvania
1853 March 27	ELLIS, Hannah W.	Female Medical College of Pennsylvania

(continued)

Year Graduated	Name	Institution
1853 March 27	*FOWLER* Ormsbee Breakspear, Almira L.	Female Medical College of Pennsylvania
1853 March 27	JOHNSON, Henrietta W.	Female Medical College of Pennsylvania
1853 March 27	*MINNIS* Homet, Maria	Female Medical College of Pennsylvania
1853 March 27	*MONTGOMERY* Nelson, Augusta R.	Female Medical College of Pennsylvania
1853 March 27	RICHARDSON, Margaret *Phillips*	Female Medical College of Pennsylvania
1853 March 27	*MOWRY*, Martha Harris (ad eundem)	Female Medical College of Pennsylvania
1853	HUNT, Harriot Kezia (hon.)	Female Medical College of Pennsylvania
1853 June	*BROWN* Winslow, Caroline	Eclectic Medical Institute
1853 June	HARRIS, Sophia *Roper*	Worcester Medical Institution
1854	BAILY, Mary Malin *Evans*	Eclectic Medical Institute
1854	*BUNKER* Stockham, Alice	Eclectic Medical Institute
1854	xCLEIS, Margaret	Eclectic Medical Institute
1854	x*CROSHAW*, Mary Eliza	Eclectic Medical Institute
1854	*JUDD* Sartain, Harriet Amelia	Eclectic Medical Institute
1854	*RUMSEY*, Julia	Eclectic Medical Institute
1854	*SMIZER*, Sarah	Eclectic Medical Institute
1854	*ENTRIKIN*, Sarah A.	Penn Medical University
1854	*GRIER*, Maria J.	Penn Medical University
1854	*MYERS*, Jane Viola	Penn Medical University
1854	RANDALL, Marenda *Briggs*	Penn Medical University
1854	x*SMITH*, Susan A.	Penn Medical University
1854 February 16	*AVERELL*, Minerva Jane	Syracuse Medical College

(continued)

Year Graduated	Name	Institution
1854 February 16	?LORD, Laura A.	Syracuse Medical College
1854 February 16	*PORTER*, Dolly Ann	Syracuse Medical College
1854 Feb 25	*BATES*, Elizabeth H.	Female Medical College of Pennsylvania
1854 Feb 25	BROWN, Lucinda *Rowley*	Female Medical College of Pennsylvania
1854 Feb 25	*ELLIGER* Piersol, Minna	Female Medical College of Pennsylvania
1854 Feb 25	*SHATTUCK*, Elizabeth G.	Female Medical College of Pennsylvania
1854 March	*BLACKWELL*, Emily	Western Reserve College Medical Department
1854 March 1	xBARRY, Elsie *Hall*	Western College of Homoeopathic Medicine
1854 March 1	xBLANCHARD, Elizabeth J.	Western College of Homoeopathic Medicine
1854 March 1	*EDSON*, Susan Ann	Western College of Homoeopathic Medicine
1854 March 3	**FLETCHER*, Sophronia	New England Female Medicine College
1854 March 3	*HARRIS, Lucy Amelia *Brown*	New England Female Medicine College
1854 March 3	**JENKS*, Mary Reed	New England Female Medicine College
1854 March 3	*THURSTON, Martha Nichols *Spaulding*	New England Female Medicine College
1854 June	*xANDERSON, L. H. H.	New York Hydropathic and Physiological School
1854 June	**COGSWELL*, Abigail S.	New York Hydropathic and Physiological School
1854 June	*xFIELD, Hannah F.	New York Hydropathic and Physiological School
1854 June	*x*FISHER*, Joanna	New York Hydropathic and Physiological School

(continued)

Year Graduated	Name	Institution
1854 June	*xHOWARD, E. B.	New York Hydropathic and Physiological School
1854 June	*x*JOHNSON*, E. M.	New York Hydropathic and Physiological School
1854 June	*LINES, Amelia *Wilkes*	New York Hydropathic and Physiological School
1854 June	*SCOTT* Seelye, Finette E.	New York Hydropathic and Physiological School
1854 June	*xSTEVENS, Jane A.	New York Hydropathic and Physiological School
1854 June 8	HOES, Minerva *Falley*	Syracuse Medical College
1855 February 3	FREASE, Cecilia Pumpelly *Ricker*	Eclectic Medical Institute
1855 February 3	*FRENCH*, Martha Ann	Eclectic Medical Institute
1855 February 22	*WALKER* Miller, Mary Edwards	Syracuse Medical College
1855 February 28	*CHAMBERLIN, Elizabeth B.	New England Female Medical College
1855 February 28	*WALCOTT Butterfield, Hannah M. *Woodward*	New England Female Medical College
1855 February 28	*BROWN* Winslow, Caroline (her 2nd MD)	Western College of Homoeopathic Medicine
1855 March 10	CLEVELAND, Emeline *Horton*	Female Medical College of Pennsylvania
1855 March 10	*NIVISON*, Samantha S.	Female Medical College of Pennsylvania
1855 March 10	*SMITH* Wilder, Mary E. (her 2nd MD)	Female Medical College of Pennsylvania
1855 March 10	THOMAS, Eliza L. *Smyth*	Female Medical College of Pennsylvania
1855 March 10	*VARNEY* Brownell, Emily A.	Female Medical College of Pennsylvania
1855 March 10	WILMARTH, Phila *Osgood*	Female Medical College of Pennsylvania

(continued)

Year Graduated	Name	Institution
1855 April 14	*xCASE, Mary A.	New York Hydropathic and Physiological School
1855 April 14	*x*COLE*, Maria	New York Hydropathic and Physiological School
1855 April 14	*de la VERGNE, Eliza	New York Hydropathic and Physiological School
1855 April 14	**SAYER* Hasbrouck, Lydia	New York Hydropathic and Physiological School
1855 April 14	*SMALLEY, C. L.	New York Hydropathic and Physiological School
1855 April 14	*x*SNOW*, Ellen M.	New York Hydropathic and Physiological School
1855 May 19	DOLLEY Laundon, Jane Elizabeth	Eclectic Medical Institute
1855 May 19	x*FINNEY*, Mary Elizabeth	Eclectic Medical Institute
1855 May 19	xHYDE, Harriet	Eclectic Medical Institute
1855 May 19	x*STRICKLAND*, Sarah	Eclectic Medical Institute
1856 February 1	x*PLEWS*, Mary Jane	Eclectic Medical Institute
1856 February 28	**COOKE* Hooper, Maria Louisa	New England Female Medical College
1856 February 28	**SALISBURY*, Sarah Whitman	New England Female Medical College
1856 March	*CALVIN*, Elizabeth	Penn Medical University
1856 March	*HOLLOWAY* Wilhite, Mary M.	Penn Medical University
1856 March	*MELLON*, Ellen J.	Penn Medical University
1856 March	THOMAS, Mary Frame *Myers*	Penn Medical University
1856 March	x*WILEMAN*, Esther C.	Penn Medical University
1856 March	x*WILHERT*, Mary M.	Penn Medical University
1856 March	*WOLFE*, Mary Ellen	Penn Medical University
1856 March	YOUNG, Sarah H.	Penn Medical University

(continued)

Year Graduated	Name	Institution
1856 March	*CHADWICK* Clapp, Sarah Ann	Western Reserve College Medicine Department
1856 March	*GREENE*, Cordelia Agnes	Western Reserve College Medicine Department
1856 March	*GRISELLE*, Elizabeth	Western Reserve College Medicine Department
1856 March	*ZAKRZEWSKA*, Marie Elizabeth	Western Reserve College Medicine Department
1856 March 1	*COLLINS* Jones, Elizabeth	Female Medical College of Pennsylvania
1856 March 1	x*HUGHES*, Debbie A.	Female Medical College of Pennsylvania
1856 March 1	*ROSS* Walcott, Laura J.	Female Medical College of Pennsylvania
1856 March 1	x*STARR*, Jane L.	Female Medical College of Pennsylvania
1856 April 10	*xBRIGGS, S. E. L. S.	New York Hygeio-Therapeutic College
1856 April 10	*xEDGERTON, A. C.	New York Hygeio-Therapeutic College
1856 April 10	*HARRIS, Rachel *Hamlin* (2nd MD, 1870)	New York Hygeio-Therapeutic College
1856 April 10	**HURD Fales, Emeline M.	New York Hygeio-Therapeutic College
1856 April 10	*McANDREW, Helen *Walker*	New York Hygeio-Therapeutic College
1856 April 10	*xWALBRIDGE, F. E. S.	New York Hygeio-Therapeutic College
1856 April 10	**WILLIS Weed, Adaline Melinda	New York Hygeio-Therapeutic College
1856 April 10	*x*WOOD*, Susan E.	New York Hygeio-Therapeutic College
1856 May	x*CODDING*, Louisa B.	Eclectic Medical Institute
1857	*KENYON* Lisk, Sarah	New York Hygeio-Therapeutic College

(continued)

Year Graduated	Name	Institution
1857	x*OWEN*, Edith Lee	Eclectic Medical Institute
1857 February 28	BAUGH, Elizabeth R. *Price*	Female Medical College of Pennsylvania
1857 February 28	*BRINTON* Carter, Hannah W.	Female Medical College of Pennsylvania
1857 February 28	*HAYHURST*, Susanna	Female Medical College of Pennsylvania
1857 February 28	*MOON* Andrews, Orianna Russell	Female Medical College of Pennsylvania
1857 February 28	x*PETERSILIA*, Lucy M.	Female Medical College of Pennsylvania
1857 February 28	*SCARLETT* Dixon, Mary J.	Female Medical College of Pennsylvania
1857 February 28	*WILSON*, Phoebe	Female Medical College of Pennsylvania
1857 March 4	*BREED* Welch, Mary Elizabeth	New England Female Medical College
1857 March 4	*BRIGHAM*, Harriet Sophia	New England Female Medical College
1857 March 4	CAPEN, Susan *Richards*	New England Female Medical College
1857 March 4	*COOKE*, Frances Sproat	New England Female Medical College
1857 March 4	HAWKS, Esther Jane *Hill*	New England Female Medical College
1857 March 4	*INMAN*, Anna	New England Female Medical College
1857 March 4	*PACKARD* Johnson, Elizabeth Ann	New England Female Medical College
1857 May 23	xBARRY, Elsie *Hall* (her 2nd MD)	Eclectic College of Medicine
1857 May 23	BRIGHAM, Sarah Cheny *Read* Randall	Eclectic College of Medicine
1857 May 23	*BROWN*, Eliza A.	Eclectic College of Medicine

(*continued*)

Year Graduated	Name	Institution
1857 May 23	COOMBS Barnes, Elizabeth *Bower*	Eclectic College of Medicine
1857 May 23	*HARRIS* Reid, Fidelia Rachel	Eclectic College of Medicine
1857 May 23	MAYO, Elzina C.	Eclectic College of Medicine
1857 May 23	x*SEELEY*, Harriet E.	Eclectic College of Medicine
1857 May 23	*SLOUT* Peterman, Salome Amy	Eclectic College of Medicine
1857 May 23	xSTILL, Emma R.	Eclectic College of Medicine
1857 May 30	COHEN, Elizabeth D. A. *Magnus*	Penn Medical University
1857 May 30	DRURY, Deborah *Smith*	Penn Medical University
1857 May 30	*HASTINGS*, Amelia	Penn Medical University
1857 May 30	*KOEHLER* Worrell, Susannah C.	Penn Medical University
1857 May 30	x*MARSDEN*, Hannah	Penn Medical University
1857 May 30	*STAMBACH* Galvin, Annie M.	Penn Medical University
1857 May 30	THOMAS, Lavinia Dolly *Bacon*	Penn Medical University
1857 May 30	WATSON, Rachel M. *Bewley*	Penn Medical University
1857 June 11	*ALLYN*, Rachel Humphrey	Worcester Medical Institution
1857 June 11	xBAKER, Livonia G.	Worcester Medical Institution
1857 June 11	EATON, Edee W. *Webster*	Worcester Medical Institution
1857 June 11	xHARRIS, Lizzie *McLean*	Worcester Medical Institution
1858	xCHAPPELL, Miriam G.	Penn Medical University

(continued)

Year Graduated	Name	Institution
1858	x*TAYLOR*, Mary Ann	Penn Medical University
1858	*YOUNG* Coleman, Margaret G.	Penn Medical University
1858 February 27	*BUCKEL*, Chloe Annette	Female Medical College of Pennsylvania
1858 February 27	FUSSELL, Rebecca *Lewis*	Female Medical College of Pennsylvania
1858 February 27	x*JONES* Price, Marie W.	Female Medical College of Pennsylvania
1858 February 27	*PARRY*, Susan	Female Medical College of Pennsylvania
1858 February 28	xHALL, D. S.	Western Homoeopathic College
1858 February 28	ALLEN, Sarah E. (degree in obstetrics)	Western Homoeopathic College
1858 March 3	*ANGELL* Curtis, Anna Sarah	New England Female Medical College
1858 March 3	*BELDEN* Taylor McCabe, Emily Norton	New England Female Medical College
1858 March 3	*VAILE*, Elizabeth Josephine	New England Female Medical College
1858 March 3	WARFIELD Walker, Sarah Elizabeth *Nichols*	New England Female Medical College
1858 March 3	*WRIGHT* Pierson, Mary	New England Female Medical College
1858 April 13	PAGE, Huldah *Allen*	New York Hygeio-Therapeutic College
1858 April 13	x*DAVIS*, Elvira L.	New York Hygeio-Therapeutic College
1858 April 13	DEWEY Maurey Newhall, Abbie Parthenia	New York Hygeio-Therapeutic College
1858 April 13	GUTHRIE, Emily M. *Smith*	New York Hygeio-Therapeutic College
1858 April 13	*HIGGINS*, Ellen J.	New York Hygeio-Therapeutic College

(continued)

Year Graduated	Name	Institution
1858 April 13	HUMPHREY, Sarah R. *Randall*	New York Hygeio-Therapeutic College
1858 April 13	*HURD* Fales, Emeline Morrow	New York Hygeio-Therapeutic College
1858 April 13	SELLECK Olmsted, Anne S.	New York Hygeio-Therapeutic College
1858 April 13	SMALLEY, C. L.	New York Hygeio-Therapeutic College
1858 April 13	STILLMAN Severance, Juliet H. *Worth*	New York Hygeio-Therapeutic College
1858 May 13	xJONES, Elizabeth	Eclectic Medical Institute
1858 May 13	WILLIAMS, Savina Leah *Fogle*	Eclectic Medical Institute
1858 May 13	xWUIST, Dora Sabina	Eclectic Medical Institute
1858 October 1	CAMPBELL, Lydia S.	New York Hygeio-Therapeutic College
1858 October 1	FARNHAM Fitzpatrick, Eliza Woods *Burhans*	New York Hygeio-Therapeutic College
1859	ANTON, Rebecca L. *Vancleve* (2nd MD, Eclectic Medical College, NYC)	Eclectic College of Medicine
1859	x*COOPER*, Martha Ella	Eclectic College of Medicine
1859	x*MORSE*, Mary Elvira	Eclectic College of Medicine
1859	xTANNER, M. J.	Eclectic College of Medicine
1859	WITHAM, Martha Butterworth	Eclectic College of Medicine
1859?	**AUSTIN*, Harriet Newell	New York Hygeio-Therapeutic College
1859	*BIRDSALL* Armstrong, Hannah	Penn Medical University
1859	CALDWELL, Sarah C.	Penn Medical University

(continued)

Year Graduated	Name	Institution
1859	x*ELSON*, Marianna	Penn Medical University
1859	*RICE*, Sarah Ann	Penn Medical University
1859	*RIDGEWAY* Robbins, Emily	Penn Medical University
1859	WILSON, Angeline M. L.	Penn Medical University
1859	CUSHING, Sarah L. *Lamb*	Starling Medical College
1859 March 2	*FIFIELD*, Almira	New England Female Medical College
1859 March 2	*HARRIS* Butler, Mary Ann	New England Female Medical College
1859 March 2	*HOMER* Arnold, Mary Ann	New England Female Medical College
1859 March 2	*TAYLOR*, Elizabeth	New England Female Medical College
1859 March 2	WETHERBEE, Sarah Abigail *Sheldon*	New England Female Medical College
1859 March 5	*ADAMS*, Harriet	Female Medical College of Pennsylvania
1859 March 5	BAILY, Mary Malin *Evans* (her 2nd MD)	Female Medical College of Pennsylvania
1859 March 5	x*MELLEN*, Elizabeth S.	Female Medical College of Pennsylvania
1859 March 5	PORTER, Maria W.	Female Medical College of Pennsylvania
1859 March 5	xSTRATTON, M. Almira	Female Medical College of Pennsylvania
1859 March 5	*UNDERWOOD* Jewell, Catherine Josephine	Female Medical College of Pennsylvania
1859 March 9	GATCHELL, Anna M. *Crane*	Western Homoeopathic College
1859 March 9	BURRITT, Frances	Western Homoeopathic College
1859 March 9	*MACLEAN* Fowle, Janette C.	Western Homoeopathic College

(continued)

Year Graduated	Name	Institution
1859 March 9	x*WALLACE*, Virginia C.	Western Homoeopathic College
1859 March 9	ELLIS, Sarah Maria *Leonard*	Western Homoeopathic College
1859 March 9	GROSS, Maria Maxwell *Tooker*	Western Homoeopathic College
1859 March 29	FOSTER Miner, Amanda L.	New York Hygeio-Therapeutic College
1859 March 29	*HALL* Barry, Susan E.	New York Hygeio-Therapeutic College
1859 March 29	HARRINGTON, Sarah G. *Farnsworth*	New York Hygeio-Therapeutic College
1859 March 29	*HYDE* Williams Maxcy, Rhoda H.	New York Hygeio-Therapeutic College
1859 March 29	LITTLEJOHN, Adeline *Sadler*	New York Hygeio-Therapeutic College
1859 March 29	McCUNE, Olive F. *Frisbie*	New York Hygeio-Therapeutic College
1859 March 29	*SHOTWELL*, Phebe A.	New York Hygeio-Therapeutic College
1859 March 29	xSIKES, Mary C.	New York Hygeio-Therapeutic College
1859 March 29	SMITH, Rebecca Lippett *Brooks*	New York Hygeio-Therapeutic College
1859 March 29	*WILEY* Warren Corbett, Elizabeth Jane (2nd MD, 1879, Michigan)	New York Hygeio-Therapeutic College
1859 March 29	xWILLIAMS, Jane A.	New York Hygeio-Therapeutic College
1859 March 29	WOOD, Olive Chesilla Arnold	New York Hygeio-Therapeutic College
1860	SEAMAN, Cleora Augusta *Stevens*	Western Homoeopathic College
1860	RABON, Janet *Bailey* (degree in obstetrics)	Western Homoeopathic College

(continued)

Year Graduated	Name	Institution
1860 February 29	BURROUGHS, DeLavenna	New England Female Medical College
1860 February 29	xHASKINS, Hannah *Hall*	New England Female Medical College
1860 February 29	JACKSON, Mercy *Ruggles* Bisbee	New England Female Medical College
1860 March 10	*ZIMMERMAN* Burnside, Eliza J.	Female Medical College of Pennsylvania
1860 March 31	CHOATE, Eunice S.	New York Hygeio-Therapeutic College
1860 March 31	ESTEE, Susan *Maxson*	New York Hygeio-Therapeutic College
1860 March 31	*FAIRCHILD*, Marion Augusta	New York Hygeio-Therapeutic College
1860 March 31	SILL HEURTLEY, Cordelia *Brown*	New York Hygeio-Therapeutic College
1860 April	ABELL, Lucy W.	Penn Medical University
1860 April	EVERETT, Susan A. *Hamblen*	Penn Medical University
1860 April	FAIRCHILD Wheaton Plantz, Laura M. *Wheeler*	Penn Medical University
1860 April	*FULLER*, Adeline J.	Penn Medical University
1860 April	GOULDING, Anna *Eames*	Penn Medical University
1860 April	*HUGHES*, Eliza Clark	Penn Medical University
1860 April	PAINTER, Hettie *Kersey*	Penn Medical University
1860 April	x*PARSONS*, Sarah E.	Penn Medical University
1860 April	PETTINGILL, Sarah Brooks *Felt*	Penn Medical University
1860 April	*WHITNEY*, Rebecca S.	Penn Medical University
1860 April	*WOOD* Watkins, Zelinda	Penn Medical University
1861	*SHEPARD* Presley, Louisa	Graefenberg Medical Institute

(continued)

Year Graduated	Name	Institution
1861	BOWDITCH, Lucinda M. *Browne*	Penn Medical University
1861	BUSTEED, Lavinia Ann *Gates*	Penn Medical University
1861	CLARK, Betsy R. *Russell*	Penn Medical University
1861	*DENNETT*, Maria J.	Penn Medical University
1861	*FERGUSON*, Willimanna	Penn Medical University
1861	*GILKERSON* Smith, Agnes Mitilda	Penn Medical University
1861	*GRENNAN*, M. Adelaide	Penn Medical University
1861	LONGSHORE, Rebecca H. *Reynolds*	Penn Medical University
1861	O'LEARY, Helen *Bartlett*	Penn Medical University
1861	*RUGGLES*, Reed Anne M.	Penn Medical University
1861	x *WOODS*, Virginia A.	Penn Medical University
1861 March 6	ARNOLD, Hannah Angeline *Batchelor*	New England Female Medical College
1861 March 6	*FLANDERS*, Martha Jane	New England Female Medical College
1861 March 6	PARKER, Louisa Fearing *Coffin*	New England Female Medical College
1861 March 6	SOMERBY Bartlett, Elizabeth *Phillips*	New England Female Medical College
1861 March 6	STONE, Eliza Leavitt *Ingersoll*	New England Female Medical College
1861 March 6	WITHERBY, Lamoille	New England Female Medical College
1861 March 13	x *DAVIES*, Frances V.	Female Medical College of Pennsylvania
1861 March 13	*KLECKNER* Saltzgiver, Sarah E.	Female Medical College of Pennsylvania
1861 March 13	*PAUL* Sandt, Sarah E.	Female Medical College of Pennsylvania
1861 March 13	*PAYNE*, Jane	Female Medical College of Pennsylvania

(continued)

Year Graduated	Name	Institution
1861 March 13	REYNOLDS, Mary J. *Smith*	Female Medical College of Pennsylvania
1861 March 13	*SPEAKMAN*, Rachel T.	Female Medical College of Pennsylvania
1861 March 29	x*BELL*, Sarah Ann	New York Hygeio-Therapeutic College
1861 March 29	BUTTS, Mary A. *Denton*	New York Hygeio-Therapeutic College
1861 March 29	*COOKINGHAM*, Carrie H.	New York Hygeio-Therapeutic College
1861 March 29	*GOODELL* Smith, Ellen Hermans	New York Hygeio-Therapeutic College
1861 March 29	SARGENT, Eveline E. *Moseley*	New York Hygeio-Therapeutic College
1861 March 29	*WILLIAMS* Maxson, Olive A.	New York Hygeio-Therapeutic College
1861 March 29	xWORTHING, Mary L.	New York Hygeio-Therapeutic College

Appendix B

Medical Graduates of the American Hydropathic Institute, 1851 and 1852

Note: An *x* preceding a name signifies that no information has been found about that person.

Term 1. Graduation December 6, 1851

xMary Ann Torbet, Alabama, practiced water-cure, 385 Broadway, New York City
xAmanda M. Cook, Massachusetts
Harriet N. Austin, New York (see biography)
xEsther C. Wildman, Ohio (prob. Esther C. Wileman, MD, Penn Medical University, 1856)
xMary G. Pusey, Pennsylvania
xMary J. Colburn, Massachusetts
xCaroline E. Youngs, Connecticut
xMargaret W. Sill, New York
Harriet A. Judd, Connecticut, later Sartain, MD, Eclectic College of Medicine, 1854.
plus eleven men
(see *Water-Cure Journal*, February 1852, 41; or Donegan, 171)

Term 2. Graduation April 4, 1852.

xCharlotte C. Sherwood, South Carolina
xIsabelle Pennell, New York
xCharlotte Killam, Connecticut
xMargaretta B. Pierce, Ohio
plus five men
(see *Water-Cure Journal* May 1852, 113)

Term 3. The next term of AHI was to be in Portchester, New York, starting November 1, 1852. It was not held.

Appendix C

Pre–Civil War Women Medical Doctors Mentioned in Books and Biographical Dictionaries

	WWW	EWA 1868	Cleave 1873	DOA 1883	Apple 1887–1931	W+L 1893	NCAB 1892–1984	Lamb 1900	King 1905	Kelly 1912	DAB 1927	NAW 1971	AMB 1984	ANB 1999
Harriot Newell Austin				.										D
Susan Hall Barry						+								
Elizabeth Blackwell	I	+		+	+	+	+	+		+	+	+	+	+
Emily Blackwell	I	+		+	+	+	+			+	+	+	+	+
Chloe Annette Buckel				.								+		+
Emeline H. Cleveland				+						+		+	+	
Sarah Adamson Dolley				+						+		+	+	
Susan Ann Edson			+	.				+						
Sarah M. Leonard Ellis			+											
Marion Augusta Fairchild						+								
Eliza Burhans Farnham	H						+	+				F		P
Lydia Folger Fowler				S								T		
Rachel Brooks Gleason				+		+				+				+
Cordelia Agnes Greene													+	+
Maria Maxwell Gross			+											
Lydia Sayer Hasbrouck	H+IV											F		D

	WWW	EWA	Cleave	DOA	Apple	W+L	NCAB	Lamb	King	Kelly	DAB	NAW	AMB	ANB
Harriot Kezia Hunt	H	+		+	+		+	+		+	+	+&F	+	+
Mercy Bisbee Jackson	H		+	+	+				+		+			
Catherine Underwood Jewell				+										
Hannah Myers Longshore	I	+		+		+	+					+	+	
Anna M. Longshore-Potts						+								
Clemence Harned Lozier	H	+		+	+		+	+	+	1928	+	+	+	+
Myra King Merrick													+	
Martha Harris Mowry						+								
Jane Viola Myers				.										
Almira Fowler Ormsbee			+	.										
Sarah Brooks Felt Pettingill			+											
Ann Preston	H	+		.	+	+	+	+		+	+	+	+	+
Mary J. Scarlett Dixon						+								
Cleora Augusta Seaman							+							
Juliet H. Stillman Severance					+									
Alice Bunker Stockham	I					+								
Mary Frame Myers Thomas				+				+				+	+	

(continued)

	WWW	EWA	Cleave	DOA	Apple	W+L	NCAB	Lamb	King	Kelly	DAB	NAW	AMB	ANB
Mary Edwards Walker	I					+	+			1928	+	F	+	
Mary Holloway Wilhite						+								
Caroline Brown Winslow			+			+								
Laura J. Ross Wolcott				+									+	
Marie Elizabeth Zakrzewska	I			+		+				+	+	+	+	+

Key to symbols:
+   physician
D   dress reformer
F   feminist
P   prison reformer
S   scientist
T   temperance advocate
·   mentioned by name only

References:

WWW *Who Was Who*. Historical volume (H), volume 1 (I), and volume 4 (IV). A. N. Marquis & Co., Chicago, 1967, 1942, 1968.

EWA James Parton et al., *Eminent Women of the Age*. Hartford, CT, 1873.

Cleave Egbert Cleave, *Cleave's Biographical Cyclopaedia of Homoeopathic Physicians and Surgeons*. Philadelphia, 1873.

DOA Phebe A. Hanaford, *Daughters of America; or, Women of the Century*. Augusta, ME, ca. 1882.

Apple *Appleton's Cyclopaedia of American Biography*. 12 vols. New York, 1887–1931.

W+L Frances E. Willard and Mary A. Livermore, *American Women: Fifteen Hundred Biographies with Over 1,400 Portraits*. 2 vols. New York, Chicago, Springfield, OH, orig. 1893. Rev. ed. 1897.

NCAB *National Cyclopedia of American Biography*. James T. White, publ. New York, 1892–1984.

Lamb John Howard Brown, ed., *Lamb's Biographical Dictionary of the United States*. Boston, 1900 et seq.

King William Harvey King, *History of Homoeopathy and Its Institutions in America*. 4 vols. New York, 1905.

Kelly Howard A. Kelly, *Cyclopedia of American Medical Biography*. 2 vols. Philadelphia, 1912. 1928 edition (1928): Howard A. Kelly and Walter L. Burrage, *Dictionary of American Medical Biographies*, New York, 1928.

DAB *Dictionary of American Biography*. 11 vols. plus supplements. New York: American Council of Learned Societies, 1927 et seq.

NAW Edward T. James, ed., *Notable American Women 1607–1950, a Biographical Dictionary*. 3 vols. Cambridge, MA, 1971.

AMB Martin Kaufman et al., *Dictionary of American Medical Biography*. 2 vols. Westport, CT / London, 1984.

ANB John A. Garraty and Mack C. Carnes, eds., *American National Biography*. 24 vols. New York, 1999.

Appendix D

Principal Locations in Which the Graduates Served Professionally

Note: Maiden surnames in italics. Surnames at graduation in uppercase.

CALIFORNIA	Immusdale	Emeline Morrow *HURD* Fales
	National City	Rebecca H. *Reynolds* LONGSHORE
	National City	Anna Mary *LONGSHORE* Potts
	Oakland	Chloe Annette *BUCKEL*
	Oakland	Emily A. *VARNEY* Brownell
	Pasadena	Fidelia Rachel *HARRIS* Reid
	San Francisco	Eliza Jane *Hall* McQUIGG
	San Francisco	Martha Nichols *Spaulding* THURSTON
	San Francisco	Elizabeth Jane *WILEY* Warren Corbett
	San Francisco	Eliza L. WILLIS
	San Francisco	Lamoille WITHERBY
	San Francisco	Sarah H. YOUNG
	San Jose	Eliza L. WILLIS
	Santa Cruz	Eliza Wood *Burhans* FARNHAM Fitzpatrick

(continued)

COLORADO	Denver	Augusta R. *MONTGOMERY* Nelson
CONNECTICUT	Greenwich	Anna E. SELLECK OLMSTED
	Winchester/Winsted	Permilia R. *BRONSON*
DISTRICT OF COLUMBIA		Lucy W. ABELL
		Susan Ann *EDSON*
		Caroline *BROWN* Winslow
GEORGIA	Covington?	Janet *MACLEAN* Fowle
ILLINOIS	?	Jane L. *STARR*
	?	Esther C. *WILEMAN*
	?	Laura J. *ROSS* Wolcott
	Aurora	Rhoda *HYDE* Williams Maxcy
	Bloomington	Eliza A. BROWN
	Bloomington	Augusta *MONTGOMERY* Nelson
	Bloomington	Catherine Josephine *UNDERWOOD* Jewell
	Chicago	Chloe Annette *BUCKEL*
	Chicago	Frances BURRITT
	Chicago	Maria Maxwell *Tooker* GROSS
	Chicago	Alice *BUNKER* Stockham
	Geneva	Anna Mary *LONGSHORE* Potts
	Hindsboro	Elizabeth *Bower* COOMBS Barnes
	Lee Center	Sarah Ann *CHADWICK* Clapp
	Molina	Sarah *Randall* HUMPHREY
	Morrison	Elzina C. MAYO

(continued)

	Peoria	Sarah *KENYON* Lisk
	Quincy	Marion Augusta *FAIRCHILD*
	Rutland	Phebe A. *SHOTWELL*
	Springfield	Amelia A. *HASTINGS*
	Wheaton	Minerva *Falley* HOES
	Winfield	Rhoda A. *HYDE* Williams Maxcy
INDIANA	Crawfordsville	Mary Mitchell *HOLLOWAY* Wilhite
	Lafayette	Alice *BUNKER* Stockham
	Lafayette	Minerva S. *Falley* HOES
	Richmond	Mary Frames *Myers* THOMAS
	Terre Haute	Angeline M. *Lockwood* WILSON Moore
IOWA	Clarence	Savina Leah *Fogle* WILLIAMS
	Davenport	Maria W. PORTER
	Delhi (and Lyons)	Adeline *Sadler* LITTLEJOHN
	Grinnell	Rachel *Hamlin* HARRIS
	Iowa City	Helen *Bartlett* O'LEARY
	Tipton and Onion Grove (now Clarence)	Lydia S. CAMPBELL
	Wilton Junction	Martha *Butterworth* WITHAM
KANSAS	Atchison City (and Topeka)	Olive C. *Arnold* WOOD
	Lawrence	Martha *Butterworth* WITHAM
	Sedgwick	Elzina C. MAYO
LOUISIANA	Natchitoches Parish	Virginia A. *WOODS*
	New Orleans	Elizabeth D. A. *Magnus* COHEN

(continued)

	New Orleans	Frances BURRITT
MAINE	Augusta	Huldah *Allen* PAGE
	Portland	Susan A. *Hamblen* EVERETT
	Waterville	Lucy Amelia *Brown* HARRIS
MARYLAND	Baltimore	Amelia A. *HASTINGS*
MASSACHUSETTS	Belchertown	Ellen *GOODELL* Smith
	Boston	Lucy W. ABELL
	Boston	Charlotte G. ADAMS
	Boston	Mercy *Ruggles* Bisbee JACKSON
	Boston	Lucinda M. *Browne* BOWDITCH
	Boston	Chloe Annette *BUCKEL*
	Boston	Lavinia Ann *Gates* BUSTEED
	Boston	Elizabeth B. CHAMBERLIN
	Boston	Nancy Elizabeth *Talbot* CLARK Binney
	Boston	Frances Sproat *COOKE*
	Boston	Edith *Webster* EATON
	Boston	Sophronia *FLETCHER*
	Boston	Anna *Eames* GOULDING
	Boston	Anna *Hall* HASKINS
	Boston	Amelia *HASTINGS*
	Boston	Harriot Kezia *HUNT*
	Boston	Mary Reed *JENKS*
	Boston	Helen *Bartlett* O'LEARY
	Boston	Louisa Fearing *Coffin* PARKER

(continued)

Boston	Martha Ann *Hayden* SAWIN
Boston	Hannah Maria *Woodward* WALCOTT
Boston	Sarah Abigail *Sheldon* WETHERBEE
Boston	Marie Elizabeth *ZAKRZEWSKA*
Brockton	Elizabeth Ann *PACKARD* Johnson
Brookfield	Annie M. *STAMBACH* Galvin
Brookline	Lucy W. ABELL
Cambridge	Adeline *Johnson* FULLER
Charlemont	Elizabeth Hannah *BATES*
Chelsea	Elizabeth *Phillips* SOMERBY Bartlett
Fitchburg	Sarah Cheny *Read* Randall BRIGHAM
Greenfield	Eliza Leavitt *Ingersoll* STONE
Haverhill	Deborah *Smith* DRURY
Holliston	Sarah Elizabeth *Nichols* WARFIELD Walker
Hopedale	Phila *Osgood* WILMARTH
Lenox	Emily Norton *BELDEN* Taylor McCabe
Lowell	Lucinda *Capen* HALL
Lowell	Rachel Humphrey *ALLYN*
Lowell	Sarah H. YOUNG
Lynn	Mary Elizabeth *BREED* Welch

(*continued*)

	Lynn	Martha Jane *FLANDERS*
	Lynn	Esther Jane *Hill* HAWKS
	Marlborough	Sarah Ann *RICE*
	Medford	Anna Sarah *ANGELL* Curtis
	Peabody	Annie M. *STAMBACH* Galvin
	Sharon	Susan *Richards* CAPEN
	South Hadley	Emily Norton *BELDEN* Taylor McCabe
	South Hadley	Mary Ann Brown *HOMER* Arnold
	Weymouth	Sarah Whitman *SALISBURY*
	Worcester	Betsy *Russell* CLARK
	Worcester	Sophia *Roper* HARRIS
	Wrentham	Hannah Angeline *Batchelor* ARNOLD
MICHIGAN	Adrian	Anna Mary *LONGSHORE* Potts
	Detroit	Sarah Maria *Leonard* ELLIS
	Kalamazoo	Laura Marion *Wheeler* FAIRCHILD Wheaton Plantz
	Lansing	Augusta *MONTGOMERY* Nelson
	Marshall	Salome A. *SLOUT* Peterman
	Ypsilanti	Helen *Walker* McANDREW
MINNESOTA	Lake City	Catherine Josephine *UNDERWOOD* Jewell
	Minneapolis	Mary Ann Brown *HOMER* Arnold

(continued)

	Pearl Lake	Zelinda *WOOD* Watkins
MISSOURI	Cameron	Zelinda *WOOD* Watkins
	Hannibal	Marion Augusta *FAIRCHILD*
	St. Louis	M. Adelaide *GRENNAN*
	St. Louis	Augusta R. *MONTGOMERY* Nelson
	St. Louis	Eveline E. *Moseley* SARGENT
	St. Louis	Angeline M. *Lockwood* WILSON Moore
NEBRASKA	Columbus	Rebecca H. *Reynolds* LONGSHORE
	Humboldt	Olive A. *WILLIAMS* Maxson
	Lincoln	Hettie *Kersey* PAINTER
NEVADA	Washoe City	Adaline Melinda *WILLIS* Weed
NEW HAMPSHIRE	Concord	Lucinda *Capen* HALL
	Manchester	Esther Jane *Hill* HAWKS
	Troy	Mary Ann *HARRIS* Butler
NEW JERSEY	Camden	Miriam G. CHAPPELL
	Hammonton	Samantha S. *NIVISON*
	Hammonton	Marenda *Briggs* RANDALL
	Orange	Henrietta W. JOHNSON
	Orange Mountain	Almira L. *FOWLER* Ormsbee Breakspear
	Rahway	Anna N. *Smith* ANDERSON
	Smithville	Agnes Mitilda *GILKERSON* Smith
	Trenton	Sarah E. *PAUL* Sandt

(continued)

NEW YORK	?	Harriet E. SEELEY
	Albion	Elizabeth Josephine *VAILE*
	Alfred	Susan *Maxson* ESTEE
	Auburn	Eunice S. CHOATE
	Binghamton	Martha Ann *FRENCH*
	Brooklyn	Amelia *Wilkes* LINES
	Brooklyn	Olive *Frisbie* McCUNE
	Brooklyn	Eliza de la VERGNE
	Canton	Lamoille WITHERBY
	Castile	Cordelia Agnes *GREENE*
	Chittenango	Mary Elizabeth *Baum* HANCHETT
	Dansville	Harriet Newell *AUSTIN*
	Delhi	Olive *Frisbie* McCUNE
	Delta/North Bay	Abigail Parthenia *DEWEY* Maurey Newhall
	Dryden	Samantha S. *NIVISON*
	Elmira	Rachel Ingall *Brooks* GLEASON
	Gardnersville	Lucinda *Rowley* BROWN
	Gowanda	Laura A. LORD
	Homer	Maria Louisa *COOKE* Hooper
	Leroy	Eliza L. WILLIS
	Lockport	Sarah *Lamb* CUSHING
	Lyons	DeLavenna *BURROUGHS*
	Madrid	Minerva Jane *AVERELL*
	Middletown	Lydia *SAYER* Hasbrouck
	Morley	Lamoille WITHERBY
	New York City	Elizabeth *BLACKWELL*

(continued)

New York City	Emily *BLACKWELL*
New York City	Sarah Maria *Leonard* ELLIS
New York City	Laura *Wheeler* FAIRCHILD Wheaton Plantz
New York City	Lydia *Folger* FOWLER
New York City	Ellen J. *HIGGINS*
New York City	Anna *INMAN*
New York City	Clemence Sophie *Harned* Lozier BAKER
New York City	Hulda *Allen* PAGE
New York City	Mary E. *SMITH* Wilder
New York City	Rachel T. *SPEAKMAN*
Newburgh	Cora (Cornelia) *Brown* SILL HEURTLEY
Oswego	Sarah Gates *Farnsworth* HARRINGTON
Oswego	Mary Edwards *WALKER* Miller
Owego	Elizabeth H. *BATES*
Palmyra	Harriet *ADAMS*
Petersburg	Susan *Maxson* ESTEE
Petersburg	Olive A. *WILLIAMS* Maxson
Pitcher	Elizabeth *TAYLOR*
Rochester	Sarah Read *ADAMSON* Dolley
Rochester	Lettice *Hyde* DOUD
Rochester	Rebecca B. WHEELER
Saratoga Springs	Martha Ann *FRENCH*
Staatsburg	Carrie H. *COOKINGHAM* (Helen Caroline?)

(continued)

	Syracuse	Dolly Ann *PORTER*
	Syracuse	Rebecca Lippett *Brooks* SMITH
	Syracuse	Mary E. *SMITH* Wilder
	Troy	Mary Malin *Evans* BAILY
	Troy	Rebecca Lippett *Brooks* SMITH
	Utica	Olive C. *Arnold* WOOD
	Utica	Rebecca Lippett *Brooks* SMITH
	Utica	Caroline *BROWN* Winslow
	Verona Springs	Angenette A. *Payne* HUNT
	Walworth	Abigail Parthenia *DEWEY* Maurey Newhall
	Walworth	Sarah Abigail *Sheldon* WETHERBEE
NORTH CAROLINA	Asheville	Anna Maria *Crane* GATCHELL
OHIO	Alexanderville	Doris Sabina WUIST
	Alliance	Eliza L. *Smyth* THOMAS
	Cleveland	Abigail S. *COGSWELL*
	Cleveland	Elizabeth *GRISELLE*
	Cleveland	Myra *King* MERRICK
	Cleveland	Janet *Bailey* RABON
	Cleveland	Finette E. *SCOTT* Seelye
	Cleveland	Cleora Augusta *Stevens* SEAMAN
	Columbus	Savina Leah *Fogle* WILLIAMS
	Dayton	Lavinia Dolly *Bacon* THOMAS

(continued)

	Elyria	Jane Elizabeth DOLLEY Laundon
	Kirtland	Mary *WRIGHT* Pierson
	Lebanon	Rebecca L. *Vancleve* ANTON
	Locust Center	Cecilia Pumpelly *Ricker* FREASE
	Maineville	Margaret *Butterworth* WITHAM
	Mount Vernon	Jane *PAYNE*
	Pomeroy	Laura *Wheeler* FAIRCHILD Wheaton Plantz
	Salem	Elizabeth *GRISELLE*
	Salem	Rachel M. *Bewley* WATSON
	Sycamore	Sarah SMIZER
	Tiffin	Julia *RUMSEY*
OREGON	Portland	Augusta R. *MONTGOMERY* Nelson
	Salem	Adaline Melinda *WILLIS* Weed
PENNSYLVANIA	Bristol	Anna N. *Smith* ANDERSON
	Christiana	Hannah *BRINTON* Carter
	Doylestown	Susan *PARRY*
	Homet's Ferry	Maria *Minnis* HOMET
	Kennett Square	Phebe *WILSON*
	Kennett Square	Phebe M. *WAY*
	Lewisburg	Maria Jane *GRIER*
	Lewisburg	Mary Ellen *WOLFE*
	Mifflinburg	Sarah E. *KLECKNER* Saltzgiver

(continued)

Norristown	Margaret *Phillips* RICHARDSON
North Coventry	Elizabeth R. *Price* BAUGH
Philadelphia	Sarah C. *CALDWELL*
Philadelphia	Elizabeth *CALVIN*
Philadelphia	Emeline *Horton* CLEVELAND
Philadelphia	Maria J. *DENNETT*
Philadelphia	Minna *ELLIGER* Piersol
Philadelphia	Hannah W. ELLIS
Philadelphia	Susanna H. *ELLIS*
Philadelphia	Marianna *ELSON*
Philadelphia	Rebecca *Lewis* FUSSELL
Philadelphia	Margaretta *Baldwin* GLEASON
Philadelphia	Susan N. *HAYHURST*
Philadelphia	Elizabeth *COLLINS* Jones
Philadelphia	Susanna C. *KOEHLER* Worrell
Philadelphia	Hannah Elizabeth *Myers* LONGSHORE
Philadelphia	Hannah *MARSDEN*
Philadelphia	Ellen J. *MELLON*
Philadelphia	Jane Viola *MYERS*
Philadelphia	Sarah Brooks *Felt* PETTINGILL
Philadelphia	Ann *PRESTON*
Philadelphia	Ann *Ruggles* REED
Philadelphia	Harriet Amelia *JUDD* Sartain
Philadelphia	Mary J. *SCARLETT* Dixon

(continued)

	Philadelphia	Elizabeth G. *SHATTUCK*
	Philadelphia	Susan A. *SMITH*
	Philadelphia	Annie M. *STAMBACH* Galvin
	Philadelphia	Phebe M. *WAY*
	Philadelphia	Eliza J. *ZIMMERMAN* Burnside
	Unionville	Rebecca *Reynolds* LONGSHORE
	West Chester	Sarah A. *ENTRIKIN*
	Wilkins	M. Almira *STRATTON*
	Williamsport	Margaret G. *YOUNG* Coleman
RHODE ISLAND	Providence	Anna Sarah *ANGELL* Curtis
	Providence	Julia A. *Bridgeham* BEVERLY
	Providence	Anna *INMAN*
	Providence	Martha Harris *MOWRY*
SOUTH CAROLINA	Beaufort	Ester Jane *Hill* HANKS
	Columbia	Jane A. WILLIAMS
TEXAS	Plantersville	Mary Ann T. *Denton* BUTTS
	San Antonio	Eveline E. *Moseley* SARGENT
TENNESSEE		Mary Ann *TAYLOR*
UTAH	Ogden	Augusta R. *MONTGOMERY* Nelson
VERMONT	Fairfax	Lucinda M. *Browne* BOWDITCH
	Northeast Kingdom	Emily A. *VARNEY* Brownell
	Plymouth Union (and N. Shrewsbury)	Mary Ann *HARRIS* Butler

(continued)

	Putney	Laura *Wheeler* FAIRCHILD Wheaton Plantz
	Woodstock	Amanda L. FOSTER Miner
	Woodstock	Marenda *Briggs* RANDALL
VIRGINIA	Scottsville	Orianna Russell *MOON* Andrews
WASHINGTON	Seattle	Adaline Melinda *WILLIS* Weed
WEST VIRGINIA	Wheeling	Eliza Clark *HUGHES*
WISCONSIN	Beaver Dam	Fidelia Rachel *HARRIS* Reid
	Kenosha	Anna Maria *Crane* GATCHELL
	Lake Geneva	Mary J. *Smith* REYNOLDS
	Milwaukee	Juliet H. *Worth* STILLMAN Severance
	Milwaukee	Laura J. *ROSS* Wolcott
	Sparta	Eveline E. *Moseley* SARGENT
AUSTRALIA	Victoria	Willimanna *FERGUSON*
CANADA WEST	Bowmanville	Mary Jane *PLEWS*
QUEBEC	Grand Ligne Mission	Zelinda *WOOD* Watkins
ENGLAND	London	Elizabeth *BLACKWELL*
	London	Lydia *Folger* FOWLER
	London	Frances G. MITCHELL
JERUSALEM		Orianna Russell *MOON* Andrews

Appendix E

Lists Showing Career Choices and Accomplishments of the Graduates

The Doctor as Author

Harriet Newell Austin
Elizabeth Blackwell
Emily Blackwell
Emeline Horton Cleveland
Susan Read Adamson Dolley
Susan A. Hamblen Everett
Marion Augusta Fairchild
Eliza Wood Burhans Farnham Fitzpatrick
Lydia Folger Fowler
Margaretta Baldwin Gleason
Rachel Brooks Gleason
Ellen Hermans Goodell Smith
Cordelia Agnes Greene
Mary Elizabeth Baum Hanchett
Esther Hill Hawks
Harriot Kezia Hunt
Anna Mary Longshore-Potts
Ann Preston
Mary J. Scarlett Dixon
Alice Bunker Stockham
Mary Frame Myers Thomas
Mary Edwards Walker Miller
Rachel M. Bewley Watson
Eliza E. L. Willis
Marie Elizabeth Zakrzewska

The Doctor as Popular Lecturer

(probably incomplete)
Abigail S. Cogswell

Susan A. Hamblen Everett
Laura M. Wheeler Fairchild Wheaton Plantz
Marion Augusta Fairchild
Eliza Wood Burhans Farnham Fitzpatrick
Lydia Folger Fowler
Rachel Brooks Gleason
Ellen Hermans Goodell Smith
Hannah Elizabeth Myers Longshore
Huldah Allen Page
Anna Mary Longshore-Potts
Clemence Sophia Harned Lozier Baker
Martha H. Mowry
Samantha Nivison
Alice Bunker Stockham
Adaline Melinda Willis Weed
Mary Mitchell Holloway Wilhite

Civil War Service

(probably incomplete)
Elizabeth Blackwell
Chloe Annette Buckel
Sarah Ann Chadwick Clapp
Emeline Horton Cleveland
Susan Ann Edson
Laura Wheeler Fairchild Wheaton Plantz
Eliza Wood Burhans Farnham Fitzpatrick
Almira Fifield
Susan Hall Barry
Fidelia Rachel Harris Reid
Esther Hill Hawks
Adeline Sadler Littlejohn
Myra King Merrick
Augusta R. Montgomery Nelson
Orianna Russell Moon Andrews
Esther (Hettie) Kersey Painter
Maria W. Porter
Mary Frame Myers Thomas
Mary Edwards Walker
Caroline Brown Winslow

The Doctor at Water-Cure or Health Institution

Harriet Newell Austin
Marion Augusta Fairchild
Cecilia Pumpelly Ricker Frease
Anna Maria Crane Gatchell
Rachel Brooks Gleason
Ellen Hermans Goodell Smith
Cordelia Agnes Greene
Maria Maxwell Tooker Gross
Lucinda Susanna Capen Hall
Sarah R. Randall Humphrey
Amelia Wilkes Lines
Helen Walker McAndrew
Samantha S. Nivison
Angenette A. Payne Hunt
Anna Mary Longshore Potts
Finette E. Scott Seelye

The Doctor as College Professor

(School doctor; instructor in anatomy, physiology, hygiene)
Emily Norton Belden Taylor McCabe, Mt. Holyoke (1864–68, resident physician and teacher of physiology)
Frances Sproat Cooke, Wheaton Seminary (later College; 1859–69 physiology lecturer)
Lydia Folger Fowler, Wheaton Seminary (assistant teacher; 1842–44)
Minerva Falley Hoes, Illinois Institute (later Wheaton College; 1855–56)
Sophronia Fletcher, Mt. Holyoke (1854–56)
Elizabeth J. Shattuck, Vassar College, 1865 (died before serving)
Rachel T. Speakman, Wellesley College, 1884–94.

The Doctor as Medical School Professor

(Those who were career academics are listed in bold)
Emily Norton Belden Taylor McCabe, New England Female Medical College, 1864–65, obstetrics and diseases of women and children
Elizabeth Blackwell, Woman's Medical College of the New York Infirmary, 1868–69, hygiene
Emily Blackwell, Woman's Medical College of the New York Infirmary, 1869–99, obstetrics and diseases of women
Emeline Horton Cleveland, Female Medical College of Pennsylvania, 1857–78, anatomy & histology; 1867, obstetrics and diseases of women and children

Frances Sproat Cooke, New England Female Medical College, 1859–66, physiology and hygiene; 1866–72, anatomy, physiology, and hygiene; 1862–65 dean

Sarah Maria Leonard Ellis, New York Medical College for Women, 1863–65, anatomy

Marion Augusta Fairchild, Washington University School of Medicine and St. Louis Medical College

Lydia Folger Fowler, Central Medical College, 1851–52, midwifery and diseases of women and children; New York Hygeio-Therapeutic College, 1862, instructor in clinical midwifery; New York Medical College for Women, 1863, pathology, principles and practice of medicine

Anna Inman, New York Medical College for Women, 1867, obstetrics

Mary R Bisbee Jackson, New England Female Medical College, 1872–73, diseases of children

Mary Reed Jenks, New England Female Medical College, 1853–62, demonstrator of anatomy; 1862–64, anatomy

Hannah E. Longshore, New England Female Medical College, 1851–52, demonstrator of anatomy, Female Medical College of Pennsylvania, 1853, demonstrator of anatomy, Penn Medical University, 1853–57

Clemence Harned Lozier, New York Medical College and Hospital for Women, 1863–82, diseases of women and children

Myra King Merrick, Homoeopathic College for Women, 1867–70?

Martha Harris Mowry, Female Medical College of Pennsylvania, 1853–54, obstetrics and diseases of women and children

Huldah Allen Page, New York Hygeio-Therapeutic College, 1859, physiology and hygiene; New York Medical College and Hospital for Women, 1863, physiology and hygiene

Ann Preston, Female Medical College of Pennsylvania, 1853–72, physiology and hygiene

Sarah Whitman Salisbury, New England Female Medical College, 1862–64, chemistry, materia medica, and therapeutics, 1864–65, anatomy

Mary J. Scarlet Dixon Female Medical College of Pennsylvania, 1862–81, anatomy

Cleora A Seaman Stevens, Homoeopathic College for Women, 1867–69?

Marie E. Zakrzewska, New England Female Medical College, 1859–62, obstetrics and diseases of women and children

Bibliography

Bibliographical references pertaining to a particular person are listed at the end of that person's biographical sketch. This bibliography is divided into the following sections:

Medical School Histories and Catalogs
General Directories
Medical Directories and Registers
Homoeopathic Directories
Biographical Dictionaries
Serials
Bibliographies
Secondary Works

Medical School Histories and Catalogs

Medical school annual announcements and catalogs of the fourteen chartered American medical schools that conferred medical degrees on women before 1862

Geneva Medical Institution

Smalley, Frank, ed. *Alumni Record and General Catalogue of Syracuse University 1872–1910 including Genesee College 1835–1871 and Geneva Medical College, 1835–1872.* Syracuse, NY, n.d.

Central Medical College

Corner, Betsey C. "Rochester's Early Medical School." [Central Medical College]. Paper read December 5, 1927, before the Medical History Club at the University of Rochester. Published in *Rochester Historical Society Publications Fund Series*, vol. 7, edited by Edward R. Foreman, 141–52. Rochester, 1928.

Eclectic Medical and Surgical Journal (Rochester), June 1850, 382. [Fowler]

Eclectic Journal of Medicine (Rochester), March 1852, 125–26. [Bronson, Doud, Sawyer]

Eclectic Journal of Medicine (Rochester), July 1852, 306. [Merrick]

Eclectic Medical Journal (Cincinnati), August 1852, 373(?).
New York Eclectic Medical and Surgical Journal (Rochester), August 1851, 62.
[Adamson & R. Gleason]

Syracuse Medical College

American Medical & Surgical Journal (Syracuse), April 1852, 93. [Hanchett, Wheeler, Willis]
American Journal of Medicine (Syracuse), June 1852, 149. [Smith Wilder]
Eclectic Medical & Surgical Journal, March 1851, 66. [M. Gleason]
Syracuse Daily Standard, March 18, 1852. [omits Wheeler]
Syracuse Daily Standard, June 8, 1852. [Smith]
Syracuse Medical Journal, April 1852. [includes Wheeler]
Syracuse Medical & Surgical Journal, July 1854, 192 [Hoes]
Syracuse Daily Standard, February 21, 1854 [Averell, Porter]
Syracuse Medical & Surgical Journal, March 1855, 193 [Walker]
Union Journal of Medicine, April 1853, 138. [Lozier]

Note: Thanks to Sarah Kozma, Onondaga Historical Association, Syracuse, NY, for some of this information.

Female Medical College of Pennsylvania

Alsop, Gulielma Fell. *History of the Woman's Medical College, 1850–1950*. Philadelphia, 1950.
Marshall, Clara. *The Woman's Medical College of Pennsylvania: An Historical Outline*. Philadelphia, 1897.
Woman's Medical College of Pennsylvania. *Register of Alumnae of the Woman's Medical College of Pennsylvania*. Philadelphia, 1940.
Woman's Medical College of Pennsylvania, Alumnae Association, *Reports of Proceedings of Annual Meetings. . . .* Philadelphia, 1875 et seq.

Note: Archives of the Female Medical College of Pennsylvania, now housed at Drexel University College of Medicine, contain useful information about several of the fifty-one graduates included in this study.

Western College of Homoeopathic Medicine (after 1857, Western Homoeopathic College)

Beckwith, David Herrick. "The Western College of Homoeopathic Medicine." In *History of Homoeopathy and Its Institutions in America*, 4 vols., edited by William Harvey King, 2:13–85 (New York, 1905).

Western Reserve College Medical Department

Goldstein, Linda L. "Women Enter Medicine in the Western Reserve: The Graduation of the First Six Woman Doctors from Western Reserve College, 1852–1856." *Pan-American Medical Woman's Journal,* March 1952.

Waite, Frederick C. "The Medical Education of Women in Cleveland (1850–1930)." *Western Reserve University Bulletin,* no. 16, September 30, 1930.

Waite, Frederick C. *Western Reserve University Centennial History of the School of Medicine,* 126–28, Cleveland, 1946.

Worcester Medical Institution

Ward, George Otis, *The Worcester Academy: Its Locations and Its Principals, 1834–1882.* Worcester, 1918.

Worcester (MA) Journal of Medicine. Edited by Calvin Newton, MD, 1852–57.

Eclectic Medical Institute (and) Eclectic College of Medicine

Catalogue of Graduates 1845 to 1881. Cincinnati, 1882. 20 pages.

Felter, Harvey Wickes. *History of the Eclectic Medical Institute, Cincinnati, Ohio, 1845–1902.* Cincinnati, 1902. [Includes ECM 1856–59.]

Note: Records of EMI and ECM are now found at the Lloyd Library & Museum in Cincinnati but include no information about the postcollegiate careers of the thirty-three women in this study.

New England Female Medical College:

Gardner, Martha, "Midwife, Doctor, or Doctress? The New England Female Medical College and Woman's Place in Nineteenth-Century Medicine and Society." Doctoral Thesis, Brandeis University, May 2002.

New England Female Medical College. Scrapbook. Francis A. Countway Library of Medicine, Harvard University. 184 pages of clippings from Massachusetts newspapers, dealing with the medical college, kept by Samuel Gregory, one of the school's founders, covering the period September 7, 1847–65.

Waite, Frederick C. *History of the New England Female Medical College 1848–1874.* Boston, 1950.

Note: Records of the New England Female Medical College are now at Boston University's Gotlieb Archives.

Penn Medical University

Abrahams, Harold J. *Extinct Medical Schools of Nineteenth-Century Philadelphia*, Philadelphia, 1966.

Annual Announcement for 1879–80. Philadelphia, 1879. [List of graduates 1853–79.]

Waite, Frederick C. *Medical Education of Women at Penn Medical University*. N.p: Froben Press, 1933. Reprinted from *Medical Review of Reviews*, June 1933.

Note: The Library of the Philadelphia College of Physicians has seven PMU annual announcements (1853–59/60). Copies of the 1857 annual announcement are also available at the Library Company of Philadelphia, the Historical Society of Pennsylvania, and the National Library of Medicine, Bethesda, MD. Thanks to Dr. Steven J. Peitzman and Ms. Lucretia McClure for this information.

New York Hygeio-Therapeutic College

Centennial Catalogue of the New York Hygeio-Therapeutic College. New York, 1876.

New York Hydropathic and Physiological School. *Catalogue . . . for 1854–5*. New York, 1855.

New York Hygeio-Therapeutic College. *Biennial Catalogue . . . for 1856–7, 1858–9, 1860–61*. New York, 1857, 1859, 1861.

New York Hygeio-Therapeutic College. *The Triennial Catalogue of the New York Hygeio-Therapeutic College for 1861, 1862, 1863–4, with an Introductory Lecture by Dr. R. T. Trall to the Medical Class of 1863–4, a Plan for Raising an Endowment of $100,000, Report to the Regents of the University, Etc.* New York, 1864.

Water-Cure Journal, New York, 1853–70.

Note: The 1854–55 and 1860–61 catalogs of this school are the only editions that list graduates; other years list students only. For those other years it is necessary to rely on the *Water-Cure Journal* and on local newspapers.

Starling Medical College

"Starling Medical College 1847–1907." In *The Ohio State University College of Medicine: A Collection of Source Material Covering a Century of Medical Progress 1834–1934*, 115. Blanchester, Ohio, 1934.

Graefenberg Medical Institute

American Journal of Medicine (Syracuse) 2 (April 1852).

Howard, Holly L. "Dr. Philip Madison Shepard and His Medical School." *De Historia Medicinae* 2 (February 1958).

Medical Association of the State of Alabama. *Transactions*, 1898.

Turner, Roy H., "Graefenberg: The Shepard Family's Medical School." *Annals of Medical History*, n.s., 5 (1933): 548–60.

General Directories

New England

The New England Business Directory. Adams, Sampson & Co., Boston, 1856, 1860.
The New England Business Directory. Sampson, Davenport & Co., Boston, 1865, 1868, 1871, 1873, 1875, 1877, 1879, 1881, 1883, 1885.

Connecticut

The Connecticut Register. Hartford: Brown & Parsons, 1850; F. A. Brown, 1855; Brown & Gross, 1867, 1868, 1874, 1879, 1882.
Jones, A. D. *The Illustrated Commercial, Mechanical, Professional and Statistical Gazetteer and Business-Book of Connecticut for 1857–8.* Vol. 1. New Haven, 1857.

Maine

Hoyt, Edmund S., *Maine State Year-Book, and Legislative Manual, for the Year 1873–4.* Portland, ca. 1873.

Massachusetts:

The Massachusetts Register . . . for 1852, 1855, 1856, 1857. Boston: George Adams, 1852, ca. 1855, ca. 1856, ca. 1857.
The Massachusetts Register . . . for the Year 1858, 1860. Boston: Adams, Sampson & Co., ca. 1858, 1860.
The Massachusetts Register. Boston: Sampson, Davenport & Co., 1865, 1867, 1868, 1872, 1875, 1878.

Boston

Boston Business and Co-partnership Directory. Boston: Dean Dudley, 1863–64.
The Boston Almanac and Business Directory. Vols. 16–58. Boston: Damrell & M. Moore and George Coolidge; later George Coolidge; later Sampson, Davenport & Co.; later Davenport, Murdock & Co., 1851–93.
Boston Directory for the Year 1857. Boston: George Adams, 1857.
Boston Directory for the Year 1866. Boston: Sampson, Davenport & Co., 1866.

Note: Special Collections at the Massachusetts State Library, at the State House in Boston, holds an extensive collection of historical city directories for most of the communities in Massachusetts.

New Hampshire

Lyon, G. Parker. *The New-Hampshire Annual Register and United States Calendar.* Concord, NH, 1855–92. [Title varies.]

The New Hampshire Annual Register and Farmers' Almanac. Claremont, NH, 1872 and 1874; Concord, NH, 1873.

The New Hampshire Business Directory for 1875. Boston: Briggs & Co., 1875.

The New Hampshire Business Directory for 1881. Boston: Briggs & Co., 1881.

The New Hampshire Register and Business Directory. Claremont, NH, 1875, 1877, 1879, 1880, 1881; White River Junction, VT, 1884, 1887; Burlington, VT, 1892.

Vermont

Atwater, W. W. *The Vermont Directory.* Rutland, 1864, 1867.

The Vermont Business Directory for the Year Commencing January 1, 1875. Boston: Briggs & Co., 1875.

Waltons' Vermont Register and Farmers' Almanac. Published variously in Montpelier, Claremont, NH; White River Junction, Rutland, Brattleboro, and Burlington, VT, 1850–1910.

New York

The New York State Business Directory. Boston: Sampson, Davenport & Co., 1867, 1874, 1882.

Pennsylvania

Boyd's Pennsylvania State Business Directory 1861. Philadelphia, 1861.

McElroy's Philadelphia City Directory for 1865. Philadelphia, 1865.

United States

The Progressive Annual, Comprising an Almanac, a Spiritual Register, and a General Calendar of Reform. New York: A. J. Davis & Co., 1862, 1863, 1864.

United States census, 1850, 1860, 1870, 1880, 1900, 1910, 1920.

Local city directories: Auburn, NY; Boston; Dayton, OH; Lincoln City, NE; Lowell, MA; Lynn, MA; New York; Philadelphia; Providence; San Francisco; Worcester, MA; and other cities as listed with individual biographies.

Medical Directories and Registers

Alphabetical Lists of Battles and Roster of Regimental Surgeons and Assistant Surgeons during the War of the Rebellion, Compiled from Official Records. Washington, DC, 1885.

American Medical Association. *American Medical Directory.* Chicago, 1906, 1909, 1912, 1921, 1923.

———. *Directory of Deceased American Physicians 1804–1929.* 2 vols. Chicago, 1993.

American Women's Hospitals. *Census of Women Physicians, November 11, 1918.* Edited by Marion Craig Potter, MD. Rochester, NY, 1918.

Butler, Samuel W. *The Medical Register and Directory of the United States.* Philadelphia, 1874, 1877.

Holloway, Lisabeth M. *Medical Obituaries: American Physicians' Biographical Notices in Selected Medical Journals before 1907.* New York & London, 1981.

The Medical and Surgical Directory of the State of Iowa [for 1878 and 1879 and for 1880 and 1881]. Clinton, Iowa: Charles H. Lothrop, 1878, 1880.

Medical and Surgical Directory [later *Register*] *of the United States.* Detroit: R. L. Polk & Co., 1886, 1890, 1893, 1896, 1898, 1900, 1902.

Official Registry & Directory of Physicians and Surgeons in the State of California. 3rd ed. San Francisco, January 1901.

State Board of Health of Illinois. *Official Registry of Physicians and Midwives.* Third annual report, 1880. Springfield, IL, 1881.

State Board of Health of the State of Illinois. *Eighteenth Annual Report . . . for the Year Ended December 31, 1895, with an Appendix Containing the Official Register of Physicians and Midwives 1896.* Springfield, IL, 1896.

Homoeopathic Directories

Bruce, W. T. *Annual Directory of the Homoeopathic Physicians Residing in New York, Pennsylvania, New Jersey, Maryland, Delaware, District of Columbia.* Quakertown, PA, 1878.

Dudley, Pemberton. *Directory of Homoeopathic Physicians of the State of Pennsylvania.* New York, 1874.

———. *Directory of Homoeopathic Physicians Residing in New Jersey, Pennsylvania, Delaware, Maryland, District of Columbia.* 2nd ed. Philadelphia, 1875.

Hoyne, T. S. *Hoyne's Annual Directory of Homoeopathic Physicians in the State of Illinois for the Year 1881.* Vol. 1, no. 9. [Containing also an alphabetical list of homoeopathic physicians in the states of Indiana, Missouri, Kansas, and Wisconsin.] Chicago, 1881.

King, William Harvey. *History of Homeopathy and Its Institutions in America.* 4 vols. New York, 1905.

Knerr, L. J. *Directory of Homoeopathic Physicians in Pennsylvania, New Jersey, Maryland, Delaware and District of Columbia.* Philadelphia, 1883.

Pettet, J. *The North American Homoeopathic Directory for 1877–78.* Cleveland, 1878.

Biographical Dictionaries

Appleton's Cyclopaedia of American Biography. 12 vols. New York, 1887–1931.

Brown, John Howard, ed. *Lamb's Biographical Dictionary of the United States.* Boston, 1900 et seq.

Cleave, Egbert. *Cleave's Biographical Cyclopaedia of Homoeopathic Physicians and Surgeons.* Philadelphia, 1873.

Dictionary of American Biography. 11 vols. plus supplements. New York: American Council of Learned Societies, 1927 et seq.

Garraty, John A., & Mack C. Carnes, eds., *American National Biography.* 24 vols. New York, 1999.

James, Edward T., ed. *Notable American Women 1607–1950, a Biographical Dictionary.* 3 vols. Cambridge, MA, 1971.

Kaufman, Martin, et al. *Dictionary of American Medical Biography.* 2 vols. Westport, CT / London, ca. 1984.

Kelly, Howard A. *Cyclopedia of American Medical Biography.* 2 vols. Philadelphia, 1912.

Kelly, Howard A., & Walter L. Burrage. *American Medical Biographies.* Baltimore, 1920.

Kelly, Howard A., & Walter L. Burrage. *Dictionary of American Medical Biographies,* New York, 1928.

National Cyclopedia of American Biography. James T. White, publ. New York, 1892–1984.

Parton, James et al., *Eminent Women of the Age.* Hartford, CT, 1873.

Who Was Who. Historical vol. and vol. 1. A. N. Marquis & Co., Chicago, 1967, 1942.

Willard, Frances E. *A Woman of the Century.* Buffalo, 1893.

Willard, Frances E., and Mary A. Livermore. *American Women: Fifteen Hundred Biographies with Over 1,400 Portraits.* 2 vols. New York, Chicago, Springfield, OH, orig. 1893. Rev. ed. 1897.

Serials

Eclectic Medical & Surgical Journal (Syracuse; Rochester), July 1849–January 1851.

American Journal of Medicine (Syracuse), January–October 1852.

Eclectic Journal of Medicine (Rochester), January–December 1852.

Syracuse Medical & Surgical Journal (Syracuse), February 1854–February 1855.

Water-Cure Journal (New York), 1845–62.

Herald of Health and Water-Cure Journal (New York) 1863.

Herald of Health (New York) 1863–64.

Herald of Health and Journal of Physical Culture (New York) 1865–92.

Bibliographies

Chaff, Sandra L., et al., eds., *Women in Medicine: A Bibliography of the Literature on Women Physicians.* Metuchen, NJ, & London, 1977.

King, William Harvey. *History of Homoeopathy and Its Institutions in America.* 4 vols. New York, 1905.

Secondary Works

Abram, Ruth J., ed. *"Send Us a Lady Physician": Women Doctors in America 1835–1920.* New York, 1920.

Braude, Ann. *Radical Spirits: Spiritualism and Women's Rights in Nineteenth Century America.* Boston: Beacon Press, 1989.

Brockett, L. P., and Mary C. Vaughan. *Woman's Work in the Civil War.* Philadelphia, 1867.

Cayleff, Susan E. *Wash and Be Healed the Water-Cure Movement and Women's Health.* Philadelphia, 1987.

Croskey, John W. *History of Blockley: A History of the Philadelphia General Hospital from Its Inception, 1731–1928.* Philadelphia, 1929.

Donegan, Jane B. *"Hydropathic Highway to Health": Women and Water-Cure in Antebellum America.* New York, Westport, CT, and London, 1986.

Drachman, Virginia G. *Hospital with a Heart Women Doctors and the Paradox of Separatism at the New England Hospital 1862–1969.* Ithaca and London, 1984.

Gevitz, Norman, ed. *Other Healers: Unorthodox Medicine in America.* Baltimore: Johns Hopkins University Press, 1988.

Haller, John S., Jr. *Medical Protestants: The Eclectics in American Medicine 1825–1939.* Carbondale, IL, 1994.

Hanaford, Phebe A., *Daughters of America; or, Women of the Century.* Augusta, ME, ca. 1882.

Hoolihan, Christopher. *An Annotated Catalogue of the Edward C. Atwater Collection of American Popular Medicine and Health Reform.* 3 vols. Rochester, 2001, 2004, 2008.

Hurd-Mead, Kate Campbell. *Medical Women of America.* New York, 1933.

Lawrence, Charles. *History of the Philadelphia Almshouses and Hospitals from the Beginning of the Eighteenth to the Ending of the Nineteenth Centuries.* Philadelphia, 1905.

Moldow, Gloria. *Women Doctors in Gilded-Age Washington.* Urbana & Chicago, 1987.

Morantz-Sanchez, Regina Markell. *Sympathy and Science: Women Physicians in American Medicine.* New York, 1985.

More, Ellen S. *Restoring the Balance: Women Physicians and the Profession of Medicine 1850–1995.* Cambridge, MA, 2010.

Schultz, Jane E. *Women at the Front: Hospital Workers in Civil War America.* Chapel Hill, NC, and London, 2001.

Silver-Isenstadt, Jean L. *Shameless: The Visionary Life of Mary Gove Nichols.* Baltimore and London: Johns Hopkins University Press, 2002.

Walsh, Mary Roth. *"Doctors Wanted No Women Need Apply."* New Haven, CT, 1977.

Weiss, Harry B., and Howard R. Kemble. *The Great American Water-Cure Craze: A History of Hydropathy in the United States.* Trenton, NJ, 1967.

Wells, Susan. *Out of the Dead House Nineteenth-Century Women Physicians and the Writing of Medicine.* Madison, WI, 2001.

Index of Names

Note: Arranged by surname at graduation. Maiden surnames, if known, are in italics. (A few maiden names are presumed and may actually be married names.)

~ indicates a second entry under the better-known surname

x indicates that there is no biographical entry

This groundbreaking reference work contains brief biographical articles for over two hundred women, most of them little known, who graduated from schools of medicine in the United States before the Civil War. The volume includes an introductory essay examining the social and religious backgrounds of the women graduates, as well as their motivations for becoming physicians and their varying degrees of success as practitioners. In addition, the essay offers information on what physician training and practice were like during the period, as well as on the need for reform that provided a setting for women's entry into the profession. The biographical entries are supplemented by a chronological table of female medical graduates and a geographical table indicating the places in which they practiced.

Edward C. Atwater is emeritus professor of medicine and the history of medicine at the University of Rochester School of Medicine.